Dementia

Editor

JOHN M. RINGMAN

NEUROLOGIC CLINICS

www.neurologic.theclinics.com

Consulting Editor
RANDOLPH W. EVANS

May 2017 • Volume 35 • Number 2

ELSEVIER

1600 John F. Kennedy Boulevard • Suite 1800 • Philadelphia, Pennsylvania, 19103-2899

http://www.theclinics.com

NEUROLOGIC CLINICS Volume 35, Number 2
May 2017 ISSN 0733-8619, ISBN-13: 978-0-323-52852-8

Editor: Stacy Eastman
Developmental editor: Donald Mumford

Neurologic Clinics (ISSN 0733-8619) is published quarterly by Elsevier Inc., 360 Park Avenue South, New York, NY 10010–1710. Months of issue are February, May, August, and November. Periodicals postage paid at New York, NY, and additional mailing offices. Subscription prices are $306.00 per year for US individuals, $607.00 per year for US institutions, $100.00 per year for US students, $383.00 per year for Canadian individuals, $736.00 per year for Canadian institutions, $423.00 per year for international individuals, $736.00 per year for international institutions, and $210.00 for Canadian and foreign students/residents. To receive student/resident rate, orders must be accompanied by name of affiliated institution, date of term, and the *signature* of program/residency coordinator on institution letterhead. Orders will be billed at individual rate until proof of status is received. Foreign air speed delivery is included in all *Clinics* subscription prices. All prices are subject to change without notice. **POSTMASTER:** Send address changes to *Neurologic Clinics*, Elsevier Health Sciences Division, Subscription Customer Service, 3251 Riverport Lane, Maryland Heights, MO 63043. **Customer Service: Telephone: 1-800-654-2452 (U.S. and Canada); 314-447-8871 (outside U.S. and Canada). Fax: 314-447-8029. E-mail: journalscustomerservice-usa@elsevier.com (for print support); journalsonlinesupport-usa@elsevier.com (for online support).**

Reprints. For copies of 100 or more of articles in this publication, please contact the Commercial Reprints Department, Elsevier Inc., 360 Park Avenue South, New York, New York, 10010-1710; Tel.: +1-212-633-3874; Fax: +1-212-633-3820, and E-mail: reprints@elsevier.com.

Neurologic Clinics is also published in Spanish by Nueva Editorial Interamericana S.A., Mexico City, Mexico.

Neurologic Clinics is covered in *Current Contents/Clinical Medicine, MEDLINE/PubMed (Index Medicus), EMBASE/Excerpta Medica, and PsycINFO, and ISI/BIOMED.*

Contributors

CONSULTING EDITOR

RANDOLPH W. EVANS, MD
Clinical Professor, Department of Neurology, Baylor College of Medicine, Houston, Texas

EDITOR

JOHN M. RINGMAN, MD, MS
Helene and Lou Galen Endowed Professor of Clinical Neurology, Department of Neurology, Keck School of Medicine of University of Southern California, Center for the Health Professionals, Los Angeles, California

AUTHORS

ABIGAIL M. ABUD, BS
Institute for Memory Impairments and Neurological Disorders, University of California, Irvine, Irvine, California

EDSEL M. ABUD, BS
Institute for Memory Impairments and Neurological Disorders, University of California, Irvine, Irvine, California

SZOFIA S. BULLAIN, MD
Assistant Professor, Department of Neurology and Institute for Memory Impairments and Neurological Disorders, University of California, Irvine, Irvine, California

HELENA C. CHUI, MD
McCarron Professor and Chair, Department of Neurology, University of Southern California, Los Angeles, California

LINA M. D'ORAZIO, PhD
Assistant Clinical Professor of Neurology, Department of Neurology, Keck School of Medicine of University of Southern California, Los Angeles, California

ADAM S. FLEISHER, MD, MAS
Dementia Neurologist, Medical Fellow, Eli Lilly and Company, Indianapolis, Indiana

DOUGLAS GALASKO, MD
Professor, Department of Neurosciences and Shiley-Marcos Alzheimer's Disease Research Center, University of California, San Diego, La Jolla, California

BIANCA GONZALEZ, PhD, MS, FNP-BC, RN
School of Nursing, University of Los Angeles, California, Los Angeles, California

KAREN H. GYLYS, PhD, RN
School of Nursing, University of Los Angeles, California, Los Angeles, California

FELIPE A. JAIN, MD
Assistant Clinical Professor of Psychiatry, Department of Psychiatry, University of California San Francisco, San Francisco, California

CLAUDIA H. KAWAS, MD
Professor, Departments of Neurology, Neurobiology and Behavior, Epidemiology, and Institute for Memory Impairments and Neurological Disorders, University of California, Irvine, Irvine, California

SARA KOLLACK-WALKER, PhD
Assoc Consultant, Scientific Comm, Global Med Comm – Bio-Medicines BU-NS, Eli Lilly and Company, Lilly Corporate Center, Indianapolis, Indiana

GRACE J. LEE, PhD
Assistant Professor, Department of Psychology, School of Behavioral Health, Loma Linda University, Loma Linda, California

COLLIN Y. LIU, MD
Department of Neurology, Keck School of Medicine at the University of Southern California, Los Angeles, California

PO H. LU, PsyD
Clinical Neuropsychologist, Executive Mental Health, Inc, Los Angeles, California

MARIO F. MENDEZ, MD, PhD
Director, Behavioral Neurology Program, Professor of Neurology and Psychiatry and Biobehavioral Sciences, David Geffen School of Medicine at University of Los Angeles, California; Director, Neurobehavior Unit, VA Greater Los Angeles Healthcare System, Los Angeles, California

BRUCE L. MILLER, MD
Professor of Neurology, University of California San Francisco School of Medicine; A.W. and Mary Margaret Clausen Distinguished Chair, Director, University of California San Francisco Memory and Aging Center, San Francisco, California

NICHOLAS T. OLNEY, MD
Clinical Fellow, Department of Neurology, University of California San Francisco Memory and Aging Center, San Francisco, California

AIMEE L. PIERCE, MD
Assistant Professor, Department of Neurology and Institute for Memory Impairments and Neurological Disorders, University of California, Irvine, Irvine, California

WAYNE W. POON, PhD
Institute for Memory Impairments and Neurological Disorders, University of California, Irvine, Irvine, California

LILIANA RAMIREZ GOMEZ, MD
Assistant Clinical Professor of Neurology, Department of Neurology, University of California San Francisco, San Francisco, California

JOHN M. RINGMAN, MD, MS
Helene and Lou Galen Endowed Professor of Clinical Neurology, Department of Neurology, Keck School of Medicine of University of Southern California, Center for the Health Professionals, Los Angeles, California

SALVATORE SPINA, MD, PhD
Assistant Professor of Neurology, University of California San Francisco Memory and Aging Center, San Francisco, California

Contents

Though the numbers of dementia cases are rising worldwide, there is evidence that incidence rates are decreasing. We now know that the neuropathological changes of Alzheimer's disease (AD) precede overt clinical signs by 15 to 20 years and we have biochemical and imaging markers that enable us to identify them. The genetic complexity of AD suggests it is not a single entity but rather represents a group of related diseases. The amyloid cascade hypothesis has led to the development of putative disease-modifying interventions but these have not yet been demonstrated to be substantively effective and additional approaches are warranted.

To date, Alzheimer disease drug candidates have produced negative results in human trials, and progress in moving new targets out of the laboratory and into trials has been slow. However, based on 3 decades of previous work, there is reason to hope that amyloid-based and other novel therapies will move at a faster pace toward successful clinical trials. This article highlights selected preclinical research topics that are rapidly advancing in the laboratory.

Cognitive abilities decline with age and older adults, as a group, are at increased risk for developing age-related cognitive disorders. Neuropsychological evaluation provides objective quantification of the type and severity of cognitive deficits that can affect the elderly population and elucidates a pattern of scores that provides diagnostic clues regarding etiology. It can also detect mild cognitive impairment that may not be evident on bedside assessment or mental status examination and provides critical information regarding the progression of cognitive changes through serial evaluations. Such information assists in counseling patients and family members and can guide therapeutic decisions.

modest symptomatic benefit but unable to slow the progression of disease.

Cerebrovascular disease (CVD) is the second leading cause of cognitive impairment in late life. Structural neuroimaging offers the most sensitive and specific biomarkers for hemorrhages and infarcts, but there are significant limitations in its ability to detect microvascular disease, microinfarcts, dynamic changes in the blood-brain barrier, and preclinical cerebrovascular disease. Autopsy studies disclose the common co-occurrence of vascular and neurodegenerative conditions, suggesting that in late life, a multifactorial approach to cognitive impairment may be more appropriate than traditional dichotomous classifications. Management of vascular risk factors remains a proven and practical approach to reducing acute and progressive cognitive impairment and dementia.

Dementia syndromes associated with Lewy bodies are subdivided into dementia with Lewy bodies (DLB), an underdiagnosed cause of dementia in the elderly, and Parkinson disease with dementia (PDD), cognitive impairment appearing in people diagnosed with Parkinson disease. Their neuropathologic substrates are the widespread distribution of aggregates of the protein α-synuclein in neurons in cortical brain regions, accompanied by variable Alzheimer pathology. Clinical features of DLB and PDD include distinctive changes in cognition, behavior, movement, sleep, and autonomic function. Diagnostic criteria for DLB and PDD incorporate these features. Current treatment options for DLB and PDD are symptomatic.

Frontotemporal dementia (FTD) is a heterogeneous disorder with distinct clinical phenotypes associated with multiple neuropathologic entities. Presently, the term FTD encompasses clinical disorders that include changes in behavior, language, executive control, and often motor symptoms. The core FTD spectrum disorders include behavioral variant FTD, nonfluent/agrammatic variant primary progressive aphasia, and semantic variant PPA. Related FTD disorders include frontotemporal dementia with motor neuron disease, progressive supranuclear palsy syndrome, and corticobasal syndrome. In this article, the authors discuss the clinical presentation, diagnostic criteria, neuropathology, genetics, and treatments of these disorders.

THE CLINICS ARE AVAILABLE ONLINE!
Access your subscription at:
www.theclinics.com

Preface

Alzheimer and the Dementias

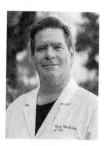

John M. Ringman, MD, MS
Editor

It is a very exciting time to be working with patients presenting with cognitive impairment and other symptoms indicating the presence of neurodegenerative illness. Though medical treatments for this group of disorders are currently limited, in the last 20 years, there has been an explosion of knowledge regarding their pathogenesis, which has led to new, more specific, diagnostic techniques and a refinement of our ability to test putative disease-modifying agents. It is an honor to edit the current issue of *Neurologic Clinics* in which experts have summarized current knowledge in diverse aspects of these conditions for the practicing neurologist and other clinicians. Here, leaders in the field update the reader on scientific progress underlying disease mechanisms in Alzheimer disease (AD) and characterize both early- and late-onset forms of AD, cognitive impairment associated with cerebrovascular disease, in the context of Lewy body disease, and the frontotemporal lobar degenerations (FTLDs). Overviews of the approach to cognitive assessment in general and the clinical and cognitive assessment of Hispanics, a growing segment of the US population, are presented. The specific and growing roles of neuroimaging in the assessment of cognitively impaired patients are also discussed. We believe readers will find that this issue enhances their approach to patients and families suffering from this devastating group of diseases.

Of course, additional important topics in dementia have been necessarily omitted. It is particularly difficult to comprehensively discuss our rapidly evolving knowledge regarding the genetic influences in AD and other neurodegenerative diseases. The reader should be aware that our growing knowledge of the diverse number of genetic variants. For a review, readers are referred to a recent article authored by leaders of the Alzheimer's Disease Genetic Consortium[1] and to Web sites in which AD risk variants are frequently updated (http://www.alzgene.org) and autosomal dominant mutations for AD and FTLD are catalogued (http://www.molgen.ua.ac.be/admutations/). To date, the most clinically relevant genetic influence in late-onset AD is the ε4 allele of the *APOE* gene, but there is still not consensus on the utility of such testing in most

Neurol Clin 35 (2017) ix–x
http://dx.doi.org/10.1016/j.ncl.2017.02.001
0733-8619/17/© 2017 Published by Elsevier Inc.

contexts. As this situation is evolving, it is important to explore the utility, feasibility, and social context of such testing, an area under active study.[2]

The current volume does not include a section devoted to treatment of the cognitive or behavioral symptoms of the dementias. The reader is referred to recent reviews regarding such pharmacological and non-pharmacological interventions.[3,4] Finally, in light of our current inability to halt or significantly reverse the diverse cognitive and behavioral manifestations of dementing illnesses, a comprehensive and multidisciplinary approach to such patients is indicated. The interested reader is referred to current guidelines regarding management[5] and reviews focusing on caregivers[6] and end-of-life care.[7] With such multidisciplinary approaches, teams of health care providers can make a significant impact on persons and families affected by this growing public health crisis.

John M. Ringman, MD, MS
Department of Neurology
Keck School of Medicine of USC
Center for the Health Professionals
1540 Alcazar Street, Suite 209F
Los Angeles, CA 90033, USA

E-mail address:
John.ringman@med.usc.edu

REFERENCES

1. Naj AC, Schellenberg GD. Alzheimer's Disease Genetics C. Genomic variants, genes, and pathways of Alzheimer's disease: an overview. Am J Med Genet B Neuropsychiatr Genet 2017;174:5–26.
2. Roberts JS, Christensen KD, Green RC. Using Alzheimer's disease as a model for genetic risk disclosure: implications for personal genomics. Clin Genet 2011;80:407–14.
3. Ihl R, Bunevicius R, Frolich L, et al. World Federation of Societies of Biological Psychiatry guidelines for the pharmacological treatment of dementias in primary care. Int J Psychiatry Clin Pract 2015;19(1):2–7.
4. Gauthier S, Cummings J, Ballard C, et al. Management of behavioral problems in Alzheimer's disease 2010;22:346–72.
5. Segal-Gidan F, Cherry D, Jones R, et al. California Workgroup on Guidelines for Alzheimer's Disease M. Alzheimer's disease management guideline: update 2008. Alzheimers Dement 2011;7:e51–9.
6. Parkinson M, Carr SM, Rushmer R, et al. Investigating what works to support family carers of people with dementia: a rapid realist review. J Public Health (Oxf) 2016. [Epub ahead of print].
7. Murphy E, Froggatt K, Connolly S, et al. Palliative care interventions in advanced dementia. Cochrane Database Syst Rev 2016;(12):CD011513.

Update on Alzheimer's and the Dementias: Introduction

John M. Ringman, MD, MS

KEYWORDS

- Alzheimer's disease • Dementia • Amyloid cascade hypothesis • Prevention
- Intervention • Genetic • Presymptomatic • Diagnostic criteria

KEY POINTS

- Incipient neuropathologic changes of Alzheimer's disease (AD) precede overt clinical signs by 15 to 20 years.
- It is becoming more evident that AD is not a single entity but rather a group of diseases at least partially differentiable by their underlying genetic architecture.
- There may be pathophysiological subtypes of AD depending on the age of disease onset.
- In light of the recognition of the long presymptomatic course of AD and its recalcitrant nature once established, there is increasing focus on its prevention.

With the growing population and overall extension of life expectancy in many parts of the world, the prevalence of dementia is becoming alarmingly high. By the middle of this century, the numbers of persons in the United States with Alzheimer's disease (AD), the most common cause of dementia, are expected to reach 13.8 million.[1] Although some studies in industrialized countries suggest a decrease in dementia incidence in recent years, possibly as the result of better control of risk factors for vascular disease,[2] the worldwide prevalence numbers are sure to continue to increase.[3] It is hopeful that better control of modifiable risk factors (eg, hypertension and hypercholesterolemia) might help to stem the epidemic,[4] but the constant influences of population growth, genetics, and aging ensure an increasing need for resources to care for affected individuals.

The characteristic neuropathology of AD (amyloid plaques [APs] and neurofibrillary tangles [NFTs]) contribute to the cause of dementia in approximately two-thirds of dementia cases and the effect of risk factor control on this pathology is less certain. Observational and interventional studies attempting to directly address these specific pathologic changes had previously been hampered by our inability to definitively

This work was supported by National Institute on Aging grant P50-05142.
Center for the Health Professionals, Department of Neurology, Keck School of Medicine of USC, 1540 Alcazar Street, Suite 209F, Los Angeles, CA 90089-0080, USA
E-mail address: John.ringman@med.usc.edu

identify them in living persons. However, over the last 15 years we have developed biochemical (eg, levels of Aβ42, tau, and p-tau in the cerebrospinal fluid) and imaging (eg, amyloid and tau PET) modalities that permit us to positively identify AD pathology during life, allowing for an augmented understanding of AD biology and its response to treatment. It is now clear that AD neuropathologic changes can precede overt clinical symptoms by 15 to 20 years, opening up the window for secondary prevention opportunities and the reconceptualization of AD from a "clinicopathologic" entity to a condition defined principally by biomarker changes. In 2011, in a joint venture between the National Institute on Aging and the Alzheimer's Association, criteria for "dementia due to AD,[5]" "mild cognitive impairment due to AD,[6]" and "preclinical AD pathology,[7]" based on the presence or absence of AD-specific and nonspecific biomarker changes were put forth. Consideration is now being given to revising these criteria further to define AD based purely on the presence of AD-specific biomarkers, at least for research purposes.

The APs and NFTs that are the "hallmarks" of AD and have been the focus of a multitude of studies into the etiologic mechanisms of the disease; however, there remains substantial uncertainty regarding what "upstream" and "downstream" events are most relevant and should be addressed with therapeutic interventions. Fueled by the discovery that the genetic mutations that cause young-onset Mendelian forms of AD (autosomal-dominant AD) lead to aberrant cleavage of amyloid precursor protein, fragments of which largely comprise the APs and cerebral amyloid angiopathy that characterize the illness, the "amyloid cascade hypothesis" was elaborated and has since dominated the field.[8] This posits that the misprocessing of amyloid precursor protein (APP) is central to causing all forms of AD, with non-Mendelian AD typically of later onset potentially being due to a decreased ability of the body to eliminate APP derivatives (eg, by inefficient transport of Aβ by apolipoprotein E variants associated with an increased risk of AD[9]). Interventions directly targeting the amyloid cascade have been demonstrated to positively affect Aβ production and deposition,[10] but have not yet shown substantive clinical efficacy.[11] Although still of substantial heuristic value, additional mechanisms occurring before, in association with, or consequent to amyloid deposition must be a growing focus of AD research. Recent, large-scale, genome-wide association studies in dementia have enabled the identification of many genetic variants, each with a relatively small influence on the ultimate risk of developing AD[12] (http://www.alzgene.org). Variants in genes with roles in inflammation, endocytosis, protein trafficking, and lipid transport have all been implicated. The degree to which any individual variant contributes to the development of a given case of "sporadic" AD certainly differs across cases, highlighting the importance of consideration of AD as the "Alzheimer's diseases" rather than as a monolithic entity.

After Alois Alzheimer's original description of AD in 1907, AD was thought of for decades as "presenile dementia," defined as when the clinicopathologic entity occurs before age 65. Cases of dementia occurring after that age, in the "senile" period, were attributed to "hardening of the arteries" or as the inevitable consequences of normal aging. In the late 20th century, the recognition of a continuum in the neuropathology between the majority of dementia cases across these ages led to a unification of the disease into a single entity.[13,14] However, in more recent years, with the help of more sophisticated genetic, imaging, and other tools, important differences between AD of young and late onset have come to light. Young-onset AD is more likely to have a nonamnestic presentation (eg, with logopenia, visuospatial deficits, or apraxia), have different atrophy patterns, and likely different genetic origins. Although the *APOE ε4* variant, particularly when present in the homozygous state, decreases the age of AD onset, it is less frequently present in those with atypical presentations. That the

APOE ε4 variant is clearly overrepresented in typical AD of onset in the 70s, but less so in this atypical young-onset group and in the extreme elderly when multiple diverse neuropathologies are commonly found, attests to the genetic heterogeneity of the disorder that may ultimately be reflected in differential response to treatment. Although the degree to which AD of young and late onset is similar and distinct is not yet comprehensively defined, age at onset does seem to be an important factor to consider when studying AD pathogenesis and response to treatment.

With increasing longevity, more neuropathologic studies, and the advent of more sophisticated diagnostic modalities, there was a shift from the concept of senile dementia having a purely vascular etiology ("hardening of the arteries") to that of a neurodegenerative disease associated with APs and NFTs.[15] Both large and small cerebral infarcts as well as diffuse cerebral ischemia can contribute to cognitive impairment and dementia though pure "vascular dementia" is relatively rare in neuropathologic studies as concurrent AD pathology is often present. Nonetheless, because AD and cerebrovascular disease share many risk factors, and in light of a growing appreciation of the relevance of cerebral amyloid angiopathy and recent animal studies suggesting how these pathologies might act in a synergistic way, there is increasing focus on dysfunction of the "neurovascular unit" as inducing or propagating AD pathology.[16] Although it remains to be defined to what degree this is the case, this approach could potentially identify new targets amenable to intervention.

As indicated, clinical trials of putative disease-modifying treatments have so far been disappointing, despite at least some evidence of target engagement. Most such studies have been initiated well into the symptomatic stage of the disease, when APs and NFTs are well-established and substantial neuronal and synapse loss has already occurred. It may be that these interventions have been "too little, too late." Our current understanding of the genetic nature of AD and our ability to measure AD pathology during the extended presymptomatic stage has provided the opportunity for secondary prevention studies. Specifically, there are currently studies ongoing in asymptomatic elderly persons with positive amyloid PET scans,[17] carrying dominantly inherited AD mutations,[18,19] and homozygous for the *APOE* ε4 genotype.[19] However, it remains to be seen if these approaches will be effective and it may be necessary to ultimately perform primary prevention studies in which the intervention occurs before any discernible AD pathology is present. Until effective disease-modifying therapies are identified, we must remain agnostic and unprejudiced in our quest to identify targets and implement intervention strategies for AD.

REFERENCES

1. Alzheimer's Association. 2016 Alzheimer's disease facts and figures. Alzheimers Dement 2016;12:459–509.
2. Satizabal CL, Beiser AS, Chouraki V, et al. Incidence of dementia over three decades in the Framingham Heart Study. N Engl J Med 2016;374:523–32.
3. Prince M, Ali GC, Guerchet M, et al. Recent global trends in the prevalence and incidence of dementia, and survival with dementia. Alzheimers Res Ther 2016;8:23.
4. Barnes DE, Yaffe K. The projected effect of risk factor reduction on Alzheimer's disease prevalence. Lancet Neurol 2011;10:819–28.
5. McKhann GM, Knopman DS, Chertkow H, et al. The diagnosis of dementia due to Alzheimer's disease: recommendations from the National Institute on Aging-Alzheimer's Association Workgroups on Diagnostic Guidelines for Alzheimer's Disease. Alzheimers Dement 2011;7:263–9.

6. Albert MS, DeKosky ST, Dickson D, et al. The diagnosis of mild cognitive impairment due to Alzheimer's disease: recommendations from the National Institute on Aging-Alzheimer's Association Workgroups on Diagnostic Guidelines for Alzheimer's Disease. Alzheimers Dement 2011;7:270–9.

7. Sperling RA, Aisen PS, Beckett LA, et al. Toward defining the preclinical stages of Alzheimer's disease: recommendations from the National Institute on Aging-Alzheimer's Association Workgroups on Diagnostic Guidelines for Alzheimer's Disease. Alzheimers Dement 2011;7:280–92.

8. Hardy J, Selkoe DJ. The amyloid hypothesis of Alzheimer's disease: progress and problems on the road to therapeutics. Science 2002;297:353–6.

9. Castellano JM, Kim J, Stewart FR, et al. Human apoE isoforms differentially regulate brain amyloid-beta peptide clearance. Sci Transl Med 2011;3:89ra57.

10. Nicoll JA, Barton E, Boche D, et al. Abeta species removal after abeta42 immunization. J Neuropathol Exp Neurol 2006;65:1040–8.

11. Doody RS, Thomas RG, Farlow M, et al, Alzheimer's Disease Cooperative Study Steering Committee, Solanezumab Study Group. Phase 3 trials of solanezumab for mild-to-moderate Alzheimer's disease. N Engl J Med 2014;370:311–21.

12. Bertram L, McQueen MB, Mullin K, et al. Systematic meta-analyses of Alzheimer disease genetic association studies: the AlzGene database. Nat Genet 2007;39:17–23.

13. Katzman R. Alzheimer's disease. N Engl J Med 1986;314:964–73.

14. Blessed G, Tomlinson BE, Roth M. The association between quantitative measures of dementia and of senile change in the cerebral grey matter of elderly subjects. Br J Psychiatry 1968;114:797–811.

15. Roman G. Vascular dementia: a historical background. Int Psychogeriatr 2003;15(Suppl 1):11–3.

16. Bell RD, Zlokovic BV. Neurovascular mechanisms and blood-brain barrier disorder in Alzheimer's disease. Acta Neuropathol 2009;118:103–13.

17. Sperling RA, Rentz DM, Johnson KA, et al. The A4 study: stopping AD before symptoms begin? Sci Transl Med 2014;6:228fs213.

18. Morris JC, Aisen PS, Bateman RJ, et al. Developing an international network for Alzheimer research: the Dominantly Inherited Alzheimer Network. Clin Investig 2012;2:975–84.

19. Reiman EM, Langbaum JB, Fleisher AS, et al. Alzheimer's Prevention Initiative: a plan to accelerate the evaluation of presymptomatic treatments. J Alzheimers Dis 2011;26(Suppl 3):321–9.

Tau Spread, Apolipoprotein E, Inflammation, and More
Rapidly Evolving Basic Science in Alzheimer Disease

Bianca Gonzalez, PhD, MS, FNP-BC, RN[a], Edsel M. Abud, BS[b],
Abigail M. Abud, BS[b], Wayne W. Poon, PhD[b],
Karen H. Gylys, PhD, RN[a,*]

KEYWORDS

- Imaging flow cytometry • Oligomer • Synapse • Cholesterol • Microglia

KEY POINTS

- Prefibrillar and fibrillar oligomeric Aβ is localized to the synaptic compartment and precedes synaptic tau pathology.
- High levels of soluble synaptic Aβ oligomers are associated with the onset of dementia.
- Recent evidence suggests that depolarization-induced synaptic release of tau, possibly carried on exosomes, is a key mechanism underlying regional spread of tau pathology.
- Recent advances highlight the strong influence of inflammation pathways and glial activation on Alzheimer disease pathology and synapse loss; these pathways may be examined with imaging flow cytometry.

To date, Alzheimer disease (AD) drug candidates have produced negative results in human trials, and progress in moving new targets out of the laboratory and into trials has been slow. However, based on 3 decades of previous work, there is reason to hope that amyloid-based and other novel therapies will move at a faster pace toward successful clinical trials. Here we highlight selected preclinical research topics that are rapidly advancing in the laboratory.

THE AMYLOID CASCADE HYPOTHESIS

In 1907, experimental observations by Alois Alzheimer led to the identification of Aβ and tau pathologies, which are the main pathologic constituents in AD (Alzheimer, 1987).

Funded by: National Institutes of Health grant numbers: P50 AG05142, P50 AG16970, R56 AG027465; NIHMS-ID: 843123.
[a] UCLA School of Nursing, Box 956919, Factor Building 6-266, Los Angeles, CA 90095, USA;
[b] Institute for Memory Impairments and Neurological Disorders, UC Irvine, 2642 Biological Sciences III, Irvine, CA 92697-4545, USA
* Corresponding author.
E-mail address: kgylys@sonnet.ucla.edu

Thereafter, familial studies identified mutations in *APP*, *PSEN1*, and *PSEN2*, that lead to misprocessing of Aβ and autosomal dominant AD (ADAD) that is typically of early onset.[1,2] These advances led to the formulation of the amyloid cascade hypothesis proposed by Hardy and Higgins in 1992.[3] According to this hypothesis, Aβ peptide, which originates from sequential proteolytic cleavage of the amyloid precursor protein (APP) by β-secretase and the γ-secretase complex, is the causative agent of Alzheimer pathology. In AD, Aβ42 is the more pathologic Aβ fragment (the predominant species being Aβ40), and more readily adopts misfolded conformers that are more prone to aggregate. Overproduction or reduced clearance of Aβ leads to the accumulation of different Aβ conformations; that is, oligomers, fibrils, that can block neuronal transmission and lead to synaptic loss and neuronal toxicity. Updated in 2002 to propose tau pathology as downstream of the original insult of Aβ accumulation,[4] and then more recently in light of newly identified genetic risk variants, the amyloid hypothesis has been re-evaluated to include apoE/cholesterol effects, inflammation, and endosomal recycling as additional cellular drivers downstream of initial Aβ deposition.[5]

Although the evidence supporting different species of Aβ as causative of AD is strong, it is widely recognized that neurofibrillary tangle (NFT) pathology is a closer correlate of neuronal death and symptom manifestation in AD. Hyperphosphorylated tau is a major component of such NFTs and therefore how Aβ might influence tau phosphorylation is an important topic. Multiple lines of evidence support elaboration of the amyloid hypothesis suggesting that soluble Aβ oligomers cause subsequent tau toxicity. In recent reports, Aβ42 oligomers have been shown to activate AMP-activated kinase (AMPK), which is associated with tau accumulation in AD neurons.[6] Using HeLa cell lines and in vivo mouse models, Mairet-Coello and colleagues[6] demonstrated that AMPKα1 phosphorylates tau on Serine 262 in response to Aβ42 oligomers. Furthermore, investigators found that blocking tau phosphorylation at Serine 262 prevents neurons from Aβ42-mediated toxicity and subsequent dendritic spine loss induced by AMPKα1 phosphorylation. Similarly, Pooler and colleagues[7] demonstrated that Aβ increases tau aggregation and propagation by using immunofluorescence labeling, cell quantification, fluorescence in situ hybridization, and real-time polymerase chain reaction analysis methods in vivo in a mouse model (rTgTauEC × APP/PS1 mice) that expresses tau and Aβ. Their results showed that Aβ increases tau spreading in the cortex as well as tau-induced neuronal toxicity.[7] The lack of tau pathology in most animal models has long been cited as a problem for the amyloid cascade hypothesis, but the current consensus view is that model systems with human rather than murine tau support this version of the amyloid hypothesis.[5]

SYNAPTIC LOSS AND ELABORATIONS ON THE AMYLOID CASCADE HYPOTHESIS

Synaptic loss has long been associated with cognitive decline in AD[8] and correlates strongly with soluble Aβ early in disease progression, differentiating high pathology control from AD cases.[9,10] As the field has moved to accept a version of the amyloid hypothesis in which the primary proximal toxin to neurons and synaptic function is soluble oligomeric Aβ,[5] we and others have demonstrated accumulations of oligomeric Aβ within presynaptic boutons.[11,12] Synaptic Aβ consists of multiple oligomeric species, both prefibrillar and fibrillar,[10,12] and insoluble Aβ fibrils also accumulate in presynaptic terminals.[13] The recent development of a PET ligand to quantify synaptic density in the living human brain should greatly advance AD molecular research as well as empower clinicians with a robust complementary diagnostic tool.[14]

Aβ deposits in plaques may in themselves be relatively benign, but are a potential source of soluble oligomeric Aβ, which directly causes neurotoxicity and neuronal death through postsynaptic interactions with glutamate receptors, cellular prion protein, neuroligin, Wnt, and insulin receptors.[15,16] Complicating work in this area is the difficulty of accurate quantification of soluble amyloid oligomers, combined with the precarious structural stability that is the nature of oligomers. Recent studies have made use of an oligomer sandwich enzyme-linked immunosorbent assay (ELISA) using an anti-Aβ antibody as both capture and detection, which accurately quantifies Aβ oligomers with n>2. With this assay, high pathology but nondemented control samples showed lower oligomer levels compared with AD samples,[17] suggesting that cognition is impaired when soluble oligomers reach a threshold.

Consistent with this hypothesis and extending it into the synaptic compartment, recent experiments by Bilousova and colleagues[10] used flow cytometry and confocal microscopy methods to measure Aβ and tau within synaptosomes of human cortex and rodent models to test the amyloid hypothesis.[10] Consistent with a synaptic amyloid cascade, synaptic Aβ accumulation occurred early in AD before the appearance of phosphorylated tau. Synaptic phosphorylated tau was not prevalent until late-stage AD compared with earlier stages in both human samples and rodent models. Most importantly, soluble Aβ oligomers in synaptic terminals were increased in early AD human synaptosomes compared with controls with high pathology and without dementia, suggesting that a threshold soluble synaptic oligomer level is associated with the onset of a dementia. Confocal images with conformation-dependent monoclonal antibodies reveal that both prefibrillar (M55 antibody) and fibrillar Aβ oligomers accumulate in AD synapses (M116 antibody; **Fig. 1**).

SPREAD OF TAU PATHOLOGY

A wide body of literature has shown that cytoskeletal protein tau accumulates in the brain leading to the formation of intracellular neurofibrillary tangles (NFTs), and it has long been known that tau pathology follows a progression suggestive of regional spread.[18] More recent evidence has moved toward a model by which tau is released from neurons and may travel to surrounding neurons transsynaptically.[19]

Recent data have greatly expanded understanding of specific cellular mechanisms driving the spread of tau pathology. For example, several lines of evidence demonstrate depolarization-dependent tau release. Pooler and colleagues[20] used KCl-treated primary neuronal cultures to stimulate AMPA receptors to propagate action potentials and measured tau release with a sandwich ELISA. Investigators found that stimulation of healthy neurons causes tau release that is dependent on intracellular calcium and mediated by exosomes and membrane vesicle secretion.[20] Yamada and colleagues[21] used in vivo microdialysis to measure tau from brain interstitial fluid of wild-type (WT) mice, demonstrating that presynaptic glutamate release drives tau release and neuronal activity increased extracellular tau.[21] Experiments by our group expanded on the results from animal model systems into humans by measuring tau release from postmortem synaptosome preparations. KCl-mediated depolarization markedly increased tau release from AD synaptosomes.[22] Flow cytometry analysis also revealed the abundance of tau within presynaptic terminals, along with increased C-terminal truncated tau in AD. Similar experiments determining the exact tau peptide released in human AD will be important in guiding development of tau immunotherapies.[23,24]

Exosomes are approximately 100-nm extracellular vesicles that are released by most cells, including those in the central nervous system (CNS), and are thought to be derived from late endosomes termed multivesicular bodies.[25] A good deal of evidence supports the hypothesis that extracellular and trans-synaptic tau spreading occurs via exosomes.[26–29] Recent studies also have implicated microglia and

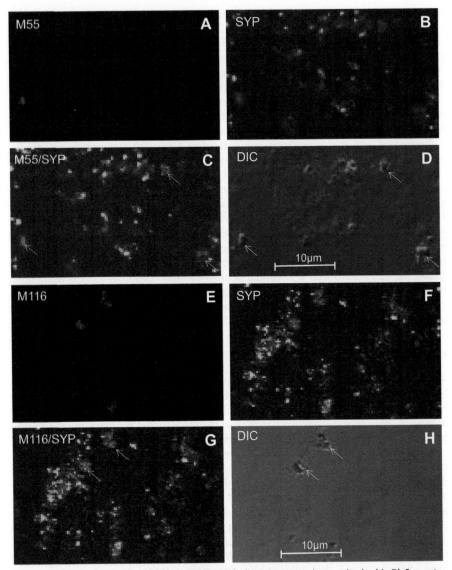

Fig. 1. Conformation-dependent antibodies label Aβ in synaptic terminals. (*A–D*) Synaptosomes were dual labeled with synaptophysin and the monoclonal antibody M55 directed against prefibrillar oligomers: (*A*) M55; (*B*) synaptophysin (SYP); (*C*) overlay image with arrows indicating colocalization; (*D*) differential interference contrast (DIC) image. (*E–H*) Synaptosomes dual labeled with synaptophysin and the monoclonal antibody M116 directed against fibrillar oligomers: (*E*) M116; (*F*) synaptophysin (SYP); (*G*) overlay image with arrows indicating colocalization; (*H*) DIC image.

microglial-derived exosomes in tau propagation.[29,30] Alternatively, exosomes also may be a mechanism for sequestration of Aβ and misfolded proteins.[31] More recently, exosome-associated total and p-tau in plasma have been suggested as predictors of incipient AD,[32] suggesting promise for exosomes as circulating biomarkers of AD. Having a size in the low nanometer range means that there are significant technical barriers in the study of these particles; however, the potential impact on AD diagnosis and treatment has made this an active and dynamic areas of focus in the field of neurodegeneration.

APOLIPOPROTEIN E AND CHOLESTEROL IN ALZHEIMER DISEASE

The *APOE* gene encodes an apolipoprotein that functions as a cholesterol carrier (apoE), and a good deal of evidence indicates that lipid metabolism modulates Aβ levels. More recently, a number of genes regulating lipid metabolism have been implicated in AD.[33] Cholesterol levels in the brain are thought to play an important role in brain neuronal homeostasis with the distribution of cholesterol playing an important role.[34] In the brain, cholesterol exists in 2 major pools: unesterified (free cholesterol), which accounts for 95% of cholesterol in the brain, and the esterified cholesterol, which constitutes 5% of total cholesterol. Free cholesterol resides in cell membranes and functions in cellular membrane fluidity, electrical transduction, structure, repair, and permeability.[35] Conversely, esterified cholesterol is found intracellularly and is sequestered into lipid droplets. Esterified cholesterol is thought to function as cholesterol storage in the brain.[36,37] High-density lipoprotein, which contains free cholesterol and esterified cholesterol, is produced by astrocytes and binds to apoE via lipidation by ABC transporters. It is subsequently transported to neurons via apoE for the purposes of membrane repair and cellular maintenance.[38,39]

Multiple studies have confirmed the role free cholesterol plays in AD models. Schneider and colleagues[40] demonstrated in neuronal cultures that reduced free cholesterol is associated with reduction in Aβ. Furthermore, when free cholesterol was increased, Aβ aggregation also increased.[40] Concurrently, Ferrera and colleagues[41] found that free cholesterol promotes Aβ-mediated neurotoxicity and is associated with a reduction of cell viability markers.[41] Additionally, Abramov and colleagues[42] used hippocampal neuronal cultures to demonstrate that increasing membrane cholesterol caused neuronal death when treated with Aβ.[42]

In neurons, lipid rafts are membrane microdomains that are enriched for free cholesterol and GM1 ganglioside and are thought to promote β-secretase cleavage of APP, producing the aggregation-prone Aβ42.[43,44] Consistent with this long-held hypothesis, experiments by Djelti and colleagues[45] observed significantly elevated free cholesterol when the mRNA of the metabolic enzyme *CYp46a1*, which regulates neuronal cholesterol content, was inhibited.[45] When investigators isolated lipid rafts from mouse hippocampi on sucrose gradients, APP and Aβ peptide levels were increased and tau phosphorylation was observed. The increased cholesterol was accompanied by endosomal enlargement, and animals exhibited cognitive deficits and neuronal death.

Historically, most neuronal cholesterol literature has focused on free cholesterol due to its abundance. However, several studies have sought to manipulate neuronal cholesterol dynamics to investigate potential mechanisms in AD. For example, inhibition of acyl-coenzyme A:cholesterol acyltransferase (ACAT1), which catalyzes cholesterol ester formation, reduces Aβ generation via alteration of the intracellular distribution of cholesterol.[34,46] For example, in mice containing the London and Swedish mutations, treatment with ACAT inhibitors reduced esterified cholesterol by 86%, and Aβ plaque level by 88% to 99%, along with a slight improvement in spatial learning in mice.[46] Similarly, Bryleva and colleagues[37] eliminated ACAT1 in triple transgenic mice and saw a 60% reduction in human APP, and observed improved cognitive function in mice with cognitive deficits. In this work, lack of ACAT1 caused an increase in 24-S-OH and cholesterol.[37] ACAT inhibition has also been shown to enhance autophagy and reduce tau in the triple transgenic AD mouse model.[47] Taken together, this evidence suggests that the ratio of esterified cholesterol to free cholesterol is a primary determinant of AD neuropathology.

Another study investigated associations between neurotoxic Aβ fibrils, intracellular vesicular trafficking, and cholesterol homeostasis by labeling esterified cholesterol and free cholesterol in rat neuronal cell cultures.[48] Neurotoxic Aβ fibril treatment increased free cholesterol, reduced esterified cholesterol, and increased vesicular exocytotic markers. These results suggest that Aβ fibrils alter cholesterol homeostasis through vesicular trafficking mechanisms and that free cholesterol may regulate vesicular trafficking that are involved in cellular cholesterol homeostasis. Another hypothesis postulates that Aβ fibrils bind membrane cholesterol and attenuate the conversion of free cholesterol to esterified cholesterol. Along this line, our group previously reported a marked increase in free cholesterol and ganglioside GM1 in Aβ-positive synaptosomes from AD cortex,[49] another result that may reflect increased rafts in synaptic membrane, or the binding of cholesterol to synaptic Aβ.

In contrast, a study conducted by Hutter-Paier and colleagues[46] showed that ACAT inhibition reduced esterified cholesterol levels by 89%, reduced accumulation of Aβ plaques by 88% to 99%, reduced insoluble Aβ by 83% to 96%, and reduced soluble Aβ by 34% in brain homogenates of transgenic mice expressing human APP.[46] Furthermore, spatial learning and memory in mice improved and correlated with reduced Aβ levels. These results suggest that reduced esterified cholesterol through ACAT inhibition may reduce AD pathogenesis. Similarly, several studies demonstrate that ACAT1 deficiency in mice (ACAT$^{-/-}$) results in reduced APP and Aβ levels.[37,47] These studies imply that reduced esterified cholesterol levels prevent Aβ accumulation in AD. Overall, the literature concerning esterified cholesterol in AD is varied. Because cholesterol pool dynamics associated with AD pathogenesis remain unclear and difficult to measure due to fast turnover of cholesterol pools, more research is needed to investigate the potential mechanisms underlying cholesterol esterification. Furthermore, functional studies and imaging studies in total cholesterol versus esterified and free cholesterol turnover need to be conducted in human models.

In recent reports, cholesterol in AD has been found to be mediated by APOE. Arold and colleagues[50] measured free cholesterol across apoE isoforms in synaptosomes from both human and targeted replacement mice expressing human apoE isoforms (apoETR). Consistent with the hypothesis that synaptic Aβ is cleared by apoE, apoE levels were increased in Aβ-positive synapses in normal samples compared with late AD samples, suggesting effective clearance in normal samples. Furthermore, the apoE2 isoform expressed higher levels of apoE and free cholesterol compared with apoE4 samples. These results suggest that the increased lipidation capacity of the apoE2 isoform is optimal for Aβ clearance compared with the apoE4 isoform.[50] Additionally, Hu and colleagues[51] demonstrated that apoETR mice expressing human apoE4 have reduced apoE-associated cholesterol and increased Aβ accumulation compared with mice expressing apoE3 and apoE2 isoforms.[51] Adding important data from human subjects, Shinohara and colleagues[52] showed that the APOE2 allele is associated with lower incidence of cognitive decline during aging using retrospective clinical data.[52] This was validated with experiments on aged apoE2TR mice that exhibited reduced synaptic loss and increased apoE levels when compared with either apoE3TR or apoE4TR mice. Additionally, free cholesterol was reduced among apoE2 mice, but not in apoE4 mice. Overall, despite the lack of consensus, there is strong experimental evidence suggesting APOE isoform mediates cholesterol dynamics contributing to pathologic changes in AD.

INFLAMMATION AND THE INNATE IMMUNE SYSTEM IN ALZHEIMER DISEASE
Apolipoprotein E and Inflammation

A wide body of evidence suggests that aggregated proteins can initiate an immune response that can exacerbate neurodegenerative conditions such as AD. Injured neurons are thought to release distress signals, initiating a strong response from microglia, the immune cells of the CNS. This inflammatory response may itself injure neurons and synapses, but may ultimately protect circuits. Much work is needed to understand the early sequence of events that occur in vivo.[53] ApoE, genetic variants of which contribute differentially to AD risk, is the predominant apolipoprotein present in the CNS. It is mainly produced by astrocytes and activated microglia in the brain.[54] Recent lines of evidence make it clear that apoE is a key mediator of the immune response to stressors both in the brain and in the periphery.[55,56]

Studying APOE effects in the periphery, Gale and colleagues[56] evaluated the innate immune response to organ injury in sepsis using whole blood from healthy APOE3/3 and APOE3/4 humans. Healthy volunteers were given lipopolysaccharide (LPS) to induce an inflammatory response. The APOE3/4 volunteers exhibited higher temperatures, tumor necrosis factor (TNF)α levels, and interleukin (IL)-6 levels compared with the APOE3/3 volunteers. This suggests that APOE genotype modulates immune response to Toll-like receptor signaling during systemic stressors in the periphery.[56] Similarly, Ringman and colleagues[57] analyzed 77 plasma signaling proteins in a small cohort of subjects with ADAD with PSEN1 or APP mutations (mean age, 33–42 years, mostly asymptomatic). Surprisingly, signaling proteins were not altered in mutation carriers, but APOE genotype affected the level of 17 proteins. They found that in persons with the e2/3 and e3/3 genotypes, apoE and superoxide dismutase (SOD1) levels were significantly higher than in e3/4 genotypes. Furthermore, IL-13, IL-3, IL-4, IL-5, and IL-12p40 levels were elevated in e3/4 compared with e3/3 and e2/3 genotypes. These results suggest that APOE genotype modulates inflammatory mediators in AD, with e4 carriers demonstrating elevated inflammatory mediators.[57]

Focused on chronic neuroinflammation, Tai and colleagues[55] reported results from transgenic mice expressing 5 familial AD mutations and human apoE isoforms (EFAD mice).[55] Results showed that impaired apoE4 function modulates Aβ-induced neuroinflammatory signaling; increases were observed in detrimental TLR4-p38α signaling, whereas the beneficial IL-4R-nuclear receptor pathway was suppressed. However, the differential modulation varied with progression of disease. In mixed glial cultures from such mice, oligomeric Ab-induced TNFα secretion was increased by apoE4 via the TLR4 pathway, suggesting TNFα and TLR4 as potential targets for APOE-modulated Aβ-induced neuroinflammation.

Furthermore, data from Rodriguez and colleagues[58] support the hypothesis that APOE genotype affects Aβ-associated neuroinflammation. Investigators studied the impact of APOE genotype on Aβ-associated microglial activity in EFAD mouse models. E4FAD mice had increased levels of Aβ plaques compared with E3FAD and E2FAD mice. Moreover, IL-1β levels and microglial reactivity were increased in E4FAD mice compared with E3FAD and E2FAD mice.[58] Overall, results from these reports strongly suggest that APOE genotype influences Aβ-mediated microglial activation and neuroinflammatory processes in AD progression.

In a series of experiments in APP transgenic mouse models, Chakrabarty and colleagues[59] studied IL-10 expression and its effects on apoE and Aβ.[59] IL-10 is a cytokine that attenuates inflammatory cascades by inhibiting inflammatory cytokines. Investigators found that IL-10 expression exacerbated AD pathology by increasing plaque burden and reduced synaptic markers, and also produced cognitive decline as measured by fear tone conditioning tasks. Importantly, IL-10 also increased apoE expression and apoE colocalization with insoluble Aβ, and both IL-10 and apoE reduced phagocytosis of Aβ by microglia.[59] Despite these studies, more work is needed to determine whether apoE isoforms differentially affect this Aβ-mediated inflammatory response in AD.

Microglia in Alzheimer Disease

Microglia are the innate immune cells of the CNS and have been known to play an essential role in mediating and responding to inflammatory signals in the brain. Like the importance of cholesterol metabolism, the evidence showing that inflammatory mediators and innate immunity are critical mediators in AD has exploded in recent years.[5] For example, it has been known for decades that inflammation plays a role in the pathogenesis of AD and early studies looking at the use of nonsteroidal anti-inflammatory drugs (NSAIDs) and AD have highlighted the inverse correlation between NSAID use and AD development.[60] Furthermore, the innate immune system has been implicated in AD; for example, complement pathway proteins were observed near plaques and tangles in 1989, and microglia have been shown to interact with and internalize senile plaques.[61,62]

Recent genome-wide association studies have identified single nucleotide polymorphisms (SNPs) in immune genes that confer an elevated risk in developing AD. Of particular interest to the field is the microglial-enriched triggering receptor expressed on myeloid cells 2 (TREM2), which has sharply highlighted the strength of the association between inflammatory pathways and innate immunity and AD.[63,64] TREM2 is a cell surface receptor expressed in microglia that signals via its co-adaptor protein TYROBP, a tyrosine kinase protein. R47H, the most frequently studied TREM2 SNP, has been shown in some meta-analysis studies to increase the risk of developing AD to the same degree as possessing a single allele of *APOE4*, which has long been the leading risk factor in late-onset AD.[5] Although the function of TREM2 is not fully defined, recent studies have shown that it plays a role in sustaining microglial phagocytosis of Aβ and neuronal debris, promoting microglia survivability, compacting Aβ plaques, and lipid sensing via apolipoproteins E and J.[65–67] Efforts in establishing the exact role that TREM2 plays in AD have identified a connection between microglia and neuronal health. In one study, a set of key observations was made by Wang and colleagues,[65] who examined TREM2$^{-/-}$ 5XFAD mice and demonstrated that the lack of TREM2 expression was associated with increased Aβ accumulation in the hippocampus and increased loss of layer-V cortical neurons compared with controls. TREM2 deficiency was shown to impair microglial colocalization with Aβ plaques and the mechanism proposed was that TREM2 acts as a sensor of anionic and zwitterionic lipids that accompany neuronal damage and Aβ accumulation.[65] The discovery of the link between microglial-TREM2 and AD has highlighted the importance in looking at microglial phagocytosis of CNS substrates, such as neuronal synapses and beta-amyloid.

Recent focus on microglial dysfunction across age-related neurologic diseases, such as Parkinson-like diseases and AD, have highlighted the heterogeneity in microglia morphology and function. In a study conducted by Bachstetter and colleagues,[68] investigators assessed microglia in human brain tissue from patients with dementia with Lewy body, hippocampal sclerosis, and AD using immunohistochemistry analysis of microglia/macrophage markers IBA1 and CD68. The investigators first found that microglia exhibited varying morphology based on disease and classified them according to 5 forms: ramified, hypertrophic, dystrophic, rod-shaped, and ameboid microglia. In agreement with previous literature, there was increased dystrophic/deteriorated microglia level in AD samples, implying hypoactivation of microglia in AD pathology.[68] Of note, rodlike microglia have been highlighted to be a morphology associated with age and many neurologic diseases, such as in vitro microglial aging, CNS injury, and a transgenic Tau-APP mouse models.[69–71] Rodlike microglia observed in close proximity with damaged and degenerating neurons have been implicated in synaptic stripping in the CNS. These studies emphasize microglial response to neurodegenerative diseases and have further highlighted their role in maintaining neuronal homeostasis.

A recent pioneering study assessed neuronal synapse health in AD using transgenic mouse models. Hong and colleagues[72] used the J20 mouse model of AD to investigate the hypothesis that synaptic loss is mediated by the complement cascade and microglia early in AD. The initiating complement protein C1q level was elevated and localized to the synapse before plaque formation, and C1q was necessary for the downstream toxic effects of soluble Aβ oligomers on synapses. Inhibition of C1q, C3, and the C3 receptor, CR3 (CD11b-CD18/MAC-1), reduced the number of activated microglia and the degree of early synapse loss. Importantly, microglial phagocytosis of Aβ-treated synaptic material was found to be in part via a CR3-dependent process. Overall, the findings of this study suggest that synaptic loss early in AD involves activation of the complement cascade and phagocytosis by microglia. Thus, these elements of innate immunity early in AD may represent novel therapeutic targets with microglia being a cell-target.[72]

To begin to further understand microglia in disease and potentially develop therapies aimed at AD, new tools and technologies must be developed. One major challenge in studying microglia in vivo has been distinguishing them from their macrophage counterparts under disease or injury states. Mounting evidence highlights the importance of peripheral-derived macrophages and their role in CNS diseases, and recent studies have suggested that macrophages may be TREM2-positive cells despite reports highlighting TREM2 being microglial-enriched in the CNS.[71,73] Recently, Bennet and colleagues[74] developed novel rabbit monoclonal antibodies to detect Tmem119 intracellular and extracellular domains in mice. Investigators were able to use Tmem119 antibody in immunohistochemical identification of microglia and FACS isolation of microglia. They found that TMEM119 immunoreactivity remains constant, independent of microglia activation state and the TMEM119 antibody can be used to isolate and study either quiescent or activated microglia.[74] However, in an SOD1 mutation model of ALS, TMEM119 mRNA levels decreased compared with WT controls. TMEM119 appears to be a superior method for identifying microglia versus other myeloid cells in the CNS and its use will advance the studying of microglia in transgenic models. Studies using in vitro models like mouse microglial cell lines have allowed for studying molecular pathways involved in phagocytosis or inflammation. A recent study looking at a mouse AD model deficient of T and B cells (Rag5xfAD) revealed increased beta-amyloid expression compared with an immune-intact AD model.[75] Renewed analysis of the gene expression data of Rag5xfAD mice revealed an increased expression of the phagocytosis regulator enzyme SHIP1 (INPP5D; **Fig. 2A**). Inhibiting SHIP1 in BV2 microglia using a SHIP1-specific inhibitor increased phagocytosis of fibrillar Aβ greater than vehicle and similar to immunoglobulin (Ig)G-stimulated increased phagocytosis (**Fig. 2B**). New tools also have been developed for studying human microglial lines using induced pluripotent lines. In collaboration, we have begun to investigate how TREM2+ induced pluripotent stem (iPS)-derived microglialike cells (iMGLs) internalize human-derived synaptosomes from patient cases. Using this platform, we

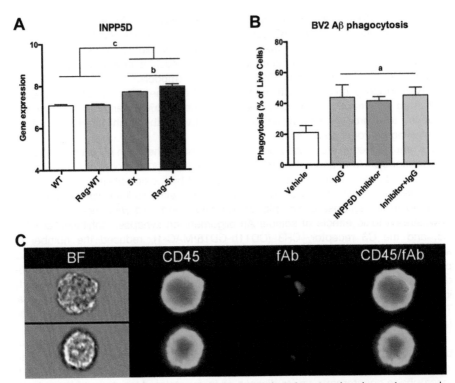

Fig. 2. Modeling and targeting microglial genes and their functional pathways in neurodegenerative diseases using in vitro models. Microglial molecular pathways implicated in AD can be modeled and their pathways interrogated using murine mouse models. (*A*) A recent study highlights that immune-deficient AD mice (Rag-5x) have elevated beta-amyloid compared with 5x littermates.[75] Analysis of deposited whole-brain mRNA data reveal elevated expression of the phagocytosis-modulator INPP5D/SHIP1. (*B*) Bar graphs of murine BV2 microglia phagocytosis of fibrillary Aβ on Amnis ImagestreamX flow cytometer. BV2 microglia preincubated with nonspecific mouse IgG, INNP5D inhibitor, or both increases microglia phagocytosis. (*C*) Representative images captured on Amnis ImagestreamX flow cytometer of BV2 microglia internalizing fibrillary beta-amyloid. Statistical analysis was determined using 1-way analysis of variance followed by Tukey's post hoc test. (*A*) n = 4 per group, (*B*) n = 2 to 4 per group; [a] $P<.001$, [b] $P<.01$, and [c] $P<.05$.

will continue to study the role of microglia-mediated inflammation in AD models as well as their role in synaptic pruning and phagocytosis in health and disease.

Astrocytes

Astrogliosis is a prominent feature of AD pathobiology. Synaptic pruning by astrocytes is not only important in brain development but may be aberrantly activated in neurodegenerative diseases, including AD. Barres and colleagues have used murine synaptosome phagocytosis assays to identify important cell surface receptors that are necessary for synaptic pruning (MERTK).[76,77] A newly developed technology, Amnis Imagestream (Seattle, WA), couples traditional flow cytometry to imaging, and will greatly facilitate studies examining pruning in development as well as neurologic diseases like AD. Astrocyte phagocytosis can be assessed by incubating astrocytes with human synaptosomes prelabeled with pHrodoRed (Lifetech, Waltham, MA), which emits fluorescence only at low pH, and is present in intracellular acidified lysosomes. Therefore, fluorescent signal is indicative of bona fide phagocytosis. As shown in **Fig. 3**A, traditional flow analysis can gate for phagocytic events within iPS-derived astrocytes that lack fluorescence in the absence of synaptosomes (left panel), but on incubation with synaptosomes emit fluorescence (right panel). In **Fig. 3**B, the imaging capability allows for the visualization of every cell and the potential to determine colocalization between the pHrodoRed-emitting synaptosomes and the MERTK receptor, which has been implicated in synaptic pruning. Quantification of colocalization indicates that essentially all cells that demonstrated phagocytic activity also expressed MERTK. The synaptosome phagocytosis assay can be used to assess astrocyte function. In **Fig. 2**C, the synaptosome phagocytosis is used to demonstrate that the ability of iPS-derived astrocytes to phagocytose synaptosomes is similar to fetal-derived astrocytes. Therefore, this assay can be used to investigate how *APOE* genotype influences astrocyte-mediated synaptic pruning during development or in response to neurotoxic insults, like Aβ or inflammatory cytokines.

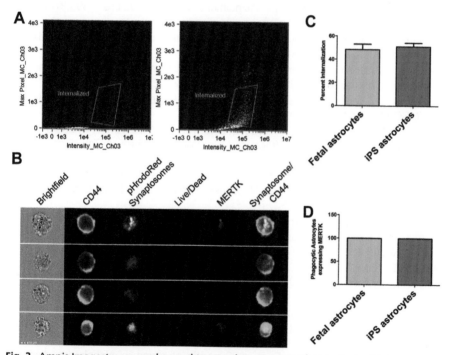

Fig. 3. Amnis Imagestream can be used to examine astrocyte phagocytosis of human synaptosomes (*A–D*). Synaptosomes were labeled with pHrodoRed (ThermoFisher) and incubated with iPS-derived astrocytes. Astrocytes are then labeled with CD44 and MERTK and cells that were CD44-positive were examined for the presence of pHrodoRed. (*A*) Flow cytometry analysis of astrocytes to gate for phagocytic events. (*B*) Representative images of iPS-derived astrocytes can evaluate viability, and can be used to examine colocalization between synaptosome-containing cellular compartments and MERTK. (*C*) iPS astrocytes can functionally phagocytose synaptosomes to the same extent as fetal astrocytes. (*D*) Essentially all iPS-derived astrocytes that demonstrate a phagocytic event express MERTK, which has been shown to be essential for astrocyte-mediated synaptic pruning.

SUMMARY

Research into AD mechanisms has produced an immense and complex body of literature, reflecting the multifactorial nature of the disease. This short review is not meant to be comprehensive, but is intended to highlight some of recent advances and directions in which the basic science is moving. Given the lack of success in amyloid and other clinical trials to date, new directions offer the possibility for translation into the clinic for prevention and treatment of a costly and devastating disease.

ACKNOWLEDGMENTS

AG16573 (W.W. Poon). We are indebted to Jenn Atwood and the Immunology Institute Flow Core.

REFERENCES

1. Levy-Lahad E, Wijsman EM, Nemens E, et al. A familial Alzheimer's disease locus on chromosome 1. Science 1995;269(5226):970–3.
2. Sherrington R, Rogaev EI, Liang Y, et al. Cloning of a gene bearing missense mutations in early-onset familial Alzheimer's disease. Nature 1995;375(6534): 754–60.
3. Hardy JA, Higgins GA. Alzheimer's disease: the amyloid cascade hypothesis. Science 1992;256(5054):184–5.
4. Hardy J, Selkoe DJ. The amyloid hypothesis of Alzheimer's disease: progress and problems on the road to therapeutics. Science 2002;297(5580):353–6.
5. Selkoe DJ, Hardy J. The amyloid hypothesis of Alzheimer's disease at 25 years. EMBO Mol Med 2016;8(6):595–608.
6. Mairet-Coello G, Courchet J, Pieraut S, et al. The CAMKK2-AMPK kinase pathway mediates the synaptotoxic effects of Abeta oligomers through Tau phosphorylation. Neuron 2013;78(1):94–108.
7. Pooler AM, Polydoro M, Maury EA, et al. Amyloid accelerates tau propagation and toxicity in a model of early Alzheimer's disease. Acta Neuropathol Commun 2015;3:14.
8. Terry RD, Masliah E, Salmon DP, et al. Physical basis of cognitive alterations in Alzheimer's disease: synapse loss is the major correlate of cognitive impairment. Ann Neurol 1991;30(4):572–80.
9. Lue LF, Kuo YM, Roher AE, et al. Soluble amyloid beta peptide concentration as a predictor of synaptic change in Alzheimer's disease. Am J Pathol 1999;155(3): 853–62.
10. Bilousova T, Miller CA, Poon WW, et al. Synaptic amyloid-beta oligomers precede p-Tau and differentiate high pathology control cases. Am J Pathol 2016;186(1): 185–98.
11. Gylys KH, Fein JA, Yang F, et al. Synaptic changes in Alzheimer's disease: increased amyloid-beta and gliosis in surviving terminals is accompanied by decreased PSD-95 fluorescence. Am J Pathol 2004;165(5):1809–17.
12. Pickett EK, Koffie RM, Wegmann S, et al. Non-fibrillar oligomeric amyloid-beta within synapses. J Alzheimers Dis 2016;53(3):787–800.
13. Capetillo-Zarate E, Gracia L, Yu F, et al. High-resolution 3D reconstruction reveals intra-synaptic amyloid fibrils. Am J Pathol 2011;179(5):2551–8.
14. Finnema SJ, Nabulsi NB, Eid T, et al. Imaging synaptic density in the living human brain. Sci Transl Med 2016;8(348):348ra396.

15. Ferreira ST, Klein WL. The Abeta oligomer hypothesis for synapse failure and memory loss in Alzheimer's disease. Neurobiol Learn Mem 2011;96(4):529–43.
16. Ferreira ST, Lourenco MV, Oliveira MM, et al. Soluble amyloid-beta oligomers as synaptotoxins leading to cognitive impairment in Alzheimer's disease. Front Cell Neurosci 2015;9:191.
17. Esparza TJ, Zhao H, Cirrito JR, et al. Amyloid-beta oligomerization in Alzheimer dementia versus high-pathology controls. Ann Neurol 2013;73(1):104–19.
18. Braak H, Braak E. Neuropathological stageing of Alzheimer-related changes. Acta Neuropathol 1991;82(4):239–59.
19. de Calignon A, Polydoro M, Suarez-Calvet M, et al. Propagation of tau pathology in a model of early Alzheimer's disease. Neuron 2012;73(4):685–97.
20. Pooler AM, Phillips EC, Lau DH, et al. Physiological release of endogenous tau is stimulated by neuronal activity. EMBO Rep 2013;14(4):389–94.
21. Yamada K, Holth JK, Liao F, et al. Neuronal activity regulates extracellular tau in vivo. J Exp Med 2014;211(3):387–93.
22. Sokolow S, Henkins KM, Bilousova T, et al. Presynaptic C-terminal truncated tau is released from cortical synapses in Alzheimer's disease. J Neurochem 2015; 133(3):368–79.
23. Pooler AM, Noble W, Hanger DP. A role for tau at the synapse in Alzheimer's disease pathogenesis. Neuropharmacology 2014;76(Pt A):1–8.
24. Herrmann A, Spires-Jones T. Clearing the way for tau immunotherapy in Alzheimer's disease. J Neurochem 2015;132(1):1–4.
25. Kowal J, Tkach M, Thery C. Biogenesis and secretion of exosomes. Curr Opin Cell Biol 2014;29:116–25.
26. Dinkins MB, Dasgupta S, Wang G, et al. Exosome reduction in vivo is associated with lower amyloid plaque load in the 5XFAD mouse model of Alzheimer's disease. Neurobiol Aging 2014;35(8):1792–800.
27. Mohamed NV, Herrou T, Plouffe V, et al. Spreading of tau pathology in Alzheimer's disease by cell-to-cell transmission. Eur J Neurosci 2013;37(12):1939–48.
28. Polanco JC, Scicluna BJ, Hill AF, et al. Extracellular vesicles isolated from the brains of rTg4510 mice seed tau protein aggregation in a threshold-dependent manner. J Biol Chem 2016;291(24):12445–66.
29. Asai H, Ikezu S, Tsunoda S, et al. Depletion of microglia and inhibition of exosome synthesis halt tau propagation. Nat Neurosci 2015;18(11):1584–93.
30. Maphis N, Xu G, Kokiko-Cochran ON, et al. Reactive microglia drive tau pathology and contribute to the spreading of pathological tau in the brain. Brain 2015; 138(Pt 6):1738–55.
31. Yuyama K, Sun H, Usuki S, et al. A potential function for neuronal exosomes: sequestering intracerebral amyloid-beta peptide. FEBS Lett 2015;589(1):84–8.
32. Fiandaca MS, Kapogiannis D, Mapstone M, et al. Identification of preclinical Alzheimer's disease by a profile of pathogenic proteins in neurally derived blood exosomes: a case-control study. Alzheimers Dement 2015;11(6):600–7.e1.
33. Sato N, Morishita R. The roles of lipid and glucose metabolism in modulation of beta-amyloid, tau, and neurodegeneration in the pathogenesis of Alzheimer disease. Front Aging Neurosci 2015;7:199.
34. Puglielli L, Konopka G, Pack-Chung E, et al. Acyl-coenzyme A: cholesterol acyltransferase modulates the generation of the amyloid beta-peptide. Nat Cell Biol 2001;3(10):905–12.
35. Petrov AM, Kasimov MR, Zefirov AL. Brain cholesterol metabolism and its defects: linkage to neurodegenerative diseases and synaptic dysfunction. Acta Naturae 2016;8(1):58–73.

36. Murphy SR, Chang CC, Dogbevia G, et al. Acat1 knockdown gene therapy decreases amyloid-beta in a mouse model of Alzheimer's disease. Mol Ther 2013; 21(8):1497–506.

37. Bryleva EY, Rogers MA, Chang CC, et al. ACAT1 gene ablation increases 24(S)-hydroxycholesterol content in the brain and ameliorates amyloid pathology in mice with AD. Proc Natl Acad Sci U S A 2010;107(7):3081–6.

38. Dietschy JM. Central nervous system: cholesterol turnover, brain development and neurodegeneration. Biol Chem 2009;390(4):287–93.

39. Mauch DH, Nagler K, Schumacher S, et al. CNS synaptogenesis promoted by glia-derived cholesterol. Science 2001;294(5545):1354–7.

40. Schneider A, Schulz-Schaeffer W, Hartmann T, et al. Cholesterol depletion reduces aggregation of amyloid-beta peptide in hippocampal neurons. Neurobiol Dis 2006;23(3):573–7.

41. Ferrera P, Mercado-Gomez O, Silva-Aguilar M, et al. Cholesterol potentiates beta-amyloid-induced toxicity in human neuroblastoma cells: involvement of oxidative stress. Neurochem Res 2008;33(8):1509–17.

42. Abramov AY, Ionov M, Pavlov E, et al. Membrane cholesterol content plays a key role in the neurotoxicity of beta-amyloid: implications for Alzheimer's disease. Aging Cell 2011;10(4):595–603.

43. Ehehalt R, Keller P, Haass C, et al. Amyloidogenic processing of the Alzheimer beta-amyloid precursor protein depends on lipid rafts. J Cell Biol 2003;160(1): 113–23.

44. Lee SJ, Liyanage U, Bickel PE, et al. A detergent-insoluble membrane compartment contains A beta in vivo. Nat Med 1998;4(6):730–4.

45. Djelti F, Braudeau J, Hudry E, et al. CYP46A1 inhibition, brain cholesterol accumulation and neurodegeneration pave the way for Alzheimer's disease. Brain 2015;138(Pt 8):2383–98.

46. Hutter-Paier B, Huttunen HJ, Puglielli L, et al. The ACAT inhibitor CP-113,818 markedly reduces amyloid pathology in a mouse model of Alzheimer's disease. Neuron 2004;44(2):227–38.

47. Shibuya Y, Niu Z, Bryleva EY, et al. Acyl-coenzyme A:cholesterol acyltransferase 1 blockage enhances autophagy in the neurons of triple transgenic Alzheimer's disease mouse and reduces human P301L-tau content at the presymptomatic stage. Neurobiol Aging 2015;36(7):2248–59.

48. Liu Y, Peterson DA, Schubert D. Amyloid beta peptide alters intracellular vesicle trafficking and cholesterol homeostasis. Proc Natl Acad Sci U S A 1998;95(22): 13266–71.

49. Gylys KH, Fein JA, Yang F, et al. Increased cholesterol in Abeta-positive nerve terminals from Alzheimer's disease cortex. Neurobiol Aging 2007;28(1):8–17.

50. Arold S, Sullivan P, Bilousova T, et al. Apolipoprotein E level and cholesterol are associated with reduced synaptic amyloid beta in Alzheimer's disease and apoE TR mouse cortex. Acta Neuropathol 2012;123(1):39–52.

51. Hu J, Liu CC, Chen XF, et al. Opposing effects of viral mediated brain expression of apolipoprotein E2 (apoE2) and apoE4 on apoE lipidation and Abeta metabolism in apoE4-targeted replacement mice. Mol Neurodegener 2015;10:6.

52. Shinohara M, Kanekiyo T, Yang L, et al. APOE2 eases cognitive decline during Aging: clinical and preclinical evaluations. Ann Neurol 2016. [Epub ahead of print].

53. Czirr E, Wyss-Coray T. The immunology of neurodegeneration. J Clin Invest 2012; 122(4):1156–63.

54. LaDu MJ, Shah JA, Reardon CA, et al. Apolipoprotein E and apolipoprotein E receptors modulate A beta-induced glial neuroinflammatory responses. Neurochem Int 2001;39(5-6):427-34.

55. Tai LM, Ghura S, Koster KP, et al. APOE-modulated Abeta-induced neuroinflammation in Alzheimer's disease: current landscape, novel data, and future perspective. J Neurochem 2015;133(4):465-88.

56. Gale SC, Gao L, Mikacenic C, et al. APOepsilon4 is associated with enhanced in vivo innate immune responses in human subjects. J Allergy Clin Immunol 2014; 134(1):127-34.

57. Ringman JM, Elashoff D, Geschwind DH, et al. Plasma signaling proteins in persons at genetic risk for Alzheimer disease: influence of APOE genotype. Arch Neurol 2012;69(6):757-64.

58. Rodriguez GA, Tai LM, LaDu MJ, et al. Human APOE4 increases microglia reactivity at Abeta plaques in a mouse model of Abeta deposition. J Neuroinflammation 2014;11:111.

59. Chakrabarty P, Li A, Ceballos-Diaz C, et al. IL-10 alters immunoproteostasis in APP mice, increasing plaque burden and worsening cognitive behavior. Neuron 2015;85(3):519-33.

60. Szekely CA, Town T, Zandi PP. NSAIDs for the chemoprevention of Alzheimer's disease. Subcell Biochem 2007;42:229-48.

61. McGeer PL, Akiyama H, Itagaki S, et al. Activation of the classical complement pathway in brain tissue of Alzheimer patients. Neurosci Lett 1989;107(1-3):341-6.

62. Haga S, Akai K, Ishii T. Demonstration of microglial cells in and around senile (neuritic) plaques in the Alzheimer brain. An immunohistochemical study using a novel monoclonal antibody. Acta Neuropathol 1989;77(6):569-75.

63. Benitez BA, Jin SC, Guerreiro R, et al. Missense variant in TREML2 protects against Alzheimer's disease. Neurobiol Aging 2014;35(6):1510.e9-26.

64. Guerreiro R, Wojtas A, Bras J, et al. TREM2 variants in Alzheimer's disease. N Engl J Med 2013;368(2):117-27.

65. Wang Y, Cella M, Mallinson K, et al. TREM2 lipid sensing sustains the microglial response in an Alzheimer's disease model. Cell 2015;160(6):1061-71.

66. Yuan P, Condello C, Keene CD, et al. TREM2 haplodeficiency in mice and humans impairs the microglia barrier function leading to decreased amyloid compaction and severe axonal dystrophy. Neuron 2016;90(4):724-39.

67. Melchior B, Garcia AE, Hsiung BK, et al. Dual induction of TREM2 and tolerance-related transcript, Tmem176b, in amyloid transgenic mice: implications for vaccine-based therapies for Alzheimer's disease. ASN Neuro 2010;2(3):e00037.

68. Bachstetter AD, Van Eldik LJ, Schmitt FA, et al. Disease-related microglia heterogeneity in the hippocampus of Alzheimer's disease, dementia with Lewy bodies, and hippocampal sclerosis of aging. Acta Neuropathol Commun 2015;3:32.

69. Caldeira C, Oliveira AF, Cunha C, et al. Microglia change from a reactive to an age-like phenotype with the time in culture. Front Cell Neurosci 2014;8:152.

70. Yuan TF, Liang YX, Peng B, et al. Local proliferation is the main source of rod microglia after optic nerve transection. Sci Rep 2015;5:10788.

71. Chen W, Abud EA, Yeung ST, et al. Increased tauopathy drives microglia-mediated clearance of beta-amyloid. Acta Neuropathol Commun 2016;4(1):63.

72. Hong S, Beja-Glasser VF, Nfonoyim BM, et al. Complement and microglia mediate early synapse loss in Alzheimer mouse models. Science 2016; 352(6286):712-6.

73. Hsieh CL, Koike M, Spusta SC, et al. A role for TREM2 ligands in the phagocytosis of apoptotic neuronal cells by microglia. J Neurochem 2009;109(4): 1144–56.

74. Bennett ML, Bennett FC, Liddelow SA, et al. New tools for studying microglia in the mouse and human CNS. Proc Natl Acad Sci U S A 2016;113(12):E1738–46.

75. Marsh SE, Abud EM, Lakatos A, et al. The adaptive immune system restrains Alzheimer's disease pathogenesis by modulating microglial function. Proc Natl Acad Sci U S A 2016;113(9):E1316–1325.

76. Chung WS, Allen NJ, Eroglu C. Astrocytes control synapse formation, function, and elimination. Cold Spring Harb Perspect Biol 2015;7(9):a020370.

77. Zhang Y, Sloan SA, Clarke LE, et al. Purification and characterization of progenitor and mature human astrocytes reveals transcriptional and functional differences with mouse. Neuron 2016;89(1):37–53.

The Role of Neuropsychology in the Assessment of the Cognitively Impaired Elderly

Po H. Lu, PsyD[a],*, Grace J. Lee, PhD[b]

KEYWORDS

- Neuropsychological assessment • Normative data • Older adults
- Cognitive functioning • Dementia • Mild cognitive impairment

KEY POINTS

- Neuropsychological evaluation employs standardized and validated instruments to assess cognitive and emotional functioning. It provides a profile of strengths and weaknesses that assists with diagnostic and treatment recommendations.
- Distinct patterns of performance have been characterized in association with normal aging, mild cognitive impairment that precedes overt dementia, and age-related neurocognitive disorders.
- Special considerations in the assessment of the elderly include physical and sensory limitations, neuropsychiatric symptoms, and serial examination. These factors can affect test performance and interpretation of the results.

INTRODUCTION

The elderly are the fastest growing segment of the population in the United States. By the year 2030, the number of adults over the age of 65 will grow to 71.5 million.[1] As a group, elderly adults are at higher risk for developing cognitive impairment, and the incidence of dementia doubles approximately every 5 years after age 65.[2] With the aging of the baby boom generation, the estimated prevalence of dementia in the United States is predicted to nearly triple, from 5.2 million in 2010 to 15 million by 2050,[3] placing an overwhelming burden on patients, caregivers, and society. These staggering statistics fuel an increasing need to understand the cognitive capacities of the elderly.

Disclosure Statement: Dr P.H. Lu receives royalties from Western Psychological Services for published tests on Effort. Dr G.J. Lee has no financial disclosures.
[a] Executive Mental Health, Inc, 10801 National Boulevard, Los Angeles, CA 90064, USA;
[b] Department of Psychology, School of Behavioral Health, Loma Linda University, 11130 Anderson Street, Loma Linda, CA 92350, USA
* Corresponding author.
E-mail address: plu@emhla.com

Neuropsychological assessment involves the utilization of standardized psychometric tests to evaluate brain function through systematic measurement of various cognitive domains and behavior. The guidelines of the American Academy of Neurology for the early detection of dementia specifically state that neuropsychological batteries are "useful instruments in identifying patients with dementia, particularly when administered to a population at increased risk of cognitive impairment."[4] This article provides an overview of the neuropsychological evaluation process, including descriptions of the domains of assessment and tests used for examining these abilities (**Table 1**). Then, the current state of knowledge on the cognitive changes associated with normal aging, preclinical stages of cognitive disorders, and common age-related dementia syndromes are summarized. The article closes with discussions of special considerations in the assessment of elderly patients.

NEUROPSYCHOLOGICAL ASSESSMENT

Neuropsychological assessment provides an objective, structured method of evaluation that encompasses an individual's cognitive and emotional functioning. Standardized measures have age-based, education-based, and/or gender-based normative data so that individual test scores can be compared with specific reference groups, thereby allowing for more accurate differentiation of normal and abnormal cognitive functioning. In this section the major components of a comprehensive neuropsychological evaluation are covered.

Clinical Interview

The clinical interview is essential to neuropsychological assessment, because it provides a context that informs how the test data are interpreted. In the interview, the neuropsychologist gathers information regarding a patient's relevant symptoms and areas of difficulty as well as how those problems have an impact on activities at home, school, work, and/or social functions. It also elicits pertinent details from a patient's medical, psychological, educational, occupational or social history that might be contributory to their symptoms or influence performance. It is often helpful to interview a spouse, adult child, or close friend who can provide collateral information, because some elderly may have difficulty providing an accurate description of their current symptoms or history due to poor memory or diminished insight. The interview also provides an opportunity for the neuropsychologist to make observations regarding a patient's mental status and behavior, including appearance, orientation, speech, thought process, attention/concentration, emotional state, insight, and judgment. These observations are considered together with a patient's background and history in interpreting the test data.

Mental Status Examination and Cognitive Screening Measures

Evaluations of elderly often include structured screening instruments and mental status rating scales. The most widely used measure is the Mini-Mental State Examination (MMSE),[5] a 30-item instrument that assesses orientation, attention and calculation, registration, and recall of words, language, and construction. Scores below 24 are typically regarded as abnormal and indicate cognitive impairment. It only takes 5 minutes to 10 minutes to administer and score, and it has high inter-rater and test-retest reliability. It yields only a gross estimate, however, of cognitive functioning and has poor sensitivity for identifying mild degrees of cognitive impairment. Furthermore, examination of memory and visuospatial function is inadequate and it lacks any assessment of executive function, which markedly limits its utility in the recognition of

Table 1
Neuropsychological tests used in the assessment of elderly

Cognitive Domain	Test
Global cognitive functioning	MMSE
	MoCA
General intelligence	WAIS-IV
	WASI-II
	TOPF
	National Adult Reading Test
	North American Adult Reading Test
	American National Adult Reading Test
Attention/processing speed	WAIS-IV Digit Span
	Trail Making Test (Part A)
	Stroop test (color naming, word reading)
	WAIS-IV Coding
	Symbol Digit Modalities Test
Language	Boston Naming Test
	FAS
	Animals
Visuospatial skills	Rey-Osterrieth Complex Figure Test (copy trial)
	WAIS-IV Block Design
	WAIS-IV Visual Puzzles
Verbal memory	California Verbal Learning Test
	Rey Auditory Verbal Learning Test
	Hopkins Verbal Learning Test
	Buschke Selective Reminding Test
	WMS-IV Logical Memory
	WMS-IV Verbal Paired Associates
Visual memory	Rey-Osterrieth Complex Figure Test (delayed recall)
	WMS-IV Visual Reproduction
	Brief Visuospatial Memory Test
Executive function	FAS
	Trail Making Test (Part B)
	Stroop test (Color-Word Interference)
	Wisconsin Card Sorting Test
	WAIS-IV Similarities
	WAIS-IV Matrix Reasoning
Neuropsychiatric symptoms	Geriatric Depression Scale
	Patient Health Questionnaire-9 (depression)
	Hamilton Rating Scale for Depression
	Geriatric Anxiety Inventory
	Hamilton Rating Scale for Anxiety
	Neuropsychiatric Inventory
Functional capacity	Functional Activities Questionnaire
	IADLS
	Everyday Cognition scale
	Direct Assessment of Functional Status

frontal or frontal-subcortical circuit disorders and focal cognitive deficits. Additionally, like most standardized cognitive tests, the MMSE is subject to tremendous influence by education and other sociocultural factors.[6]

The Montreal Cognitive Assessment (MoCA)[7] is another screening instrument that expands on the abilities assessed by the MMSE, including additional items assessing frontal-executive functions, cued/recognition memory, and visuospatial function. Consequently, the MoCA is more sensitive than the MMSE in detecting mild cognitive impairment (MCI).[8] Other mental status rating scales include the Alzheimer's Disease Assessment Scale,[9] Dementia Rating Scale,[10] and Blessed Dementia Scale,[11] but these instruments have more limited utility in assessing non-Alzheimer pathologies.

General Intellectual Functioning

A full neuropsychological evaluation should include an assessment of general intellectual functioning, often accomplished through the Wechsler Adult Intelligence Scale–Fourth Edition (WAIS-IV),[12] or an abbreviated version like the Wechsler Abbreviated Scale of Intelligence–Second Edition (WASI-II).[13] Knowledge of a patient's intellectual capabilities provides a reference point for interpreting neuropsychological test performance. Scores in the average range might be considered within normal limits for the general population but may represent a significant decline for someone with superior cognitive reserve. Similarly, for an individual with low average intellectual capacity, below-average scores on neuropsychological tests should not be overinterpreted as an acquired deficit but may instead reflect the limits of his/her intellectual capacity.

Premorbid intellectual functioning can be estimated for patients whose illness has already had an impact on their overall intellectual functioning. Consideration of demographic variables, such as education and occupational history, can provide a gross estimate of premorbid abilities, but performance-based approaches are also available. Tasks involving breadth of word knowledge or fund of general knowledge (as measured by the WAIS-IV Vocabulary and Information subtests) are highly correlated with Full Scale IQ scores and are resilient to the effects of cerebral insult or early stages of dementia. Premorbid abilities can also be estimated using tests requiring pronunciation of irregularly spelled words (eg, "island" and "cellist") because it reflects previous familiarity and past educational exposure rather than the ability to phonetically decipher the words. Examples of measures using this procedure include the Test of Premorbid Functioning (TOPF)[14] and the American National Adult Reading Test.[15]

Attention and Information Processing Speed

Attention is the ability to focus and direct cognitive processes to a specific task while resisting distraction; concentration is the ability to focus and sustain attention over time. Attention is commonly measured by the digit span test. The examiner recites a series of number sequences of increasing length, and the patient repeats back each number sequence in the same order. Most healthy elderly can correctly recite 5 to 7 digits.[12] More complex tests of sustained attention and cognitive processing speed include tasks involving rapid number sequencing (Trail Making Test Part A[16]), word reading and color naming (Stroop test[17]), and symbol copying (WAIS-IV Coding[11] and Symbol Digit Modalities Test[18]). Assessment of attention and processing speed is critical as poor attention/slow information processing can adversely affect performance in other cognitive domains, thus confounding the interpretation of specific cognitive deficits.

Language

Language disturbances in the elderly often manifest as word-finding difficulties. As such, assessment of language functions usually involves object naming tasks (eg, Boston Naming Test[19]), which measure their ability to retrieve semantic information on command. Verbal fluency tasks (eg, FAS and animals[20]) are also used to assess language via the spontaneous generation of words that begin with specified letters of the alphabet or belong to a semantic category. In addition to formal testing, qualitative information regarding speech and language is also gathered by listening to a patient's discourse during clinical interview and examining the patient's reading, writing, repetition, and comprehension abilities over the course of the assessment.

Visuospatial Skills

Visuospatial functions encompass perceptual and constructional abilities, which are typically assessed through copying/drawing and building/assembly tasks. On copying/drawing tasks, patients are asked to copy visual stimuli, such as overlapping pentagons, a 3-D cube, or more complex designs with multiple details (Rey-Osterrieth Complex Figure Test[21]). Building/assembly tasks involve constructing blocks to match abstract designs (WAIS-IV Block Design) or putting together individual puzzle pieces to produce a whole object (WAIS-IV Visual Puzzles). Observation of abnormal spatial relationships, absence of detail, stimulus-boundedness, loss of 3-D perspective, or neglect of one part of the drawing can help distinguish between perceptual failures, spatial confusion, and apraxia.

Learning and Memory

Memory problems are a common complaint among the elderly population, which include a tendency for misplacing items, difficulty remembering appointments, and forgetfulness for details of conversations and events. Memory has multiple dimensions, including the ability to store and retain information as well as later retrieval of desired information. Amnestic disorders, resulting from mesial limbic and hippocampal dysfunction, involve deficits in consolidation, storage, and retention of information; thus, the desired information is not accessible even with the use of recognition cues. Retrieval deficits, associated with frontal-subcortical disturbance, are characterized by difficulties in spontaneously recalling encoded information but memory performance improves with category cues and/or recognition testing. Memory tests typically follow a common format that includes (1) learning trials in which a patient is temporarily exposed to a stimulus and must then recall the stimulus immediately thereafter and (2) recalling the same information again after a delay period, for example, 20 minutes to 30 minutes later. Many tests may also include a cued recall or recognition portion that can aid in retrieval, thereby distinguishing between amnestic versus retrieval deficits.

Verbal memory is most often assessed through word list–learning tasks in which patients are read a list of words, often over repeated trials, and asked to recall as many as they can both immediately and after a delay period. Other verbal memory tests involve recall of short stories that are read aloud by an examiner. List-learning tasks are often more challenging because patients are exposed to large amounts of unstructured information, whereas in story recall, patients are provided with a meaningful context and structure that often facilitates learning and memory.

Visual memory involves learning and recall of visual stimuli, usually in the form of simple and complex line figures, where a patient draws the figure immediately after exposure and reproduces the figure again after a specified time interval. Varying formats include presenting a series of figures one at a time for 10 seconds each (Wechsler Memory Scale–Fourth Edition [WMS-IV] Visual Reproduction[22]) or presenting a page containing several figures for 10 seconds with multiple trials (Brief Visual Memory Test–Revised[23]). The Rey-Osterrieth Complex Figure Test has delayed recall trials in which patients must reproduce the figure from memory either 3 minutes or 30 minutes after the copy trial. Other visual memory tasks not involving a constructional component include recognition of faces and remembering details of pictures.

Executive Functioning

Executive functions can be conceptualized as a complex set of capacities, including volition, planning, initiation, and mental flexibility, which are involved in controlling other cognitive processes, thus enabling a person to engage successfully in goal-directed, socially appropriate behavior. The prefrontal cortex and its connections through the caudate nuclei are the biological substrates underlying executive functions.

Neuropsychological assessment of executive functioning encompasses abilities involving divided attention, mental flexibility, and set shifting (Trail Making Test Part B[16] and Wisconsin Card Sorting Test[24]), generative ideation through measures of verbal fluency[20] and design fluency,[25] and the ability to inhibit overlearned, automatic responses (Stroop test[17]). Abstract reasoning is a related executive function usually assessed through interpreting similarities between words (WAIS-IV Similarities) or deciphering patterns in a visual array or grid of figures (WAIS-IV Matrix Reasoning). Impaired insight and judgment is also an indicator of executive dysfunction.

Computerized Neuropsychological Testing

Innovations and advances in digital technology hold promise for new opportunities in neuropsychological assessment. Computerized testing offers several advantages over traditional paper-and-pencil neuropsychological evaluation; the latter requires highly trained psychometricians and clinicians to conduct and score the tests, thus presenting a heavy burden on cost and time. Furthermore, response times can be precisely measured at a level of sensitivity not possible in traditional administrations. Other advantages include minimization of human errors in data recording, observer bias, and transcription. Potential obstacles include the general lack of adequately established psychometric standards[26] and unfamiliarity with computer usage in the elderly population, although some studies have reported reduced stress and increased acceptability in association with computerized cognitive testing compared with paper-and-pencil assessment.[27]

In recent years, several computerized neuropsychological test batteries have been developed to detect cognitive decline in the elderly (reviewed by Wild and colleagues 2008[26]). Among these test batteries, Cogstate[28] seems to have gained momentum among aging/dementia researchers and clinicians. Cogstate comprises several subtests that measure simple/choice/complex reaction time, continuous learning, working memory, matching, incidental learning, and associative learning. The stimuli are presented in playing card format with minimal reliance on verbal abilities. The various tasks in the Cogstate battery have been shown effective in detecting subtle memory changes in individuals with MCI (discussed later).[29] Despite these positive findings, the suitability of computerized and online measures for the assessment, monitoring, and diagnosis of cognitive disorders in the elderly population remain equivocal due to insufficient psychometric quality, standardization, and normative data.[30] Researchers and clinicians should exercise caution when deciding on the use of computerized tests as a measurement option for detecting cognitive decline in the elderly; clarity of instructions, length of administration, and ease of interface should be critical considerations.

CHANGES IN COGNITION ASSOCIATED WITH NORMAL AGING

Cognitive changes associated with increased age have been well established through decades of extensive neuropsychological research. In cross-sectional studies, reflecting interindividual age differences, linear and steady decline in performance over time are evident across multiple cognitive domains, including processing speed, memory, visuospatial skills, language abilities, and executive/frontal systems functioning.[31] In contrast, simple attention, semantic knowledge, vocabulary, and autobiographical remote memory are resistant to the regressive effects of aging.[32] Longitudinal studies, however, reveal a different profile because most cognitive abilities follow a quadratic pattern of performance across the lifespan.[33] According to the data from the Seattle Longitudinal Study, perceptual speed peaks in the late 30s then declines linearly and precipitously thereafter, whereas verbal memory, spatial orientation, and inductive reasoning seem to plateau in midlife, from ages 40 to 60, followed by steady decline after age 60. In contrast, verbal abilities remain stable until 81 years of age, then decline modestly into the 90s.[33]

One of the most influential theories of cognitive aging posits that slowing in cognitive processing speed, the leading cognitive marker of aging, underlies the age-associated decrements in most higher-order cognitive functions, including memory and executive functioning.[34] Specifically, the age-associated variance in episodic memory is reduced by 80% to 95% after controlling for the variance in cognitive processing speed. This age-related slowing in processing speed seems largely mediated by white matter/myelin integrity,[35] which allows for the integration of information across spatially distributed networks supporting cognitive and motor functions. The connectivity and quality of white matter pathways are, therefore, of paramount importance for maintaining the speed, frequency, and neural network synchrony that underlie coherent information processing in the human brain.[36]

CLINICAL DIAGNOSIS OF DEMENTIA AND PRECLINICAL STAGES OF DEMENTIA

The neurodegenerative changes associated with age-related cognitive disorders, such as Alzheimer disease (AD), begin well before the manifestation of observable clinical symptoms.[37] The earliest changes typically occur in medial temporal lobe structures (eg, hippocampus and entorhinal cortex) that are critical for episodic memory.[38] As the pathologic changes gradually accumulate and spread to the association cortices of the temporal, frontal, and parietal lobes, many higher-order cognitive abilities are affected, including visuospatial/visuoperceptual skills, language, and executive functioning. When the cognitive deficits become global and severe enough to interfere with social and occupational functioning or instrumental activities of daily living (IADLs), a clinical diagnosis of dementia or major neurocognitive disorder is made based on criteria established by the *Diagnostic and Statistical Manual* (Fifth Edition).[39] More subtle but significant cognitive deficits, however, are likely to be experienced by a patient well before the expression of overt dementia. During this preclinical stage, the cognitive changes, although abnormal, do not impair daily functioning and may not be detectable through observation or bedside screening tests, thus making it a challenge for clinicians to document meaningful cognitive impairment.

Significant research efforts have been directed at characterizing cognitive changes that occur during the preclinical phase with the goal of identifying persons at significantly elevated risk of developing dementia. The concept of MCI[40] was introduced in an effort to define this transitional stage between normal aging and dementia. The diagnostic criteria include (1) the presence of a memory complaint on behalf of the patient or from an informant, (2) normal activities of daily living, (3) normal global cognitive function, and (4) abnormal cognitive function compared with age and education norms. Individuals meeting criteria for MCI progress to dementia at much higher rates than normal elderly controls (10%–12% vs 1%–2% per year).[40]

Even though individual clinicians and investigators may rely on clinical judgment and global assessment tools to diagnose MCI, criteria 4, highlights the need for formal neuropsychological testing to establish "evidence of lower performance in one or more cognitive domains that is greater than would be expected for the patient's age and educational background."[40] The operational definition for identifying the boundary between normal aging and MCI is somewhat arbitrary, but most studies have adopted cutoff scores of 1.0 SD or 1.5 SDs below age-adjusted normative means on neuropsychological measures as the threshold for defining abnormal cognitive function in MCI.[41,42] Several empirical studies have recognized that neuropsychological testing is a highly informative technique for predicting progression to AD in older patients with MCI.[43] Recent efforts have been made to adjust the cutoffs to detect MCI at an earlier stage (early MCI)[44] or characterize prodromal phases of the disease before the manifestation of any significant abnormalities.[45] Identifying cognitive changes during the preclinical phase of dementia is important because therapeutic interventions initiated in prodromal stages may potentially prevent or delay progression to clinical dementia.

NEUROPSYCHOLOGICAL FEATURES OF COMMON DEMENTIA SYNDROMES AFFECTING THE ELDERLY

Neuropsychological assessment can reveal distinct patterns of cognitive impairment that help illuminate the etiology and diagnosis underlying the deficits affecting elderly patients. Several possible underlying etiologies, both reversible and irreversible, can contribute to dementia. Common reversible causes of cognitive impairment include depression or other psychiatric disorder, nutritional deficiencies (ie, vitamin B_{12} deficiency), adverse drug reactions, and metabolic disorders. Irreversible causes of dementia include AD, cerebrovascular disease, Lewy body disease (DLB), frontotemporal dementia, and Parkinson disease. The co-occurrence of these pathologies is common, particularly in the extreme elderly, sometimes making the clinical distinction among them difficult.[46]

AD is the most common form of dementia, accounting for 60% to 80% of dementia cases.[47] Because of the prominent neurodegeneration of the hippocampus, dementia due to AD is characterized primarily by a profound and progressive decline in memory. Specifically, AD patients demonstrate amnestic deficits on tests of memory, with abnormal rapid forgetting and poor immediate recall, delayed recall, and recognition. Patients with AD also exhibit disturbances in semantic knowledge and language deficits on object naming and semantic fluency tasks. These changes are usually insidious and gradual in onset and get progressively worse over time. They may also show mild to moderate changes in visuospatial and executive functions, but attention and processing speed tend to remain intact.

Vascular dementia (VaD), another common form of dementia, is caused by cerebrovascular events, including stroke, transient ischemic attacks, and other ischemic changes in the brain related to hypertension, hyperlipidemia, and other cerebrovascular risk factors.[48] VaD is typically characterized by a frontal-subcortical pattern of neuropsychological deficits, namely slow processing speed and executive dysfunction, although the specific deficits observed can depend on the location of a focal underlying vascular insult. On memory tests, VaD patients usually exhibit problems with learning/encoding and retrieval rather than an amnestic pattern of deficit.

Both Parkinson disease dementia (PDD)[49] and DLB[50] are characterized by the presence of α-synuclein inclusions known as Lewy bodies in the brainstem (eg, the substantia nigra) and cerebral cortex. Therefore, both disorders share a similar neuro-psychological profile, with prominent changes in attention, executive function, and vi-suospatial skills. Language remains relatively preserved, and the pattern of memory scores indicates encoding and/or retrieval problems rather than an amnestic disorder. In addition to cognitive disturbances, a common feature of DLB and, to some extent, PDD is the presence of well-formed visual hallucinations and significant day-to-day fluctuations in alertness and cognitive functioning. The defining difference between DLB and PDD is the temporal relationship in the emergence of parkinsonism relative to cognitive symptoms. Both DLB and PDD patients exhibit extrapyramidal symp-toms, such as masked facies, bradykinesia, and gait impairment. PDD is diagnosed when Parkinson disease is the primary disorder and the extrapyramidal symptoms develop first (more than 1 year prior to the onset of cognitive deficits), whereas DLB is suggested when cognitive deficits occur first or within 1 year of the onset of parkin-sonism. The degree to which pure DLB, PDD, and DLB with concurrent AD pathology represent distinct disorders or points on a spectrum is currently a matter of controversy.[51]

Behavioral variant frontotemporal dementia (bvFTD)[52] and primary progressive aphasia (PPA)[53] are forms of dementia that tend to manifest at a younger age, with a typical age of onset between 50 and 65. BvFTD is a disorder characterized primarily by behavioral disturbances, such as disinhibition, apathy, loss of empathy or warmth, perseverative or compulsive behaviors, and dietary changes. Deficits on neuropsy-chological testing are not always present in the early stages, but changes in executive function are expected first, whereas memory and visuospatial functions are well pre-served until late stages. Unlike other forms of dementia, clinical diagnosis of bvFTD emphasizes a patient's behavioral changes rather than the cognitive profile. Distur-bances in language are the most prominent symptom of PPA, which includes agram-matic and semantic variants of the disorder. Patients with agrammatic PPA demonstrate significant difficulty with speech production, although verbal compre-hension remains intact. On neuropsychological testing, these individuals typically perform poorly on tasks requiring verbal production, such as rapid word reading or co-lor naming (Stroop) or sentence repetition (WMS-IV Logical Memory), which can, in turn, affect their performance on tests of verbal memory; however, visual memory and visuospatial skills remain intact. Semantic PPA is characterized by a loss of se-mantic knowledge, which leads to deficits in verbal comprehension, word knowledge, and object naming, whereas speech production remains intact and fluent.

SPECIAL CONSIDERATIONS IN THE ASSESSMENT OF THE ELDERLY
Physical Limitations

In the assessment of the elderly, there are several physical and sensory changes asso-ciated with aging that should be considered in the selection of test materials and inter-pretation of test results. Between 30% and 50% of older adults experience gradual age-related hearing loss,[54] which can compromise test performance on measures of auditory attention and auditory verbal memory as well as other tasks if instructions were not fully heard. The use of hearing aids and personal sound amplifiers may partially circumvent this deficit, but this issue and its potential confound should be documented and considered in the interpretation of test results. Similarly, visual capa-bility deteriorates with age and approximately half of individuals over age 65 have vi-sual acuity of 20/70 or less,[55] adversely affecting any tests that require processing of visual information. Older age is also associated with a greater likelihood of physical disabilities, such as neuromuscular disorders or severe arthritis, that may have a negative impact on performance on graphomotor tasks. Elderly patients may also require more frequent rest breaks to combat fatigue and escalating frustration if they feel challenged by the testing process.

Neuropsychiatric Symptoms

Neuropsychiatric symptoms are common in cognitive disorders, affecting up to 92% of persons with AD and as many as 50% of patients with MCI.[56,57] These numbers are even higher for disorders involving profound behavioral and personality alterations (eg, bvFTD and DLB). Mood and behavioral disturbances related to life stressors (eg, retirement, bereavement from death of family members and friends, and financial concerns) can also occur in healthy older adults without cognitive impairment. Estimates of prevalence for depression in the elderly living in the community can be as high as 13.5%.[58] In a large-scale population-based study, common neuropsychiatric symptoms expressed by cognitively intact elderly persons include depression (7.2%), anxiety (5.8%), and irritability (4.6%).[57] Neuropsychiatric symptoms can exacerbate cognitive deficits, cause distress to patients and their caregivers, adversely affect prognosis, and diminish quality of life. MCI and demented patients with neuropsychiatric symptoms, especially disinhibited and aggressive behavior, require more intensive care and supervision, representing higher caregiver burden and cost of care. Measuring these symptoms is of clinical importance because they may be remediable with appropriate nonpharmacologic and, when necessary, pharmacologic interventions.

A comprehensive neuropsychological examination typically includes an assessment of mood and emotional functioning through clinical interview and objective rating scales. Self-report screening measures, such as the Geriatric Depression Scale,[59] Geriatric Anxiety Inventory,[60] and Patient Health Questionnaire (depression module),[61] offer well-established psychometric properties and simplicity in instructions and content, making them more suitable for older adults and mild to moderately cognitively impaired individuals. Self-report scales, however, may not be reliable in more severely demented patients due to reduced or loss of insight. The Neuropsychiatric Inventory[62] is a caregiver/informant-based instrument that measures the presence, frequency, and severity for 12 domains of behavioral disturbances. It samples a broad range of neuropsychiatric difficulties but its reliance on proxy report for behavioral symptoms requires the presence of a knowledgeable family member or caregiver.

Serial Examination

As detailed previously, cognitive abilities decline with increasing age, even in healthy elderly individuals, demonstrating a need to monitor and track their cognitive and functional status to accurately detect the onset of cognitive changes that signal the beginning of an evolving neurodegenerative process. In MCI patients, it is estimated that approximately 10% to 12% progress to dementia each year.[40] However, 4% to 53% of MCI patients may revert to normal cognition,[63] depending on the specific population, suggesting that potentially reversible factors, not neurodegenerative disease, may be contributing to deficits at baseline. Longitudinal neuropsychological evaluations serve an important role in documenting the rate and progression of cognitive deterioration over time, establishing the accuracy of the diagnosis, and prognosticating about future difficulties, thus guiding care and treatment interventions. In cases involving nonprogressive cognitive disorders, serial tracking of cognitive functioning is helpful in measuring treatment response or establishing evidence of cognitive stability or improvement after recovery from a stroke or traumatic head injury.

The Repeatable Battery for the Assessment of Neuropsychological Status (RBANS)[64] is a brief battery of tests designed to detect cognitive impairments associated with AD and other neurologic disorders through longitudinal assessment of language, attention, visuospatial skills, immediate memory, and delayed memory. It takes approximately 30 minutes to administer, reducing the risk of fatigue and burden placed on elderly patients. It seems to have good diagnostic accuracy in detecting AD-related cognitive impairments[65] but has yielded mixed findings in terms of its sensitivity in detecting MCI.[66,67] Low scores on the RBANS memory and language indices, however, have been associated with reduced medial temporal lobe volume in MCI patients,[68] providing some evidence of neuroanatomic specificity. The RBANS also provides equivalent alternative forms that can be used in serial evaluations to examine the longitudinal progression of cognitive decline while minimizing practice effects, which refer to improvements in test performance due to prior exposure to the same test material.[69] Practice effects have traditionally been viewed as a potential confound in interpreting test results[70]; however, in patients with a cognitive disorder, examination of this cognitive phenomenon, or the lack thereof, may have diagnostic utility because several studies have reported the absence of practice effects in individuals with MCI and dementia,[71,72] presumably due to impaired memory.

Functional Capacity

Clinical and legal professionals often rely on neuropsychologists to render opinions regarding the decision-making capacity of older adults. Evaluations of decisional capacity made on the basis of a clinical interview and/or global mental status examination may not be reliable.[73] Neuropsychologists are ideally positioned to apply standardized assessment procedures to address questions of diminished capacity. The Uniform Guardianship and Protective Proceedings Act[74] defines an incapacitated individual as someone who is "unable to receive and evaluate information or make or communicate decisions to such an extent that the individual lacks the ability to meet essential requirements for physical health, safety, or self-care, even with appropriate technological assistance." A neuropsychologist can design and construct a test battery tailored to target these standards.

Assessment of basic activities of daily living or IADLs (eg, abilities to manage finances, health, and functioning in the home and community) is an important component of neuropsychological assessment for diagnostic clarification (eg, MCI vs dementia) and making recommendations regarding independent living, placement in assisted living facility, or conservatorship. Ability to perform IADLs can be assessed through direct query of the patient and preferably a collateral informant. Neuropsychological test results, in particular measures of executive functioning, demonstrate good ecological validity and are significantly correlated to functional abilities.[75] Informant-based objective measures, such as the Functional Activities Questionnaire[76] and the Everyday Cognition scale,[77] have been developed to assess daily functioning. Performance-based measures, such as the Direct Assessment of Functional Status,[78] are also available in which a patient's ability to perform ADLs is directly observed through specific tasks, but this process requires significant amount of time commitment and equipment that are likely prohibitive in most clinical settings.

Cognitive Training and Intervention

During feedback regarding the results of neuropsychological testing, patients often express interest in cognitive training or other interventions that can potentially improve existing deficits or postpone cognitive decline. Cognitive training programs use various cognitive exercises and strategies, including computerized approaches, to help enhance memory functioning as well as attention, processing speed, and executive functioning. There have been several systematic reviews evaluating the effectiveness of various cognitive intervention studies in healthy older adults and people with MCI.[79,80] Although the magnitude of the effect remains equivocal, researchers in this field have been generally optimistic regarding the benefits of cognitive interventions on multiple cognitive domains. The issue of whether the effects observed in the laboratory setting translate to improvement in everyday functioning remains unresolved, however, and needs to be addressed in future studies using ecologically valid outcome measures.

SUMMARY

Despite advances in neuroimaging technology, there is still no way of directly observing the fully integrated functioning of the human brain. Clinicians, therefore, continue to rely on evaluation of the behavioral expression of brain dysfunction. Neuropsychological assessment has multiple clinical applications, ranging from comprehensive characterization of a wide range of cognitive abilities and identifying a cognitive profile that can assist with diagnosis to predicting future deterioration and functional capacity in older adults. These assessments offer valuable and critical information that complement neurologic and neuroimaging procedures in providing the most comprehensive examination and care of elderly patients.

REFERENCES

1. He W, Sengupta M, Velkoff VA, et al. 65+ in the United States: 2005. Washington, DC: National Institute on Aging; U.S. Census Bureau; 2005.
2. Jorm AF, Jolley D. The incidence of dementia: a meta-analysis. Neurology 1998; 51(3):728–33.
3. Hebert LE, Weuve J, Scherr PA, et al. Alzheimer disease in the United States (2010-2050) estimated using the 2010 census. Neurology 2013;80(19): 1778–83.
4. Petersen RC, Stevens JC, Ganguli M, et al. Practice parameter: early detection of dementia: mild cognitive impairment (an evidence-based review). Report of the Quality Standards Subcommittee of the American Academy of Neurology. Neurology 2001;56(9):1133–42.
5. Folstein MF, Folstein SE, McHugh PR. "Mini-mental state". A practical method for grading the cognitive state of patients for the clinician. J Psychiatr Res 1975; 12(3):189–98.
6. Espino DV, Lichtenstein MJ, Palmer RF, et al. Ethnic differences in mini-mental state examination (MMSE) scores: where you live makes a difference. J Am Geriatr Soc 2001;49(5):538–48.
7. Nasreddine ZS, Phillips NA, Bedirian V, et al. The Montreal Cognitive Assessment, MoCA: a brief screening tool for mild cognitive impairment. J Am Geriatr Soc 2005;53(4):695–9.
8. Dong Y, Lee WY, Basri NA, et al. The Montreal Cognitive Assessment is superior to the Mini-Mental State Examination in detecting patients at higher risk of dementia. Int Psychogeriatr 2012;24(11):1749–55.
9. Rosen WG, Mohs RC, Davis KL. A new rating scale for Alzheimer's disease. Am J Psychiatry 1984;141(11):1356–64.
10. Mattis S. Dementia rating scale. Odessa (FL): Psychological Assessment Resources; 1988.
11. Blessed G, Tomlinson BE, Roth M. The association between quantitative measures of dementia and of senile change in the cerebral grey matter of elderly subjects. Br J Psychiatry 1968;114(512):797–811.

12. Wechsler D. Wechsler adult intelligence scale - fourth edition (WAIS-IV). San Antonio (TX): Psychological Corporation; 2008.

13. Wechsler D. Wechsler abbreviated scale of intelligence - second edition (WASI-II). San Antonio (TX): Psychological Corporation; 2011.

14. Wechsler D. Advanced clinical solutions for WAIS-IV and WMS-IV (ACS). San Antonio (TX): Psychological Corporation; 2009.

15. Grober E, Sliwinski M. Development and validation of a model for estimating premorbid verbal intelligence in the elderly. J Clin Exp Neuropsychol 1991;13(6): 933–49.

16. Reitan R, Wolfson D. The halstead-reitan neuropsychological test battery. Tucson (AZ): Neuropsychology Press; 1985.

17. Golden CJ, Hammeke TA, Purisch AD. Diagnostic validity of a standardized neuropsychological battery derived from Luria's neuropsychological tests. J Consult Clin Psychol 1978;46(6):1258–65.

18. Smith A. Symbol digit modalities test (SDMT). Los Angeles (CA): Western Psychological Services; 1982.

19. Kaplan E, Goodglass H, Weintraub S. Boston naming test. Philadelphia: Lea & Fabiger; 1983.

20. Benton AL, Hamsher KD. Multilingual aphasia examination. Iowa City (IA): AJA Associated; 1989.

21. Meyers JE, Meyers KR. Rey complex figure test and recognition trial professional manual. Odessa (FL): Psychological Assessment Resources; 1995.

22. Wechsler D. Wechsler memory scale - fourth edition (WMS-IV). San Antonio (TX): The Psychological Corporation; 2009.

23. Benedict R, Schretlen D, Groninger L, et al. Revision of the brief visuospatial memory test: studies of normal performance, reliability, and validity. Psychol Assess 1996;8:145–53.

24. Heaton RK, Chelune GJ, Talley JL, et al. Wisconsin card sorting test manual: revised and expanded. Odessa (FL): Psychological Assessment Resources; 1993.

25. Delis D, Kaplan E, Kramer J. Delis-Kaplan executive function system. San Antonio (TX): The Psychological Corporation; 2001.

26. Wild K, Howieson D, Webbe F, et al. Status of computerized cognitive testing in aging: a systematic review. Alzheimers Dement 2008;4(6):428–37.

27. Collerton J, Collerton D, Arai Y, et al. A comparison of computerized and pencil-and-paper tasks in assessing cognitive function in community-dwelling older people in the Newcastle 85+ Pilot Study. J Am Geriatr Soc 2007;55(10):1630–5.

28. Westerman R, Darby D, Maruff P, et al. Computer-assisted cognitive function assessment in pilots: how and why? ADF Health 2001;2:29–36.

29. Weaver Cargin J, Maruff P, Collie A, et al. Mild memory impairment in healthy older adults is distinct from normal aging. Brain Cogn 2006;60(2):146–55.

30. Gates NJ, Kochan NA. Computerized and on-line neuropsychological testing for late-life cognition and neurocognitive disorders: are we there yet? Curr Opin Psychiatry 2015;28(2):165–72.

31. Mitrushina M, Boone KB, Razani J, et al. Handbook of normative data for neuropsychological assessment. 2nd edition. New York: Oxford University Press; 2005.

32. Salmon DP. Neuropsychology of aging and dementia. Handb Clin Neurol 2008; 88:113–35.

33. Schaie KW. What can we learn from longitudinal studies of adult development? Res Hum Dev 2005;2(3):133–58.

34. Salthouse TA. The processing-speed theory of adult age differences in cognition. Psychol Rev 1996;103(3):403–28.

35. Lu PH, Lee GJ, Tishler TA, et al. Myelin breakdown mediates age-related slowing in cognitive processing speed in healthy elderly men. Brain Cogn 2013;81(1): 131–8.

36. Bartzokis G, Lu PH, Heydari P, et al. Multimodal magnetic resonance imaging assessment of white matter aging trajectories over the lifespan of healthy individuals. Biol Psychiatry 2012;72(12):1026–34.

37. Dubois B, Hampel H, Feldman HH, et al. Preclinical Alzheimer's disease: definition, natural history, and diagnostic criteria. Alzheimers Dement 2016;12(3): 292–323.

38. Braak H, Braak E. Neuropathological stageing of Alzheimer-related changes. Acta Neuropathol 1991;82(4):239–59.

39. American Psychiatric Association. Diagnostic and statistical manual of mental disorders. 5th edition. Washington, DC: American Psychiatric Publishing; 2013.

40. Petersen RC, Smith GE, Waring SC, et al. Mild cognitive impairment: clinical characterization and outcome. Arch Neurol 1999;56(3):303–8.

41. Ganguli M, Dodge HH, Shen C, et al. Mild cognitive impairment, amnestic type: an epidemiologic study. Neurology 2004;63(1):115–21.

42. Lopez OL, Jagust WJ, DeKosky ST, et al. Prevalence and classification of mild cognitive impairment in the Cardiovascular Health Study Cognition Study: part 1. Arch Neurol 2003;60(10):1385–9.

43. Schmand B, Eikelenboom P, van Gool WA, Alzheimer's Disease Neuroimaging Initiative. Value of neuropsychological tests, neuroimaging, and biomarkers for diagnosing Alzheimer's disease in younger and older age cohorts. J Am Geriatr Soc 2011;59(9):1705–10.

44. Aisen PS, Petersen RC, Donohue MC, et al. Clinical core of the Alzheimer's disease neuroimaging initiative: progress and plans. Alzheimers Dement 2010; 6(3):239–46.

45. Goldman WP, Morris JC. Evidence that age-associated memory impairment is not a normal variant of aging. Alzheimer Dis Assoc Disord 2001;15(2):72–9.

46. White LR, Edland SD, Hemmy LS, et al. Neuropathologic comorbidity and cognitive impairment in the Nun and Honolulu-Asia Aging Studies. Neurology 2016; 86(11):1000–8.

47. Thies W, Bleiler L. 2013 Alzheimer's disease facts and figures. Alzheimers Dement 2013;9(2):208–45.

48. Sachdev P, Kalaria R, O'Brien J, et al. Diagnostic criteria for vascular cognitive disorders: a VASCOG statement. Alzheimer Dis Assoc Disord 2014;28(3):206–18.

49. Emre M, Aarsland D, Brown R, et al. Clinical diagnostic criteria for dementia associated with Parkinson's disease. Mov Disord 2007;22(12):1689–707 [quiz: 1837].

50. McKeith IG, Dickson DW, Lowe J, et al. Diagnosis and management of dementia with Lewy bodies: third report of the DLB Consortium. Neurology 2005;65(12): 1863–72.

51. Lippa CF, Duda JE, Grossman M, et al. DLB and PDD boundary issues: diagnosis, treatment, molecular pathology, and biomarkers. Neurology 2007;68(11): 812–9.

52. Rascovsky K, Hodges JR, Knopman D, et al. Sensitivity of revised diagnostic criteria for the behavioural variant of frontotemporal dementia. Brain 2011; 134(Pt 9):2456–77.

53. Gorno-Tempini ML, Hillis AE, Weintraub S, et al. Classification of primary progressive aphasia and its variants. Neurology 2011;76(11):1006–14.

54. Plomp R. Auditory handicap of hearing impairment and the limited benefit of hearing aids. J Acoust Soc Am 1978;63(2):533–49.
55. Owsley C, McGwin G Jr, Ball K. Vision impairment, eye disease, and injurious motor vehicle crashes in the elderly. Ophthalmic Epidemiol 1998;5(2):101–13.
56. Cummings JL, Mega M, Gray K, et al. The neuropsychiatric inventory: comprehensive assessment of psychopathology in dementia. Neurology 1994;44(12): 2308–14.
57. Lyketsos CG, Lopez O, Jones B, et al. Prevalence of neuropsychiatric symptoms in dementia and mild cognitive impairment: results from the cardiovascular health study. JAMA 2002;288(12):1475–83.
58. Beekman AT, Copeland JR, Prince MJ. Review of community prevalence of depression in later life. Br J Psychiatry 1999;174:307–11.
59. Yesavage JA, Brink TL, Rose TL, et al. Development and validation of a geriatric depression screening scale: a preliminary report. J Psychiatr Res 1982;17(1): 37–49.
60. Pachana NA, Byrne GJ, Siddle H, et al. Development and validation of the geriatric anxiety inventory. Int Psychogeriatr 2007;19(1):103–14.
61. Kroenke K, Spitzer RL, Williams JB. The PHQ-9: validity of a brief depression severity measure. J Gen Intern Med 2001;16(9):606–13.
62. Cummings JL. The Neuropsychiatric Inventory: assessing psychopathology in dementia patients. Neurology 1997;48(5 Suppl 6):S10–6.
63. Kryscio RJ, Schmitt FA, Salazar JC, et al. Risk factors for transitions from normal to mild cognitive impairment and dementia. Neurology 2006;66(6):828–32.
64. Randolph C, Tierney MC, Mohr E, et al. The repeatable battery for the assessment of neuropsychological status (RBANS): preliminary clinical validity. J Clin Exp Neuropsychol 1998;20(3):310–9.
65. Duff K, Humphreys Clark JD, O'Bryant SE, et al. Utility of the RBANS in detecting cognitive impairment associated with Alzheimer's disease: sensitivity, specificity, and positive and negative predictive powers. Arch Clin Neuropsychol 2008;23(5): 603–12.
66. Karantzoulis S, Novitski J, Gold M, et al. The repeatable battery for the assessment of neuropsychological status (RBANS): utility in detection and characterization of mild cognitive impairment due to Alzheimer's disease. Arch Clin Neuropsychol 2013;28(8):837–44.
67. Duff K, Hobson VL, Beglinger LJ, et al. Diagnostic accuracy of the RBANS in mild cognitive impairment: limitations on assessing milder impairments. Arch Clin Neuropsychol 2010;25(5):429–41.
68. England HB, Gillis MM, Hampstead BM. RBANS memory indices are related to medial temporal lobe volumetrics in healthy older adults and those with mild cognitive impairment. Arch Clin Neuropsychol 2014;29(4):322–8.
69. Beglinger LJ, Gaydos B, Tangphao-Daniels O, et al. Practice effects and the use of alternate forms in serial neuropsychological testing. Arch Clin Neuropsychol 2005;20(4):517–29.
70. Busch R, Chelune G, Suchy Y. Using norms in neuropsychological assessment of the elderly. In: Attix D, Bohmer K, Welsh-Bohmer K, editors. Geriatric neuropsychology: assessment and intervention. New York: Guilford Press; 2006. p. 133–57.
71. Duff K, Chelune G, Dennett K. Within-session practice effects in patients referred for suspected dementia. Dement Geriatr Cogn Disord 2012;33(4):245–9.
72. Machulda MM, Pankratz VS, Christianson TJ, et al. Practice effects and longitudinal cognitive change in normal aging vs. incident mild cognitive impairment

and dementia in the Mayo Clinic Study of Aging. Clin Neuropsychol 2013;27(8): 1247–64.

73. Marson DC, McInturff B, Hawkins L, et al. Consistency of physician judgments of capacity to consent in mild Alzheimer's disease. J Am Geriatr Soc 1997;45(4): 453–7.

74. National Conference of Commisioners on Uniform State Laws. 1997.

75. Razani J, Casas R, Wong JT, et al. Relationship between executive functioning and activities of daily living in patients with relatively mild dementia. Appl Neuropsychol 2007;14(3):208–14.

76. Pfeffer RI, Kurosaki TT, Harrah CH Jr, et al. Measurement of functional activities in older adults in the community. J Gerontol 1982;37(3):323–9.

77. Farias ST, Mungas D, Reed BR, et al. The measurement of everyday cognition (ECog): scale development and psychometric properties. Neuropsychology 2008;22(4):531–44.

78. Loewenstein DA, Amigo E, Duara R, et al. A new scale for the assessment of functional status in Alzheimer's disease and related disorders. J Gerontol 1989; 44(4):P114–21.

79. Lustig C, Shah P, Seidler R, et al. Aging, training, and the brain: a review and future directions. Neuropsychol Rev 2009;19(4):504–22.

80. Reijnders J, van Heugten C, van Boxtel M. Cognitive interventions in healthy older adults and people with mild cognitive impairment: a systematic review. Ageing Res Rev 2013;12(1):263–75.

Assessment of the Hispanic Cognitively Impaired Elderly Patient

Liliana Ramirez Gomez, MD[a],*, Felipe A. Jain, MD[b],
Lina M. D'Orazio, PhD[c]

KEYWORDS

- Hispanics • Cognitive impairment • Dementia • Neuropsychological assessment

KEY POINTS

- Hispanics exhibit a higher prevalence of dementia and present with more severe symptoms than non-Hispanic whites but receive less medical care.
- Hispanics tend to attribute symptoms of dementia, in particular nonamnestic behavioral manifestations, to other causes, such as psychosocial stress or aging.
- It is important to consider sociocultural variables (eg, language use, education, acculturation, and socioeconomic level) during the clinical evaluation of Hispanic patients.
- Cognitive and neuropsychological assessment instruments should be used with caution and scored according to cultural Hispanic demographic factors and specific norms.

INTRODUCTION

Hispanics are the largest and fastest growing ethnic minority group in the country, comprising approximately 17% of the US population, with a projected increase to 31% by 2060. Estimates indicate that 7.1% of the US population older than 65 years in 2012 were Hispanic, and this is expected to increase to 19.8% in 2050.[1] Unfortunately, health care services for optimally evaluating and treating elderly Hispanic patients with cognitive complaints remain limited. Challenges regularly faced by Hispanic elders include limited access to or resistance to seeking medical care, language barriers, and other factors contributing to delay in diagnosis and treatment.[2] Specific to the assessment of cognitive functioning, there is an increasing appreciation of the

Disclosure Statement: The authors have nothing to disclose.
[a] Department of Neurology, University of California, San Francisco, 400 Parnassus Avenue, A871, San Francisco, CA 94143, USA; [b] Department of Psychiatry, University of California, San Francisco, 401 Parnassus Avenue, Box 0984, San Francisco, CA 94143, USA; [c] Department of Neurology, Keck School of Medicine of USC, 1520 San Pablo Street, HCCII, Suite 3000, Los Angeles, CA 90033, USA
* Corresponding author.
E-mail address: liliana.ramirezgomez@ucsf.edu

Neurol Clin 35 (2017) 207–229
http://dx.doi.org/10.1016/j.ncl.2017.01.003
0733-8619/17/© 2017 Elsevier Inc. All rights reserved.

neurologic.theclinics.com

need to consider the role of sociocultural variables (eg, language use, education, acculturation, and socioeconomic level) in the neurologic and neuropsychological assessment of patients of Hispanic origin.

This article provides an overview of dementia in Hispanics living in the United States and describes disparities in access to care. Because a valid assessment requires attention to specific cultural factors, cultural norms are described and clinicians familiarized with how to apply cognitive assessment instruments and neuropsychological tests to Hispanic patients. Case examples are presented to illustrate these points.

DEFINITION OF HISPANIC: WHO IS HISPANIC?

"Hispanic" derives from the Roman *Hispania*, referring to the entire Iberian Peninsula, and includes descendants of both Spanish language and Portuguese language speaking groups. Currently, the US Census classifies Hispanics into 4 groups: Mexican, Puerto Rican, Cuban, and a fourth inclusive category of "other" that has been used to describe individuals from Central and South America and of other Caribbean, Spanish, and Portuguese origin or ancestry. Hispanics derive from multiple racial groups, including Caucasian, Amerindian, African, and any combination thereof. A vast majority of Hispanics in the United States are of Spanish-speaking ancestry, and of these a minority are monolingual Spanish speakers, with the latter group divided among elderly immigrants and recent arrivals to the United States. This article focuses on Hispanics of Spanish language ancestry. For information on Portuguese speakers, please refer to the chapter on Brazilian/Portuguese.[3]

EPIDEMIOLOGY OF DEMENTIA IN HISPANICS
Prevalence

The prevalence of dementia among Hispanics is 1.5 times greater than that of non-Hispanic whites.[4] A recent report, "Latinos, & Alzheimer's Disease: New Numbers Behind the Crisis," estimated that the number of AD cases in Hispanics older than 65 years of age in the United States is expected to rise from 481,000 in 2015 to as many as 3.5 million by 2060.[5]

Incidence

Although early studies of Caribbean Hispanics on the East Coast suggested that the incidence of dementia was higher in Hispanics compared with other non-Hispanic whites,[6,7] more recent research has not confirmed these findings in other cohorts: a study performed in a Mexican American cohort of Hispanics in Northern California showed a similar incidence in both groups.[8] Consistent with these latter results, a recent large population-based study showed that the incidence of dementia was higher in African Americans and American Indian/Alaska Natives and intermediate for Hispanics and whites, with Asian Americans having the lowest risk. Hispanics and non-Hispanic whites also had comparable cumulative 25-year risks of developing dementia at age 65, 32% and 30%, respectively.[9] In conclusion, the epidemiologic evidence that Hispanics have an increased incidence of dementia based solely on their ethnic background is mixed.

DEMOGRAPHIC AND CLINICAL RISK FACTORS
Education

Poor quality or low educational attainment has been identified as a risk factor for the development of dementia,[10] possibly due to diminished cognitive reserve, associations with reduced ability to afford health care or obtain treatments,[11] or a higher likelihood of having an occupation that is less mentally stimulating.[12] Educational attainment among elderly Hispanics in the United States varies widely in total years and quality of schooling. According to the US Census Bureau in 2012,[13] among Hispanics living in the United States, 60.9% had earned a high school diploma, and only 12.6% completed a bachelor's degree or more. This is in contrast to the US population as a whole, which had 85.3% and 27.9% completion rates, respectively. For Hispanic elders raised in rural areas of Latin America, it is not uncommon to have completed only an elementary level of education (typically between 3 and 6 years or less), if any at all.[14] Barriers to accessing formal education include financial hardship and family responsibilities as well as systemic barriers, such as shortages of facilities and teachers.[15] The quality of education in these situations is often undermined by inconsistent attendance and lack of regulated standards for academic advancement.[14]

Poverty

Hispanics are more likely to be of low socioeconomic status: the poverty rate among Hispanics in 2012 was 25.6%, and 33% did not speak English "well."[13] A study in a cohort of Hispanics participating in the Sacramento Area Latino Study on Aging supported the conclusion that early exposures to social disadvantage increase the risk of late-life dementia.[16] This suggests that intraethnic factors, such as differences in socioeconomic status, may be important.

Bilingualism and Dementia

Several studies[17–19] but not all[20,21] have found that bilingualism may be protective or delay the onset of dementia. The discrepancies among studies might be explained by moderating factors. In a cohort of Hispanics in Southern California, bilingualism and education level were interacting predictors of age of dementia onset, with increasing degrees of bilingualism delaying diagnosis of AD in Hispanics with low education but not in those with high education.[22]

Vascular Risk Factors

Vascular risk factors have been associated with an increased risk for cognitive impairment and dementia.[23] Different cardiovascular risk profiles have been identified among subgroups of Hispanics in the United States,[24] therefore resulting in a different risk profile for dementia between individuals with the same ethnicity but different regions of origin. Hypertension is higher in some Hispanic subpopulations, including Puerto Ricans and Dominicans relative to non-Hispanic whites but not elevated in other Hispanic subpopulations. In general, diabetes, obesity, and low levels of physical activity are increased in Hispanics compared with non-Hispanic whites. Smoking prevalence, however, is generally lower in Hispanics than non-Hispanic whites.[25]

Genetic Risk Factors

Genetic risk factors for AD, although increasingly characterized in non-Hispanic whites, are understudied in Hispanics. The strongest and best-characterized genetic risk factor for late-onset AD (LOAD), the ε4 allele of the *APOE* gene, confers a 3-times greater risk for disease in non-Hispanic whites. The risk conferred by this allele in Hispanics seems to be less and may be nonexistent in persons of Mexican origin.[26,27] The contributions of other genetic variants to LOAD risk in persons of Mexican origin are largely unstudied. Future genetic studies of AD in Mexico need to account for the significant genetic heterogeneity present.[28]

Among Hispanics, the genetics of LOAD have been studied the most in persons of Caribbean origin (Dominican Republic and Puerto Rico). These studies have confirmed risk variants identified in non-Hispanic whites and identified novel ones.[29] The risk conferred by these variants is small and, therefore, although important in elucidating mechanisms of disease pathogenesis, these findings are not currently of clinical utility.

Although autosomal dominant AD of young onset is rare, accounting for approximately 1% of AD cases, the identification of specific founder mutations in Hispanics makes it relevant to question the specific geographic origin of Hispanics with onset of AD symptoms before age 65. These include mutations in the *PSEN1* gene, such as the E280A mutation in persons from Colombia, the G206A mutation in Caribbean Hispanics mostly originating from Puerto Rico, and the A431E mutation that has been identified in people whose family roots originate in or near the state of Jalisco in Mexico.[30]

CLINICAL CHARACTERISTICS SPECIFIC TO HISPANIC PATIENTS
Onset

Hispanic patients tend to have earlier age at onset.[31,32] The reasons are not completely understood but may be explained by the complex interactions between biological and cultural factors.[32,33]

Severity at Presentation

At initial presentation, Hispanics present with more severe cognitive impairment[31] and have a higher rate of behavioral symptoms overall compared with other groups.[34] A systematic review of ethnic differences in the use of dementia treatment care and research among different ethnic groups in the United States and Australia revealed that Hispanics had a longer duration of memory loss at the time of referral to specialized dementia services with a difference in Mini-mental State Examination (MMSE) of 3.5 points (95% CI, 2.87–4.09) even after controlling for level of education.[35]

Longevity

Hispanics tend to live longer with the disease compared with non-Hispanic whites.[36] Reasons for this are unclear but might be related to care provided by close-knit family relationships with large extended families.

DISPARITIES IN CARE
Barriers to Access

Hispanics experience ethnic and racial disparities in regard to access to care[37] and diagnosis of dementia.[35] Studies have shown that in minorities the diagnosis of dementia is often delayed and inadequate.[33] Hispanics are less likely to receive diagnostic services even when their condition is more advanced.[35] They are also less likely to seek care: a study of elderly Hispanics with memory or cognitive problems in a community sample found that the most common reasons for not pursuing clinical evaluation were related to personal beliefs (38%), which included mistrust of health care professionals,[38] language proficiency (33%), and economic status (13%).[39]

Health Literacy

Hispanics also have challenges with health literacy, specifically, navigating the health care system, understanding and incorporating recommendations given by their health care providers, and knowing when to seek care. Lower levels of education and socioeconomic status in addition to language barriers have been proposed as contributing to the lower levels of health literacy in Hispanics.[40]

Treatment

There are several objective disparities in the treatment of Hispanic patients. In addition to receiving less overall health care, that which they do receive is of poorer quality.[41] For example, Hispanics are less likely than non-Hispanic whites to receive specific pharmacologic treatments for dementia, such as acetylcholinesterase inhibitors or memantine.[42–44] Hispanic patients are less likely to be enrolled in clinical research trials and thus generalizability of the results to Hispanics may be reduced.[45] At the end of life, Hispanic Medicare beneficiaries are less likely to use hospice care.[46]

EVALUATION OF COGNITIVE IMPAIRMENT

CASE VIGNETTE 1: DIAGNOSTIC DILEMMA DUE TO LACK OF ACCULTURATION

Rosa is a 75-year-old right-handed Hispanic woman from Ecuador, with 1 year of formal education, who moved to the United States at the age of 55 after her husband died from cancer. Her daughter decided to bring her to the United States to take closer care for her. After moving to the United States, Rosa lived in relative isolation due to her limited ability to speak and understand English. She did not know how to drive and relied on her daughter to take her places. Rosa spent most of her time at home. She enjoyed watching telenovelas (soap operas) and helping with the house chores. Over the course of a few months, her daughter noted that Rosa became more withdrawn and was not interested in participating in family activities. Her sleep was disturbed and often she was awake late at night. Her ability to cook declined and her dishes were not as "tasty" as they used to be. Her daughter brought her for a primary care evaluation because she thought that her mother was suffering from depression.

After an evaluation by her primary care doctor (who did not speak Spanish; translation was provided by her daughter), Rosa was prescribed with a medication for depression, but her symptoms did not improve and she became more irritable. Rosa became suspicious that her son-in-law was cheating on her daughter. In one instance Rosa called the police because she was hearing loud voices inside the house and she thought that her son-in-law was assaulting her daughter, which was not confirmed by a police investigation. The environment seemed hostile to Rosa and she did not feel secure at her home. She continued to experience hallucinations of her son-in-law assaulting her daughter and being mistrustful of the neighbors, to the point that she had to be taken to the emergency department (ED).

In the ED, Rosa was noted to be very agitated and paranoid and received treatment with antipsychotics. She was discharged home after a basic work-up but without an established etiology for her symptoms. She was given a prescription for risperidone and a referral to see an outpatient psychiatrist. A few weeks later, before she was able to see the psychiatrist, she fell at home and suffered a hip fracture that required surgical treatment. After that incident, her daughter noted that Rosa had difficulties with her memory and a significant decline in her activities of daily living. When Rosa was seen by a non–Spanish-speaking psychiatrist, she was diagnosed with late-onset psychosis and her prescription for risperidone was refilled.

Rosa was later referred to a neurologist who was able to conduct an evaluation in Spanish. Additional history uncovered changes in memory that had been present for several years and were slowly progressive prior to the onset of her mood changes. Rosa endorsed insomnia and decreased enjoyment of activities. On risperidone, there were no hallucinations or delusions. She scored 16/30 on the MMSE. Neurologic examination revealed mild bilateral cogwheel rigidity in her wrists but was otherwise nonfocal. Basic laboratory work-up was normal. Brain MRI revealed moderate diffuse atrophy more prominent in bilateral parietotemporal regions, but neither space-occupying lesions nor evidence of vascular brain injury was present. She was referred for neuropsychological evaluation but there were no local providers who could perform an evaluation in Spanish. She was diagnosed with possible Alzheimer disease (AD). At that point her daughter quit her job and became the primary caregiver for her mother.

Rosa's case demonstrates patient and provider-specific factors that contributed to misdiagnosis and inappropriate treatment. Patient factors include lack of acculturation and adherence to Hispanic values of deference to authority, which prohibited Rosa's daughter from advocating more for her mother regarding a lack of diagnosis in the ED. Provider factors at the ED and primary care level include language barriers, lack of cognitive testing, and unfamiliarity with culture specific explanations of cognitive deficits. These factors important for evaluation are outlined in more detail.

Importance of Acculturation

Acculturation is the cultural and psychological change resulting from intercultural contact and exposure to the language and traditions of a new environment. This includes changes in customs, language, economic status, political life, social behavior, attitudes toward the acculturation process, and cultural identity.

In the previous example, Rosa demonstrated a low level of acculturation to the American mainstream due to not learning English and remaining socially isolated, without developing a network of friends in her new country. This left her reliant solely on her daughter's support without a larger network of social interactions in which her dementia might have been recognized earlier. The language barrier between her and her clinicians led to delays in diagnosis and inappropriate treatment.

Acculturation is a process that evolves at both individual and group levels; therefore, levels of acculturation vary widely among Hispanics in the United States. Level of acculturation to the US mainstream is an especially critical variable in neuropsychological assessment due to the documented cultural biases in the most heavily used measures of cognitive functioning.[47] These cultural biases have been found to contribute to racial disparities in performance among English-speaking American populations[48] as well as to significant differences between Hispanics and non-Hispanics in the United States.[49] Therefore, understanding the multifaceted effect of acculturation in neurologic and neurocognitive assessment is an essential part of culturally competent treatment of Hispanics.

Limitations related to the assessment of acculturation in Hispanics include problems with conceptualization, construct validity, and heterogeneity among Hispanic subgroups in the United States. Some of the scales used to evaluate level of acculturation rely heavily on measures of language or the use of proxy measures, such as generational status, age at arrival, and length of residency in the United States. These measures come at the expense of other essential aspects of acculturation, such as attitudinal, behavioral, and identity-related dimensions and ecological contexts, such as the interaction of environmental and neighborhood influences.[50] Additional research is needed to refine the scales that are currently used and to determine their validity across different Hispanic subgroups.[51] For a review of acculturation measures used with Hispanics, see Huynh and colleagues[52] and Substance Abuse and Mental Health Services Administration.[53]

Language

Of the 37.5 million Hispanics living in the United States who reported speaking Spanish at home, only 56.3% spoke English "very well" and 9% did not speak English at all.[54] The percentage of the total population 5 years and over that spoke Spanish grew from 12.0% in 2005 to 12.9% in 2011.[54]

Relative competence in a language involves not only the ability to speak but also to read, write, and think in the language. Hispanics have varying degrees of mastery of English and Spanish. It is important to assess both verbal and reading English language proficiency when treating Hispanic patients and providing written instructions and prescriptions. Additionally, Spanish labels and package inserts can be provided by pharmacies, and it is incumbent on providers to notify pharmacies of the need for Spanish instructions at the time of providing prescriptions.

The large number of Spanish language speakers with less than full English fluency also indicates the need for the availability of psychological assessment measures in Spanish as well as specialized assessment approaches for Spanish-English bilinguals.

A few case reports have described patients who regressed to the use of their primary language before developing symptoms of dementia.[55] It has been postulated that losing the second language attained is a sign of cognitive impairment or progression to dementia. In cases of Hispanics, they may lose their English language ability even if they had a strong command of the language in their younger years.

Use of Interpreters and Spanish-Speaking Providers

The use of Spanish interpreters in clinical practice has been associated with increased patient satisfaction.[56,57] A study performed with a Latino cohort in Southern California demonstrated that patients had increased satisfaction when the provider was able to communicate directly in Spanish, especially when individuals were less likely to speak or understand English.[58] Although specific studies have not been conducted in specialized neurologic clinics, these results are likely to extrapolate to the use of interpreters in neurologic examinations. In general, the use of interpreters who are trained and experienced with neurologic and psychological cases is preferred over using nonprofessional interpreters, like family, who may not have sufficient grasp of the language or medical terminology or who may have secondary motivations to influence the outcomes of the assessment.[59]

In contrast, interpreter-mediated neuropsychological testing of monolingual Spanish speakers is discouraged.[60] Research on the impact of interpreter-mediated cognitive testing with monolingual Spanish speakers demonstrated that interpreter use significantly affected scores especially for verbally mediated tasks, such as vocabulary and similarities subtests of the Wechsler Adult Intelligence Scale-III.[60] As a result, neuropsychological assessment is best conducted by a bilingual (ideally bicultural) psychologist or psychological technician.

Hispanic Values

Values, such as *respeto* (respect), *familismo*, and *personalism*, influence presentation. Respeto is characterized by the appreciation for hierarchical roles in the family, honoring the opinion and desires of the elder family members. This extends to health care providers, who are almost invariably treated with deference. Familismo is one of the main characteristics in the Hispanic culture; it places the family as an important source of support not only financially but also emotionally. The concept of familismo has been described as putting family first. It means for many Hispanics sacrificing on behalf of their close relatives.[61] This is often manifest as multiple family members presenting with a patient to their medical visits and taking active roles in their loved one's care. Personalism implies creating a relationship with the health care provider that feels friendly, caring, and warm. Providers should be aware that an attitude of intense efficiency may be interpreted as lack of caring, and building a relationship with Hispanic patients and their families requires not only time but also the ability to communicate in a warmly caring and compassionate manner.

Symptom Explanation

Hispanics may attribute some of the initial symptoms related to dementia (eg, memory loss or apathy) to normative cognitive changes associated with aging or to psychosocial stress, ultimately underestimating the clinical significance of mild declines in memory, executive functions, or language.[31,62] Additionally, Hispanics often do not realize that behavioral symptoms may be due to dementia. As a result, behavioral changes or disturbances in other cognitive domains can be minimized or overlooked. Education on disease development and early signs of decline is useful to patients and their families to increase the likelihood of their seeking medical evaluation earlier in the disease process.

Cognitive Screening Tools

Bedside cognitive screening tools provide a brief structured approach and are widely used for screening of patients that present with cognitive complaints in neurology, geriatrics, and other general medical practices. They are used during the initial encounter to assess degree of cognitive impairment and which cognitive domains are mostly affected and during subsequent follow-up visits to track progression over time. The goal is to assess multiple cognitive domains, such as attention, concentration, judgment, language, memory, and visuospatial and executive function, based on a structured or semistructured approach, often with normative criteria to determine if cognitive deficits are present and when further testing is needed. Cognitive screening tools in general have good sensitivity but lack specificity, especially for diagnosis at early stages of cognitive decline (ie, mild cognitive impairment [MCI]). Obtaining more detailed neuropsychological evaluation is recommended when there is not sufficient diagnostic clarity on initial evaluation.[63] The application of common cognitive screening tools to Hispanics is reviewed (**Table 1**).

Mini-mental State Examination

The MMSE is a 30-item measure designed to assess orientation, attention, memory, recall, language, and the ability to follow written and verbal commands.[64] Advantages of the MMSE include its ease of use, familiarity to physicians, and moderate sensitivity for the diagnosis of dementia. It is also helpful in staging and tracking progression over time. Results should be interpreted with caution because research has indicated that scores are heavily affected by age, education, and cultural background. In Hispanics, the MMSE underestimates cognitive capacities and has a higher false-positive ratio. Mungas and colleagues[65] developed an age-based and education-based correction algorithm to adjust MMSE scores for individuals with low levels of education, which may be helpful for select individuals. In terms of translation, there have been issues related to certain items resulting in different cultural and idiomatic nuances that may affect validity for detecting dementia across African Americans and Hispanics, when standard cutoffs are based on white samples.[65]

Table 1 Screening tools for the mental status evaluation	
Screening Tool	**Special Considerations for Hispanics**
MMSE	Underestimates cognitive capacity in Hispanics. Has a higher false-positive ratio. Age-based and education-based correction is recommended for use with low levels of education
Mini-Cog	Detects clinically significant cognitive impairment as well as or better than MMSE. Less biased by low education.
MoCA	Has been translated into Spanish. Greater sensitivity for the diagnosis of MCI or dementia than the MMSE. May underestimate cognitive capacity in Hispanics with <6 y of formal education.

Mini-Cog

The Mini-Cog consists of a clock drawing task and 3-item recall. It was developed as a brief test for discriminating demented from nondemented persons and is widely used as a screening tool for dementia. The Mini-Cog detects clinically significant cognitive impairment as well as or better than MMSE in multiethnic elderly individuals, including Hispanics. It is also easier to administer to non-English speakers and in general is less biased by low education, literacy, or ethnic background.[66,67] One major limitation is that, because of its brevity, the Mini-Cog is not a good tool for screening patients that present at early stages of cognitive decline, that is, MCI.[68]

Montreal Cognitive Assessment

The Montreal Cognitive Assessment (MoCA) was designed to assess for MCI, and the suggested normal range for the MoCA is 26 to 30 points, with a 1-point education correction for those individuals who have less than 12 years of education.[69] It is freely available on the Internet (www.mocatest.org) and has been translated to multiple languages, including Spanish. It evaluates several domains, including attention, orientation, language, verbal memory, visuospatial, and executive function. It offers greater sensitivity for the diagnosis of MCI or dementia than the MMSE as well as the ability to sample cognitive domains more widely than the MMSE.[70] The MoCA screens attention and components of executive function and probes language and memory in more detail than the MMSE. Limited research on the Spanish version has been done. A study conducted with a Hispanic cohort in Southern California indicated that an additional 4-point adjustment was needed for 0 to 5 years of education, but overall the Spanish version maintained adequate psychometric properties in this population.[71] Other studies in Hispanics have also suggested that individuals with less than 6 years of education exhibit poorer performance on the test predominantly in the domain of visuospatial executive performance.[72] A validation study performed in a cohort from Colombia demonstrated consistency in the psychometric properties of the Spanish version of the test.[73] Given these findings, clinicians can use the MoCA but interpret scores cautiously in Hispanics, particularly those of low educational attainment.

Additional cognitive screening instruments have been translated into Spanish and are available for the evaluation of Spanish-speaking patients who present with cognitive complaints. These include an abbreviated version of the Cognitive Abilities Screening Instrument[74]; the Modified Mini-Mental State test, which in addition to the MMSE incorporates 4 items on long-term memory, abstract thinking, category fluency, and delayed recall[75,76]; and the Saint Louis University Mental Status Examination.[77,78]

CASE 2: APPLICATION OF NEUROPSYCHOLOGICAL EVALUATION TO A HISPANIC PATIENT

Maria is a 63-year-old left-handed Hispanic woman from Nicaragua. She presented to clinic with her daughter who just had a baby a month ago. Maria graduated from high school in her native country and migrated to the United States in her early 20s. She learned English in English as a second language (ESL) classes after migration and developed enough fluency to work part time in sales. She raised 4 children as a single mother. Two years prior to presentation, Maria began demonstrating several notable behavior changes appreciated by her daughter. For example, she began to express sexual interest in younger men and made explicit erotic advances. She also started to spend significant amounts of money shopping online and began hoarding toilet paper. Maria's premorbid personality was described as a modest, caring, and responsible mother. She was initially diagnosed with late-onset bipolar disorder and quit her job at that time. She later developed stereotyped behaviors, including clapping her hands when feeling excited, and increased irritability. She began to revert to Spanish (her native language) more often and was noted to have significant word-finding difficulties. She also developed a tendency to wander and once got lost around the neighborhood. Her daughter had to quit her job 6 months prior to Maria's presentation to find a specialized dementia clinic to care for her mother. There was no significant past medical or family history of other relatives with neurodegenerative conditions. Physical examination was significant for obesity (per her daughter there was significant weight gain during the previous 2 years). Maria scored 22/30 on the MoCA and demonstrated difficulties with executive function and delayed recall. Neurologic examination did not reveal any focal findings. The diagnostic impression was of early-onset AD versus behavioral variant frontotemporal dementia and the patient was referred for neuropsychological evaluation for detailed cognitive testing to help clarify the diagnosis. Neuropsychological testing was completed by a psychometrician proficient in Spanish and results were initially interpreted by a neuropsychologist with limited experience working with Hispanic older adults. At first, results were interpreted with cutoffs for white patients, which indicated significant amnestic impairment thought to support the AD. On consultation with a colleague who specialized in assessment of Spanish-speakers, however, specific Hispanic cultural factors and Maria's educational background were taken into account and testing results were compared with normative data matched for age, ethnicity, language, and years of education—results were found more consistent with a behavioral variant frontotemporal dementia.

This case illustrates the complex presentation of cognitive and behavioral changes in early-onset dementias. Although Maria had symptoms suggestive of a frontotemporal dementia with socially inappropriate behaviors, simple repetitive movements (clapping), ritualistic behavior (hoarding), and deficits in executive function, her memory decline and reduction in the use of English (her second language) initially were weighted more highly on evaluation. In this case, neuropsychological evaluation and consultation with a psychologist with expertise in Spanish and cross-cultural testing issues helped clarify the nature of the dementia.

NEUROPSYCHOLOGICAL ASSESSMENT

A comprehensive neuropsychological assessment is used to identify cognitive dysfunction that can inform diagnostic decisions and prognoses. With the growing population of Hispanics/Latinos in the United States, the need for linguistically and culturally valid neuropsychological assessment tools has become acutely apparent.[79] Most neuropsychological measures are heavily language dependent and have been shown culturally biased, favoring the population within which they were developed, which has historically been limited to the United States and Europe.[15,80] Fortunately, research and development of cognitive measures for use with Spanish speakers has increased during the past few decades.[81] Some of these efforts have been focused on translating and adapting existing English measures, whereas others have been dedicated to the development of new measures specifically designed for use with Spanish-speaking populations. Currently, there are several neuropsychological batteries available for use with Spanish speakers (**Table 1** includes those for use with older adults) as well as several guides for cognitive assessment of Spanish speakers informed by reviews of the neuropsychology literature (eg, Ardila and colleagues,[82] 1994; Benuto,[83] 2012; Ferraro,[3] 2015; and Pontón and León-Carrión,[84] 2001). Explicit training, however, in working with these measures and interpretation of the results with an expert who understands the interplay between cultural context and test performance are still required. A selection of issues to consider for a comprehensive neurologic assessment with Spanish-speaking elderly is highlighted.

The Neuropsychological Examiner

Finding the appropriate neuropsychologist to work with Spanish speakers enhances the validity of the assessment results. A bilingual, bicultural neuropsychologist with extensive experience in assessing Spanish-speaking older adults from a range of demographic backgrounds and acculturation levels is ideally positioned to design and administer a battery of measures to appropriately estimate cognitive functioning and to interpret the results it yields.[85] Additionally, cultural competence in working with this population is critical to establishing rapport (discussed previously), which may require allowing for longer sessions, multiple visits, and involving a patient's family. The neuropsychologist should also possess a strong foundation in psychometrics to critically consider neurocognitive measures for appropriateness and to understand how to adjust assessment approaches to accommodate the needs of the patient while respecting the bounds of standardized testing. Resources for finding a Spanish-speaking neuropsychologist with the stated expertise are discussed later.

Culture and Neuropsychological Assessment

Culture dictates how members of a given society behave, feel, and think; therefore, it inevitably plays a central role in cognitive assessment. Ardila[47] outlined several culturally driven values that can influence the neuropsychological assessment, including interpersonal values (working one-on-one with a stranger; distance between the examiner and the patient; beliefs about age, gender authority, and respect; communication style, and so forth) and performance-specific values (eg, stance on competition, definition of doing "one's best," speed vs accuracy, and standardized testing procedures).[47] These values can affect test performance; therefore, it is essential to gather detailed information on a patient's cultural background and level of acculturation during the clinical interview, which may require additional time. The information gathered should inform how a patient is prepared for testing as well as test selection and administration. For example, an examiner can explain the nature and purpose of standardized testing to a patient in advance, emphasizing what is meant by "doing your best" and working "as quickly as possible," and doing so in a warm and respectful manner. Additionally, selecting tests that have been culturally adapted, rather than a Spanish translation of an existing measure, is recommended whenever possible.

Education

Neuropsychological assessment is largely an assessment of school-based skills that rely on certain levels of literacy and familiarity with the testing situation. Therefore, when working with Spanish-speaking elderly with limited education and/or literacy, care must be taken to select tests that can assist in distinguishing between organic cognitive deficits and poor performance due to lack of experience with academic-style examinations. A detailed educational history of the quality and quantity of a patient's education and performance on mental status screening tools should facilitate test selection. Tests with less emphasis on verbal abilities should always be considered, although relying solely on nonverbal tests is ill advised because many of these tests have been found susceptible to education effects.[86] Tests with education-stratified norms, especially ones that go as low as 0 to 3 years (eg, Evaluación Neuropsicological Breve en Español [NEUROPSI]),[87] should be kept on hand.

Bilingualism

There is a growing body of research that has found significant disparities in cognitive testing performance between bilinguals and monolinguals.[88,89] First, there is the issue of test language selection. Pontón[85] offers a useful decision tree for determining whether to test a bilingual individual in Spanish or the other language spoken. Second, research has indicated that bilingual individuals are in a constant state of dually active language processing, which may enhance performance on tasks of executive control (eg, mental control and inhibition) while compromising language processing speed.[90] For this reason, it is important to use normative data collected from bilinguals when possible (eg, Mitrushina and colleagues[91]) and to administer a balance of timed and untimed measures when testing bilinguals, especially on measures of language fluency. Additionally, comparison of performance in both languages and use of appropriate norms may assist interpretation of results. For an in-depth review of neuropsychological assessment with bilingual individuals, see Rivera Mindt and colleagues.[90]

Interpretation using normative data
The greatest challenge in neuropsychological assessment of elderly Hispanics once test selection and administration are complete is finding the appropriate normative data to interpret results. Using the norms from populations that are representative of a patient's demographic and sociocultural background is essential given the documented disparities on cognitive test performance by language proficiency, education, economic status, and acculturation level.[92] Hispanics with normal cognitive functioning are at increased risk of being misdiagnosed with dementia compared with non-Hispanic whites due, in part, to the use of nonrepresentative norms and diagnostic cutoff scores.[93] Although norms for non–English-speaking ethnic minorities remain limited,[2] the available norms for Spanish-speakers and Spanish-English bilinguals are growing, albeit slowly. Due to the vast diversity within the Hispanic population, however, selection of appropriate norms remains challenging and interpretation based on multiple demographic variables may be needed. Norms can be found in test manuals, published research, and compendiums (eg, Mitrushina and colleagues[91]), and the burden of responsibility for norm selection falls on the examiner. Justification and caveats to interpretation, such as using nonrepresentative normative data, should always be clearly documented.

Tables 2 and **3** contain information on some neuropsychological batteries and domain-specific tests that can be used with Hispanic older adults.

CAREGIVERS AND RESOURCES

CASE 3: ROLE OF FAMILY AND SOCIAL SUPPORT

Ruby is an 83-year-old right-handed Hispanic woman from Cuba who came accompanied by her 6 children for evaluation of slowly progressive cognitive decline. She migrated to the United States when she was a teenager and attended college and graduated from law school in the United States. She worked with her father managing a food processing company and was the chief executive officer of the company after her father passed. She retired a couple years ago after she was noted to have cognitive decline and was no longer able to manage the complex finances of the company. She was diagnosed with AD two years prior to presentation. Since then, her 6 children have been taking care of her and rotate every few weeks. The patient has a cheerful attitude and feels pleased with the care she receives. Her family hope to be able to provide care for her at home and do not want to institutionalize her. They were able to hire a companion to care for her mother who spends time with her during the day. They also hired a night nurse who provides supervision and care through the night.

Table 2
Neuropsychological batteries used to assess Hispanic elderly

Battery	Cognitive Domains	Special Considerations
Consortium to Establish a Registry for Alzheimer's Disease (Fillenbaum et al,[98] 2007; Fillenbaum et al,[99] 2008; and Morris et al,[100] 1989)	MMSE Semantic fluency Confrontation naming list-learning task Constructional praxis Delayed word list recall Word list recognition	• Specially designed for assessing AD • Translation from English with cultural modifications • Empirical support for use with Hispanics when AD is suspected; less beneficial for differential diagnosis of other dementias • Education and gender effects • Confrontation naming subtest (15-item Boston Naming Test) found to have weak sensitivity to detect AD
Spanish and English Neuropsychological Assessment Scales (Mungas et al,[101] 2004)	Verbal conceptual thinking Nonverbal conceptual thinking Verbal attention span Visual attention span Confrontation naming association Word list learning (fixed word list) Word list learning II (progressing word list)	• Specially designed for assessing elderly Spanish and English speakers • Extensive empirical support for use with Spanish-speaking or English-speaking Hispanics • Strong education and language fluency effects; authors provide updated norms • Two-list learning tasks, one with a 15-word list presented over 5 trials, one with 3 words presented in the first trial, with 3 additional words each trial after for 5 trials • Original 4-h and brief battery 2-h versions available • Available free of charge from Dr Mungas
Batería III Woodcock-Muñoz (Woodcock et al,[102] 2007)	Crystallized intelligence Fluid reasoning Visual processing Short-term memory Delayed memory Processing speed Auditory processing	• Empirical support for use with Hispanics • Norms from Mexico, Central America, Spain, and US • Spanish equivalent of Woodcock-Johnson III

(continued on next page)

Table 2
(continued)

Battery	Cognitive Domains	Special Considerations
Neuropsychological Screening Battery for Hispanics (Pontón et al,[103] 1996)	Phonemic fluency Confrontation naming Verbal memory (word list) Visuoconstruction Nonverbal memory Complex mental tracking Processing speed Working memory Nonverbal reasoning Psychomotor speed	• Developed to collect norms from Hispanics for commonly used English measures and to create cultural adaptations of these measures • Uses modified version (Pontón-Saz) of Boston Naming Test • Includes Color Trails Test instead of Trail Making Test • Norms from Mexico, Central American, Puerto Rico, and Cuba; up to age 75
NEUROPSI (Ostrosky-Solís et al,[87] 1999)	Orientation Attention Verbal memory Nonverbal memory Semantic fluency Phonemic fluency Confrontation naming	• Empirical support for use with Hispanics • Norms from 950 Spanish-speakers from Mexico; aged up to 85 y • Developed to collect norms from Hispanics for commonly used English measures and to create cultural adaptations of these measures • Appropriate for use when education is limited; not recommended for those with education >10 y • Brief: up to 90 min for cognitively impaired
Batería Neuropsicológica de Funciones Ejecutivas y Lobulós Frontales (Flores Lázaro et al,[104] 2008, and Flores et al,[105] 2012)	Verbal abstract reasoning Verbal fluency Processing speed/inhibition Nonverbal abstract Reasoning (tower test, mazes) Serial verbal learning Serial visual learning Visuospatial working memory Verbal working memory Serial addition/subtraction	• Designed to test executive functions and collect information for frontal behavioral syndromes • Norms up to age 79 • Brief: 60 min • Manual does not provide norms by subtest

Table 3
Domain-specific measures used to assess Hispanic elderly

Domain	Test	Appropriate for Limited/Low Education
Premorbid verbal IQ	Word Accentuation Test–Chicago (Kreuger et al,[106] 2006)	
Verbal memory and learning	WHO-UCLA Auditory Verbal Learning Test (Pontón et al,[103] 1996)	X
	Hopkins Verbal Learning Test (Cherner et al,[107] 2007)	X
	Spanish English Verbal Learning Test (Gonzalez et al,[108] 2002)	X
	NEUROPSI list learning and narrative memory subtests (Ostrosky-Solís et al,[87] 1999)	X
Nonverbal memory and learning	Rey-Osterrieth Complex Figure recall (Meyers and Meyers,[109] 1995, and Ostrosky-Solís et al,[87] 1999)	
	Brief Visual Memory Test–Revised (Cherner et al,[107] 2007)	X
	Raven's Progressive Matrices (Raven and Court,[110] 1998)	X
	Batería Neuropsicológica de Funciones Ejecutivas y Lobulós Frontale (Lázaro et al,[104] 2008)	
	Wisconsin Card Sorting Test (Heaton et al,[111] 1993)	
	Clock drawing	X
Executive functioning	Trail Making Test	
	Color Trails Test (D'Elia et al,[112] 1996)	X
	Stroop Color and Word Test (Golden, 1978,[117] and Peña-Casanova et al,[113] 2009)	
	NEUROPSI color-word interference subtest (Ostrosky-Solís et al,[87] 1999)	
	Tower of London (Peña-Casanova et al,[113] 2009)	
	NEUROPSI digit span or spatial span (Ostrosky-Solís et al,[87] 1999)	X
Attention	NEUROPSI conflicting instruction test (Ostrosky-Solís et al,[87] 1999)	X
	Color Trails Test (D'Elia et al,[112] 1996)	X
	Stroop Color and Word Test (Golden 1978,[117] and Peña-Casanova et al,[113] 2009)	
	NEUROPSI color-word interference subtest (Ostrosky-Solís et al,[87] 1999)	
	Modified/Pontón-Saz Boston Naming Test (Pontón et al,[103] 1996)	X
	Texas Spanish Naming Test (Marquez de la Plata et al,[114] 2008)	X
	Controlled Oral Word Association Test (Pontón et al,[103] 1996)	X
Language	NEUROPSI phonemic fluency: letter P (Ostrosky-Solís et al,[87] 1999)	X
	NEUROPSI category fluency (animals) (Ostrosky-Solís et al,[87] 1999)	X
	Semantic fluency test (Rosselli et al,[115] 2009)	X
Visuospatial	Rey-Osterrieth Complex Figure Drawing Test (Meyers and Meyers,[109] 1995, and Ostrosky-Solís et al,[87] 1999)	
	NEUROPSI simplified Rey-Osterrieth Complex Figure Drawing Test (Ostrosky-Solís et al,[87] 1999)	X
	Benton Judgment of Line Orientation (Benton et al,[116] 1983)	X

This case illustrates some of the Hispanic values discussed previously, such as familismo and respeto. It emphasizes the importance of family relationships and their relevance to coping with the caregiver role. It shows how Hispanics prefer to take care of their relatives with dementia at home.

Caregivers

In the Hispanic community, often the main caregivers are family members due to not only economical restraints, such as a lack of the ability to afford paid caregivers that provide respite care, but also cultural preferences. Hispanics have a higher percentage of family caregivers compared with other ethnic groups, and this role falls often to a female family member (ie, spouse or daughter).[94,95] Some Hispanics may view placement in a nursing home as a sign of abandonment and lack of love or care for their elders. Many Hispanics prefer to shoulder the burden of caring for their loved ones at home even when they may not have the ideal circumstances to care for them. Some of the approaches Hispanics use to manage challenging behaviors in relatives with dementia include acceptance, love, patience, adaptability, and establishing routines of care.[94] There are usually strong family connections and these play an important role as well. Hispanics tend to live in clusters and the physical proximity allows sharing the responsibility among several family members (ie, children and even grandchildren and nieces or nephews). Despite these supports, caregiver burnout is also an important factor to take into account in Hispanic populations. Hispanic caregivers have a higher rate of depressive symptoms compared with caregivers from other ethnicities.[96] A recent study of Hispanic dementia caregivers in New York demonstrated that decreased satisfaction with social support was associated with increased rates of caregiver burnout and depressive symptoms. It also showed that a majority of caregivers were daughters and had low income.[97] Another study with Hispanic caregivers in San Diego, California, defined some of the challenges they faced, including "issues with providers, problems with family members, limited knowledge of resources, emotional distress, and financial strain."[94]

Resources for the Cognitive Evaluation of Hispanics in the United States

In recent years, centers that provide culturally and linguistically appropriate neuropsychological evaluations and interventions to Latino patients have emerged. Examples include the Cultural Neuropsychology Initiative at the University of California, Los Angeles (UCLA) Semel Institute for Neuroscience and Human Behavior, the UCLA Resnick Neuropsychiatric Hospital, and the Multicultural Neuropsychology Program at the Massachusetts General Hospital. These programs are not yet widely available through the United States and are limited mostly to academic centers. There are also neuropsychologists in private practice who have a special interest in working with Hispanic patients. The Hispanic Neuropsychological Society (http://hnps.org) has a link to help find a Spanish-Speaking neuropsychologist within a certain area (http://hnps.org/find-a-spanish-speaking-neuropsychologist-2/). The development of more centers that are competent in cross-cultural neuropsychology should help fill the gap in the evaluation and management of a growing population of older Hispanics with cognitive complaints in the United States.

SUMMARY

Hispanics are the largest minority group in the United States and, with a growing number older than 65 years of age, increasing resources that are culturally informed will be required for the provision of appropriate services for evaluation and care. Health care providers who work with Hispanics should not only understand potential differences in the clinical presentation of cognitive impairment and dementia in different ethnic populations but also the differences in perception of dementia and its impact on the daily lives of patients and their caregivers. Neuropsychological assessments should be performed and interpreted with particular attention to cultural, linguistic, and educational factors. To advance multicultural services that provide culturally sensitive care for patients from ethnic minority groups, there should not only be an increase in awareness that cultural factors are important but also a commensurate increase in the culturally competent training of providers.

REFERENCES

1. U.S. Census Bureau. The next four decades: the older population in the United States: 2010 to 2050. Available at: https://www.census.gov/prod/2010pubs/p25-1138.pdf. Accessed August 15, 2016.
2. Rivera Mindt M, Byrd D, Saez P, et al. Increasing culturally competent neuropsychological services for ethnic minority populations: a call to action. Clin Neuropsychol 2010;24(3):429–53.
3. Ferraro FR. Minority and cross-cultural aspects of neuropsychological assessment: enduring and emerging trends. Studies on neuropsychology, neurology and cognition. 2, illustrated, revised edition. Hove (United Kingdom): Psychology Press; 2015.
4. Alzheimer's Association. 2015 Alzheimer's disease facts and figures. Alzheimers Dement 2015;11(3):332–84.
5. Latinos & Alzheimer's Disease: new numbers behind the crisis. 2016. USC Edward R. Roybal Institute on Aging and the LatinosAgainstAlzheimer's Network.
6. Gurland BJ, Wilder DE, Lantigua R, et al. Rates of dementia in three ethnoracial groups. Int J Geriatr Psychiatry 1999;14(6):481–93.
7. Tang MX, Cross P, Andrews H, et al. Incidence of AD in African-Americans, Caribbean Hispanics, and Caucasians in northern Manhattan. Neurology 2001;56(1):49–56.
8. Haan MN, Mungas DM, Gonzalez HM, et al. Prevalence of dementia in older latinos: the influence of type 2 diabetes mellitus, stroke and genetic factors. J Am Geriatr Soc 2003;51(2):169–77.
9. Mayeda ER, Glymour MM, Quesenberry CP, et al. Inequalities in dementia incidence between six racial and ethnic groups over 14 years. Alzheimers Dement 2016;12(3):216–24.
10. Barnes DE, Yaffe K. The projected effect of risk factor reduction on Alzheimer's disease prevalence. Lancet Neurol 2011;10(9):819–28.
11. Sharp ES, Gatz M. Relationship between education and dementia: an updated systematic review. Alzheimer Dis Assoc Disord 2011;25(4):289–304.
12. McDowell I, Xi G, Lindsay J, et al. Mapping the connections between education and dementia. J Clin Exp Neuropsychol 2007;29(2):127–41.
13. U. S. Census Bureau. National Population Projections. 2014. Available at: https://www.census.gov/population/projections/data/national/2014.html. Accessed April 1, 2016.
14. Strutt AM, Burton VJ, Resendiz CV, et al. Neurocognitive assessment of Hispanic individuals residing in the United States: current issues and potential solutions. In: Ferraro FR, editor. Minority and cross-cultural aspects of neuropsychological assessment: enduring and emerging trends. 2nd edition. New York: Taylor & Francis; 2016. p. 201–28.

15. Ponton MO, Ardila A. The future of neuropsychology with Hispanic populations in the United States. Arch Clin Neuropsychol 1999;14(7):565–80.
16. Zeki Al Hazzouri A, Haan MN, Kalbfleisch JD, et al. Life-course socioeconomic position and incidence of dementia and cognitive impairment without dementia in older Mexican Americans: results from the Sacramento area Latino study on aging. Am J Epidemiol 2011;173(10):1148–58.
17. Bialystok E. Reshaping the mind: the benefits of bilingualism. Can J Exp Psychol 2011;65(4):229–35.
18. Yang S, Yang H, Lust B. Early childhood bilingualism leads to advances in executive attention: Dissociating culture and language. Bilingualism: Language and Cognition 2011;14(03):412–22.
19. Bialystok E, Abutalebi J, Bak TH, et al. Aging in two languages: Implications for public health. Ageing Res Rev 2016;27:56–60.
20. Lawton DM, Gasquoine PG, Weimer AA. Age of dementia diagnosis in community dwelling bilingual and monolingual Hispanic Americans. Cortex 2015;66:141–5.
21. Zahodne LB, Schofield PW, Farrell MT, et al. Bilingualism does not alter cognitive decline or dementia risk among Spanish-speaking immigrants. Neuropsychology 2014;28(2):238–46.
22. Gollan TH, Salmon DP, Montoya RI, et al. Degree of bilingualism predicts age of diagnosis of Alzheimer's disease in low-education but not in highly educated Hispanics. Neuropsychologia 2011;49(14):3826–30.
23. Middleton LE, Yaffe K. Targets for the prevention of dementia. J Alzheimers Dis 2010;20(3):915–24.
24. Daviglus ML, Talavera GA, Aviles-Santa ML, et al. Prevalence of major cardiovascular risk factors and cardiovascular diseases among Hispanic/Latino individuals of diverse backgrounds in the United States. JAMA 2012;308(17):1775–84.
25. Rodriguez CJ, Allison M, Daviglus ML, et al. Status of cardiovascular disease and stroke in Hispanics/Latinos in the United States: a science advisory from the American Heart Association. Circulation 2014;130(7):593–625.
26. Campos M, Edland SD, Peavy GM. Exploratory study of apolipoprotein E epsilon4 genotype and risk of Alzheimer's disease in Mexican Hispanics. J Am Geriatr Soc 2013;61(6):1038–40.
27. Villalpando-Berumen JM, Mejia-Arango S, Aguilar-Salinas CA, et al. Apolipoprotein E epsilon4, Alzheimer's disease, and cognitive performance in elderly Mexican Mestizos. J Am Geriatr Soc 2008;56(4):677–82.
28. Moreno-Estrada A, Gignoux CR, Fernandez-Lopez JC, et al. Human genetics. The genetics of Mexico recapitulates Native American substructure and affects biomedical traits. Science 2014;344(6189):1280–5.
29. Lee JH, Cheng R, Barral S, et al. Identification of novel loci for Alzheimer disease and replication of CLU, PICALM, and BIN1 in Caribbean Hispanic individuals. Arch Neurol 2011;68(3):320–8.
30. Ringman JM, Coppola G. New genes and new insights from old genes: update on Alzheimer disease. Continuum (Minneap Minn) 2013;19(2 Dementia):358–71.
31. Livney MG, Clark CM, Karlawish JH, et al. Ethnoracial differences in the clinical characteristics of Alzheimer's disease at initial presentation at an urban Alzheimer's disease center. Am J Geriatr Psychiatry 2011;19(5):430–9.
32. Fitten LJ, Ortiz F, Fairbanks L, et al. Younger age of dementia diagnosis in a Hispanic population in southern California. Int J Geriatr Psychiatry 2014;29(6):586–93.

33. Chin AL, Negash S, Hamilton R. Diversity and disparity in dementia: the impact of ethnoracial differences in Alzheimer disease. Alzheimer Dis Assoc Disord 2011;25(3):187–95.

34. Hinton L, Haan M, Geller S, et al. Neuropsychiatric symptoms in Latino elders with dementia or cognitive impairment without dementia and factors that modify their association with caregiver depression. Gerontologist 2003;43(5):669–77.

35. Cooper C, Tandy AR, Balamurali TB, et al. A systematic review and meta-analysis of ethnic differences in use of dementia treatment, care, and research. Am J Geriatr Psychiatry 2010;18(3):193–203.

36. Mehta KM, Yaffe K, Perez-Stable EJ, et al. Race/ethnic differences in AD survival in US Alzheimer's Disease Centers. Neurology 2008;70(14):1163–70.

37. Sue S, Zane N, Nagayama Hall GC, et al. The case for cultural competency in psychotherapeutic interventions. Annu Rev Psychol 2009;60:525–48.

38. Mahoney DF, Cloutterbuck J, Neary S, et al. African American, Chinese, and Latino family caregivers' impressions of the onset and diagnosis of dementia: cross-cultural similarities and differences. Gerontologist 2005;45(6):783–92.

39. Ortiz F, Fitten J. Barriers to healthcare access for cognitively impaired older Hispanics. Alzheimer Dis Assoc Disord 2000;14(3):141–50.

40. Becerra BJ, Arias D, Becerra MB. Low health literacy among immigrant Hispanics. J Racial Ethn Health Disparities 2016. [Epub ahead of print].

41. Betancourt JR, Green AR, Carrillo JE, et al. Defining cultural competence- a practical framework for addressing racial: ethnic disparities in health and health care. Public Health Rep 2003;118:293–302.

42. Hernandez S, McClendon MJ, Zhou XH, et al. Pharmacological treatment of Alzheimer's disease: effect of race and demographic variables. J Alzheimers Dis 2010;19(2):665–72.

43. Zuckerman IH, Ryder PT, Simoni-Wastila L, et al. Racial and ethnic disparities in the treatment of dementia among Medicare beneficiaries. J Gerontol B Psychol Sci Soc Sci 2008;63(5):S328–33.

44. Gilligan AM, Malone DC, Warholak TL, et al. Racial and ethnic disparities in Alzheimer's disease pharmacotherapy exposure: an analysis across four state Medicaid populations. Am J Geriatr Pharmacother 2012;10(5):303–12.

45. Oh SS, Galanter J, Thakur N, et al. Diversity in clinical and biomedical research: a promise yet to be fulfilled. PLoS Med 2015;12(12):e1001918.

46. Alzheimer's Association. 2010 Alzheimer's disease facts and figures. Alzheimers Dement 2010;6:1–74.

47. Ardila A. Cultural values underlying psychometric cognitive testing. Neuropsychol Rev 2005;15(4):185–95.

48. Manly JJ, Byrd DA, Touradji P, et al. Acculturation, reading level, and neuropsychological test performance among African American elders. Appl Neuropsychol 2004;11(1):37–46.

49. Gasquoine PG. Variables moderating cultural and ethnic differences in neuropsychological assessment: the case of Hispanic Americans. Clin Neuropsychol 1999;13(3):376–83.

50. Lopez-Class M, Castro FG, Ramirez AG. Conceptions of acculturation: a review and statement of critical issues. Soc Sci Med 2011;72(9):1555–62.

51. Lara M, Gamboa C, Kahramanian MI, et al. Acculturation and Latino health in the United States: a review of the literature and its sociopolitical context. Annu Rev Public Health 2005;26:367–97.

52. Huynh QL, Howell RT, Benet-Martinez V. Reliability of Bidimensional Acculturation Scores: A Meta-Analysis. J Cross Cult Psychol 2009;40(2):256–74.

53. Substance Abuse and Mental Health Services Administration. Improving cultural competence. Treatment improvement protocol (TIP) series No. 59. HHS Publication No (SMA) 14–4849. Rockville (MD): Substance Abuse and Mental Health Services Administration. Originating office. Quality improvement and workforce development. Branch division of Services improvement; 2014.

54. Ryan C. Language use in the United States: 2011. In: BUREAU USC, editor. Census.gov: U.S. Department of Commerce; 2013. Available at: http://2010-2014.commerce.gov/blog/2013/08/06/new-census-bureau-interactive-map-shows-languages-spoken-america.html.

55. McMurtray A, Saito E, Nakamoto B. Language preference and development of dementia among bilingual individuals. Hawaii Med J 2009;68(9):223–6.

56. Schutt RK, Mejia C. Health care satisfaction: effects of immigration, acculturation, language. J Immigr Minor Health 2016;30:1–7.

57. Moreno G, Morales LS. Hablamos Juntos (Together We Speak): interpreters, provider communication, and satisfaction with care. J Gen Intern Med 2010; 25(12):1282–8.

58. Eskes C, Salisbury H, Johannsson M, et al. Patient satisfaction with language-concordant care. J Physician Assist Educ 2013;24(3):14–22.

59. VanderWielen LM, Enurah AS, Rho HY, et al. Medical interpreters: improvements to address access, equity, and quality of care for limited-English-proficient patients. Acad Med 2014;89(10):1324–7.

60. Casas R, Guzman-Velez E, Cardona-Rodriguez J, et al. Interpreter-mediated neuropsychological testing of monolingual Spanish speakers. Clin Neuropsychol 2012;26(1):88–101.

61. Gelman CR. Familismo and its impact on the family caregiving of Latinos with Alzheimer's disease: a complex narrative. Res Aging 2014;36(1):40–71.

62. Hinton L, Franz CE, Yeo G, et al. Conceptions of dementia in a multiethnic sample of family caregivers. J Am Geriatr Soc 2005;53(8):1405–10.

63. Knopman DS, DeKosky ST, Cummings JL, et al. Practice parameter: diagnosis of dementia (an evidence-based review). Report of the Quality Standards Subcommittee of the American Academy of Neurology. Neurology 2001;56(9):1143–53.

64. Folstein MF, Folstein SE, McHugh PR. "Mini-Mental State" a practical method for grading the cognitive state of patients for the clinician. J Psychiatr Res 1975;12: 189–98.

65. Mungas D, Marshall SC, Weldon M. Age and education correction of Mini-Mental State Examination for English- and Spanish-speaking elderly. Neurology 1996;46:700–6.

66. Borson S, Scanlan J, Brush M, et al. The Mini-Cog: a cognitive 'Vitals Signs' measure for dementia screening in multi-lingual elderly. Int J Geriatr Psychiatry 2000;15:1021–7.

67. Borson S, Scanlan JM, Watanabe J, et al. Simplifying detection of cognitive impairment: comparison of the Mini-Cog and Mini-Mental State Examination in a multiethnic sample. J Am Geriatr Soc 2005;53(5):871–4.

68. Carnero-Pardo C, Cruz-Orduna I, Espejo-Martinez B, et al. Utility of the mini-cog for detection of cognitive impairment in primary care: data from two spanish studies. Int J Alzheimers Dis 2013;2013:285462.

69. Nasreddine ZS, Phillips NA, Bedirian V, et al. The Montreal cognitive Assessment, MoCA: a Brief Screening Tool for Mild Cognitive impairment. J Am Geriatr Soc 2005;53:695–9.

70. Roalf DR, Moberg PJ, Xie SX, et al. Comparative accuracies of two common screening instruments for classification of Alzheimer's disease, mild cognitive impairment, and healthy aging. Alzheimers Dement 2013;9(5):529–37.

71. Zhou Y, Ortiz F, Nuñez C, et al. Adjustment of moca scores in a spanish-speaking population with varied levels of education. Alzheimers Dement 2014; 10(4):P727–8.

72. Rossetti HC, Lacritz LH, Cullum CM, et al. Normative data for the Montreal Cognitive Assessment (MoCA) in a population-based sample. Neurology 2011;77(13):1272–5.

73. Gil L, Vega JG, Ruiz de Sanchez C, et al. Validation of the Montreal Cognitive Assessment – Spanish Version test (MoCA-S) as a screening tool for mild cognitive impairment and mild dementia in Bogotá, Colombia. Alzheimers Dement 2013;9(4):P452–3.

74. Teng EL, Hasegawa K, Homma A, et al. The Cognitive Abilities Screening Instrument (CASI): a practical test for cross-cultural epidemiological studies of dementia. Int Psychogeriatr 1994;6(1):45–58 [discussion: 62].

75. Lyness SA, Lee AY, Zarow C, et al. 10-minute delayed recall from the modified mini-mental state test predicts Alzheimer's disease pathology. J Alzheimers Dis 2014;39(3):575–82.

76. Teng EL, Chui HC. The Modified Mini-Mental State (3MS) examination. J Clin Psychiatry 1987;48(8):314–8.

77. Tariq SH, Tumosa N, Chibnall JT, et al. Comparison of the Saint Louis University mental status examination and the mini-mental state examination for detecting dementia and mild neurocognitive disorder–a pilot study. Am J Geriatr Psychiatry 2006;14(11):900–10.

78. Kansagara D, Freeman M. A systematic evidence review of the signs and symptoms of dementia and brief cognitive tests available in VA. Washington, DC: Department of Veterans Affairs (US); 2010.

79. Manly JJ. Critical issues in cultural neuropsychology: profit from diversity. Neuropsychol Rev 2008;18(3):179–83.

80. Ardila A. The impact of culture on neuropsychological test performance. Int handbook cross-cultural Neuropsychol. Hove (United Kingdom): Psychology Press; 2007. p. 23–44.

81. Leany BD, Benuto LT, Thaler NS. Neuropsychological assessment with Hispanic clients. In: Benuto TL, editor. Guide to psychological assessment with Hispanics. Boston: Springer US; 2013. p. 351–76.

82. Ardila A, Rosselli M, Puente AE. Neuropsychological evaluation of the Spanish speaker. Germany: Springer Science & Business Media; 1994.

83. Benuto LT. Guide to psychological assessment with Hispanics. Germany: Springer Science & Business Media; 2012.

84. Pontón MO, León-Carrión José, editors. Neuropsychology and the Hispanic patient: a clinical handbook. Hove (United Kingdom): Psychology Press; 2001.

85. Pontón MO. Research and assessment issues with Hispanic populations. Neuropsychology and the Hispanic patient: a clinical handbook. Hove (United Kingdom): Psychology Press; 2001. p. 39–58.

86. Rosselli M, Ardila A. The impact of culture and education on non-verbal neuropsychological measurements: a critical review. Brain Cogn 2003;52(3):326–33.

87. Ostrosky-Solís F, Alfredo A, Monica R. NEUROPSI: a brief neuropsychological test battery in Spanish with norms by age and educational level. J Int Neuropsychol Soc 1999;5(5):413–33.

88. Paradis M. Differential use of cerebral mechanism in bilinguals. Hove (United Kingdom): Psychology Press; 2003.

89. Paradis M. Bilingualism and neuropsychiatric disorders. J Neurolinguistics 2008;21(3):199–230.

90. Rivera Mindt M, Arentoft A, Kubo Germano K, et al. Neuropsychological, cognitive, and theoretical considerations for evaluation of bilingual individuals. Neuropsychol Rev 2008;18(3):255–68.

91. Mitrushina M, Boone KB, Razani J, et al. Handbook of normative data for neuropsychological assessment. Oxford (United Kingdom): Oxford University Press; 2005.

92. Boone KB, Victor TL, Wen J, et al. The association between neuropsychological scores and ethnicity, language, and acculturation variables in a large patient population. Arch Clin Neuropsychol 2007;22(3):355–65.

93. Le Carret N, Lafont S, Mayo W, et al. The effect of education on cognitive performances and its implication for the constitution of the cognitive reserve. Dev Neuropsychol 2003;23(3):317–37.

94. Turner RM, Hinton L, Gallagher-Thompson D, et al. Using an Emic lens to understand how Latino families cope with dementia behavioral problems. Am J Alzheimers Dis Other Demen 2015;30(5):454–62.

95. Family Caregiver Alliance. Caregivers statistics demographics. 2015. Available at: https://www.caregiver.org/caregiver-statistics-demographics. Accesed August 15, 2016.

96. Covinsky KE, Newcomer R, Fox P, et al. Patient and caregiver characteristics associated with depression in caregivers of patients with dementia. J Gen Intern Med 2003;18(12):1006–14.

97. Luchsinger JA, Tipiani D, Torres-Patino G, et al. Characteristics and mental health of Hispanic dementia caregivers in New York city. Am J Alzheimers Dis Other Demen 2015;30(6):584–90.

98. Fillenbaum GG, Kuchibhatla M, Henderson VW, et al. Comparison of performance on the CERAD neuropsychological battery of Hispanic patients and cognitively normal controls at two sites. Clin Gerontologist 2007;30(3):1–22.

99. Fillenbaum GG, van Belle G, Morris JC, et al. Consortium to Establish a Registry for Alzheimer's Disease (CERAD): the first twenty years. Alzheimers Dement 2008;4(2):96–109.

100. Morris JC, Heyman A, Mohs RC, et al. The Consortium to Establish a Registry for Alzheimer's Disease (CERAD). Part I. Clinical and neuropsychological assessment of Alzheimer's disease. Neurology 1989;39(9):1159–65.

101. Mungas D, Reed BR, Crane PK, et al. Assessment Scales (SENAS): further development and psychometric characteristics. Psychol Assess 2004;16(4):347–59.

102. Woodcock R, Muñoz-Sandoval A, McGrew K, et al. Bateria III Woodcock-Munoz. Itasca (IL): Riverside Publishing Co; 2007.

103. Pontón MO, Satz P, Herrera L, et al. Normative data stratified by age and education for the Neuropsychological Screening Battery for Hispanics (NeSBHIS): Initial report. J Int Neuropsychol Soc 1996;2(02):96–104.

104. Flores Lazaro JC, Ostrosky-Solis F, Lozano Gutierrez A. Batería de funciones frontales y ejecutivas: presentación. Revista Neuropsicología, Neuropsiquiatría y Neurociencias 2008;8(1):141–58.

105. Flores Lazaro JC, Ostrosky-Solis F, Lozano Gutierrez A. BANFE: Bateria Neuropsicologica de Funciones Ejecutivas y Lobulos Frontales. Mexico, D.F.:: Manual Mod- erno.; 2012.

106. Krueger KR, Lam CS, Wilson RS. The Word Accentuation Test - Chicago. J Clin Exp Neuropsychol 2006;28(7):1201–7.
107. Cherner M, Suarez P, Lazzaretto D, et al. Demographically corrected norms for the Brief Visuospatial Memory Test-revised and Hopkins Verbal Learning Test-revised in monolingual Spanish speakers from the U.S.-Mexico border region. Arch Clin Neuropsychol 2007;22(3):343–53.
108. Gonzalez HM, Mungas D, Haan MN. A verbal learning and memory test for English- and Spanish-speaking older Mexican-American adults. Clin Neuropsychol 2002;16(4):439–51.
109. Meyers JE, Meyers KR. Rey Complex Figure Test and recognition trial professional manual. Odessa: Psychological Assessment Resources; 1995.
110. Raven J, Court J. Raven's progressive matrices and vocabulary scales. Oxford (United Kingdom): Oxford Psychologists Press; 1998.
111. Chelune RK, Meyers GJ, Talley JL, et al. Wisconsin card sort test manual: revised and expanded. Odessa (FL): Psychological Assessment Resources Inc; 1993.
112. D'Elia L, Satz P, Uchiyama C, et al. Color trails test. Odessa (FL): Psychological Assessment Resources; 1996.
113. Peña-Casanova J, Quinones-Ubeda S, Quintana-Aparicio M, et al. Spanish Multicenter Normative Studies (NEURONORMA Project): norms for verbal span, visuospatial span, letter and number sequencing, trail making test, and symbol digit modalities test. Arch Clin Neuropsychol 2009;24(4):321–41.
114. Marquez de la Plata C, Vicioso B, Hynan L, et al. Development of the Texas Spanish Naming Test: a test for Spanish speakers. Clin Neuropsychol 2008; 22(2):288–304.
115. Rosselli M, Tappen R, Williams C, et al. Level of education and category fluency task among Spanish speaking elders: number of words, clustering, and switching strategies. Neuropsychol Dev Cogn B Aging Neuropsychol Cogn 2009; 16(6):721–44.
116. Benton AL, Hamsher K, Varney NR. Judgment of line orientation. New York: Oxford University Press; 1983.
117. Golden CJ. Stroop color and word test: A manual for clinical and experimental uses. Chicago (IL): Stoelting Co; 1978.

The Role of Neuroimaging in the Assessment of the Cognitively Impaired Elderly

Sara Kollack-Walker, PhD[a],*, Collin Y. Liu, MD[b],
Adam S. Fleisher, MD, MAS[c]

KEYWORDS

- Brain imaging • MRI • CT • PET • SPECT • Dementia

KEY POINTS

- Dementia is defined as a progressive loss of cognition and several distinct causes have been identified.
- Different causes of dementia are associated with unique patterns of symptoms and abnormalities within the brain.
- Brain imaging can provide an essential window into the pathologic processes occurring in vivo within the brain of a patient experiencing cognitive complaints and potentially aid in the differential diagnosis of dementia.

INTRODUCTION

Elderly individuals often experience issues with memory. For many, such cognitive complaints reflect the normal process of aging and are characterized by relatively minor changes in brain structure and function. For some, cognitive complaints can reflect other issues, such as hypothyroidism or medication side effects, dictating the need to run additional tests to rule out these causes. However, for others, cognitive complaints may reflect an ongoing neurodegenerative process that can lead to an increasing trajectory of worsening in both cognition and daily function, as well as, perhaps difficulty with motoric abilities. Therefore, memory complaints may indicate a propensity for the future development of dementia.

According to the latest *Diagnostic and Statistical Manual of Mental Disorders, 5th Edition* criteria, dementia is classified as a major neurocognitive disorder interfering

Drs Kollack-Walker and Fleisher are employees of Eli Lilly and Company.
This study was funded by Eli Lilly and Company. This study was also supported by ADRC NIA P50-AG05142 in grant support.
[a] Scientific Comm, Global Med Comm – Bio-Medicines BU-NS, Eli Lilly and Company, Lilly Corporate Center, Indianapolis, IN 46285, USA; [b] Department of Neurology, Keck School of Medicine at the University of Southern California, 1520 San Pablo Street, HCC-2, Suite 3000, Los Angeles, CA 90033, USA; [c] Eli Lilly and Company, Lilly Corporate Center, Indianapolis, IN 46285, USA
* Corresponding author.
E-mail address: Kollack-Walker_Sara@lilly.com

Neurol Clin 35 (2017) 231–262
http://dx.doi.org/10.1016/j.ncl.2017.01.010
0733-8619/17/© 2017 Elsevier Inc. All rights reserved.

neurologic.theclinics.com

with both cognitive function and performance of everyday activities. Cognitive function refers to memory, speed, language, judgment reasoning, planning, and other thinking abilities.[1] Several distinct causes of dementia have been identified[2,3] (**Table 1**). Alzheimer disease (AD) is a degenerative brain disease and is the most common cause of dementia. Estimates of the frequency of dementias include AD, 60% to 80%; vascular dementia (VaD), 15% to 20%; dementia with Lewy bodies (DLB), 10% to 30%; and frontotemporal lobar degeneration (FTLD), other rarer causes, and occasionally reversible conditions (5%).[4,5] Of interest, several studies report that individuals with dementia can have brain abnormalities associated with more than a single cause of dementia, a condition termed mixed dementia, which is particularly common in the extreme elderly.[6–9] In most cases, AD is combined with VaD with rates ranging from 2% to 58%,[6] although a lower percentage of patients can also show evidence for combinations of AD with DLB, and AD with VaD and DLB. Different causes of dementia are associated with unique patterns of symptoms and abnormalities within the brain, and several of these causes are summarized in **Table 2**.[10,11]

AD is characterized by the abnormal accumulation of beta-amyloid (Aβ) neuritic plaques and neurofibrillary tangles (NFT) containing hyperphosphorylated tau identified in the brain on autopsy.[12] Several studies have shown that these changes begin in individuals 20 or more years before symptoms appear.[13–15] Mild cognitive impairment (MCI) is thought to serve as a potential precursor to AD and is defined as a loss of cognitive function that exceeds common age-associated changes but does not meet the diagnostic criteria for dementia (eg, everyday activities are preserved).[16] Although MCI is largely regarded as defining a population at-risk for AD, MCI can develop for reasons other than AD and not all patients diagnosed with MCI will go on to develop dementia. More recently, significant interest has been focused on understanding the earliest preclinical or prodromal phase of AD.[17,18] The revised criteria and guidelines for AD diagnosis[19–22] identify 2 stages: (1) MCI due to AD and (2) dementia due to AD. In addition, for research purposes, the guidelines also propose a preclinical phase of AD that occurs before symptoms develop, such as memory loss, during which biomarkers of amyloid deposition and/or neurodegeneration can be identified.

The differential diagnosis of dementia is predominantly based on clinical criteria and neuropsychological testing. The evaluation of a patient with cognitive complaints typically involves several steps: (1) obtaining a detailed medical history, (2) running blood tests to rule out other causes of cognitive impairment, (3) performing neuropsychological tests to assess deficits in cognition and functioning, and (4) structural brain imaging. However, a number of clinicians describe patients who have overlapping symptoms that complicate a clear diagnosis of dementia based on clinical criteria alone.[23,24] Moreover, several reviews of published studies report a relatively low sensitivity and specificity of neuropsychological evaluations for identifying pathologically confirmed AD dementia.[25,26] In the more recent study, Beach and colleagues reviewed 23 studies regarding current clinical AD diagnostic methods and reported sensitivity estimates ranging between 41-100% (median of 87%) and specificity estimates ranging between 37-100% (median of 58%).[26] In addition, using clinical and neuropathological data from the National Alzheimer's Coordinating Center (2005-2010), these authors reported sensitivity estimates ranging from 70.9-87.3% and specificity estimates ranging from 44.3-70.8% for clinical diagnosis of "probable" or "possible" AD in identifying AD histopathology across 4 levels of neuropathological criteria.[26] Thus, in this latter study, up to 30% of patients who were thought to have AD did not show evidence of postmortem histopathology consistent with AD, while at least 40% of patients diagnosed with non-AD dementia did show characteristic

Table 1
Potential causes of dementia

Neurodegenerative[a]	Vascular[b]	Toxic/Metabolic[c]	Infectious[d]	Autoimmune/ Inflammatory[e]	Structural[f]	Other[g]
Alzheimer's disease (AD)	Multi-infarct (large, small)	Medication-induced	Neurosyphilis	Multiple sclerosis	Brain tumor	Traumatic brain injury (TBI)
Frontotemporal lobar degeneration (FTLD)	Single strategic infarct	Vitamin deficiency (B12, folate)	HIV-related	Behcet's disease	Normal-pressure hydrocephalus	Pseudodementia from depression
Parkinson's disease (PD)	Lacunar state	Thyroid/adrenal disease	Creutzfeldt-Jakob disease (CJD)	Lupus		Hippocampal sclerosis
Dementia with Lewy bodies (DLB)	Binswanger's disease	Alcohol-related	Chronic meningitis	Sarcoidosis		Mitochondrial encephalopathies
Huntington's disease (HD)	CADASIL	Altered levels electrolytes	Viral encephalitis			Other extrapyramidal disorders
	Cerebral amyloid angiopathology	Organ failure (liver, kidney)	Postencephalitic			Vascular-Other
		Heavy metal toxicity	Lyme's disease			Epileptiform

[a] Three major clinical syndromes observed for FTLD: (1) behavioral variant FTLD (bvFTLD), (2) primary progressive aphasia (PPA) – 3 variants: (i) progressive nonfluent/agrammatic variant (agPPA). (ii) logopenic variant (lvPPA),and (iii) semantic variant (svPPA), (3) disturbances motor function – (i) amyotrophic lateral sclerosis (ALS, also known as Lou Gehrig's disease), (ii) corticobasal syndrome (CBS), and (iii) progressive supranuclear palsy (PSP).

[b] Vascular dementia: multiple large/small vessel infarcts, single strategic infarct, Lacunar state, Binswanger's disease, CADASIL (Cerebral autosomal dominant arteriopathy with subcortical infarcts and leukoencephalolpathy). Cerebral amyloid angiopathology (Congophilic angiopathy).

[c] Toxic/Metabolic: Medication-induced dementia, Vitamin deficiency (B12, folate), Thyroid disease, Adrenal disease-Cushing's disease, Addison's disease, Alcohol-related, Hypo- or hypermagnesemia, Hypo- or hypercalcemia, Renal failure, Liver failure, Porphyria, Domoic acid poisoning.

[d] Infectious: Prion diseases-Creutzfeldt-Jakob Disease, Gerstmann-Straussler-Scheinker Disease, Kuru, New variant Creutzfeldt-Jakob Disease, Neurosyphilis, AIDS dementia (HIV-related), Chronic meningitis-Fungal, Tuberculosis, Lyme disease, Viral encephalitis, Whipple's disease.

[e] Autoimmune/Inflammatory disorders: Multiple sclerosis, Behcet's disease, Lupus erythematosus, Sarcoidosis, Temporal arteritis and other nervous system vasculitides.

[f] Structural: Brain tumors, Normal-pressure hydrocephalus.

[g] Other: Traumatic brain injury (TBI)-dementia related to closed-head injury-Chronic Traumatic Encephalopathy (CTE, also known as Dementia pugilistica), Chronic subdural hematoma, Hippocampal sclerosis, Mitochondrial encephalopathies, Other extrapyramidal disorders-Wilson's disease, Hallervorden-Spatz disease. Vascular-Chronic subdural hematoma (spontaneous, iatrogenic), Postsubarachnoid hemorrhage, Epileptiform-Partial complex status epilepticus, Absence status.

Table 2
Characteristics of AD and other major dementias

Dementia	Characteristic Features
Alzheimer's Disease (AD)	Early symptoms: difficulty remembering recent conversations, names or events, and possibly apathy and depression. Later symptoms: impaired communication, disorientation, confusion, poor judgment, behavioral changes, difficulty speaking, swallowing and walking. Neuropathology: accumulation of β-amyloid peptide as plaques outside of neurons and tau neurofibrillary tangles inside of neurons.
Vascular Dementia (VD)	Early symptoms: impaired judgment or impaired ability to make decisions, plan or organize; can have changes in cognition, and difficulty with motor function, such as slow gait and poor balance. Neuropathology: blood vessel blockage or damage leading to infarcts (strokes) or bleeding in the brain; the location, number and size of the injuries determines the clinical symptoms experienced.
Dementia with Lewy bodies (DLB)	Early symptoms: sleep disturbances, well-formed visual hallucinations and slowness, gait imbalances or other parkinsonian movement features. Neuropathology: accumulation of Lewy bodies as abnormal aggregations of the protein α-synuclein. Some symptoms also common in AD, confounding diagnosis (though may reflect multiple pathologies, mixed dementia). Cognitive impairment distinguishes DLB from Parkinson's disease.
Mixed Dementia	Evidence for presence of multiple pathologies underlying observed dementia: AD combined with VD (most common), AD combined with DLB, AD combined with VD and DLB.

Frontotemporal Lobar Degeneration (FTLD) (Inclusive of several dementias, previously referred to as Pick's disease)	Early symptoms: marked changes in personality and behavior, and/or difficulty producing or comprehending language, memory typically spared early in disease.
	Neuropathology: accumulation of either tau protein, transactive response DNA-binding protein inclusions (TDP-43), or fused in sarcoma (FUS) protein.
	There are 3 major subtypes; 2 are further subdivided into specific variants or disorders:
	1. Behavior variant frontotemporal dementia (bvFTD): characterized by prominent changes in personality, interpersonal relationships and conduct.
	2. Primary progressive aphasia (PPA): affects language skills, speaking, writing and comprehension; there are 3 variants:
	   i. *Progressive nonfluent/agrammatic variant* (agPPA) – individual's speaking is hesitant, labored or ungrammatical
	   ii. *Logopenic variant* (lvPPA) – individual presents deficits in word-search and phonological working memory (difficulty repeating complex sentences)
	   iii. *Semantic variant* (svPPA) – individual loses ability to understand or formulate words in a spoken sentence.
	3. Disturbances of motor function:
	   i. *Amyotrophic Lateral Sclerosis* (ALS) – a motor neuron disease that causes muscle weakness or wasting; also known as Lou Gehrig's disease
	   ii. *Corticobasal Degeneration* (CBD) – causes arms and legs to become uncoordinated or stiff
	   iii. *Progressive Supranuclear Palsy* (PSP) – causes muscle stiffness, difficulty walking and changes in posture, also affects eye movements.

(continued on next page)

Table 2
(continued)

Dementia	Characteristic Features
Parkinson's Disease (PD) Dementia (PDD)	Symptoms: problems with movement – slowness, rigidity, tremor, changes in gait. Neuropathology: α-synuclein protein aggregates within in the substantia nigra, leading to degeneration of nerve cells that produce dopamine. As PD progresses, it can result in dementia that is secondary to either the accumulation of Lewy bodies in cortex (similar to DLB) or accumulation of β-amyloid clumps and tau fibrillary tangles (similar to AD).
Creutzfeldt-Jakob disease (CJD)	Symptoms: rapidly fatal disorder with impaired memory, coordination problems and behavioral changes. Neuropathology: presence of misfolded protein (prion) that causes other proteins within the brain to misfold and malfunction. May be hereditary, sporadic (unknown etiology), or caused by a known prion infection; a specific form called variant Creutzfeldt-Jakob disease is thought to be caused by mad cow disease.
Normal Pressure Hydrocephalus	Symptoms: difficulty walking, memory loss and inability to control urination. Neuropathology: impaired reabsorption of cerebrospinal fluid and consequent build-up of fluid in the brain, increasing intracranial pressure.

From Alzheimer's Association. 2016 Alzheimer's disease facts and figures. Alzheimers Dement 2016;12:459–509; Gorno-Tempini ML, Hillis AE, Weintraub S, et al. Classification of primary progressive aphasia and its variants. Neurology 2011;76:1006–14.

AD histopathological findings.[26] Brain imaging can provide an essential window into the pathological processes occurring *in vivo* within the brain of a patient experiencing cognitive complaints, and potentially aide in the differential diagnosis of dementia. There is some evidence to suggest that brain imaging may be superior to neuropsychological testing for early and reliable diagnosis of AD.[27,28]

BIOMARKERS

A biomarker is a biological feature used to measure a biological state, such as the presence or progression of a disease or the possible effects of treatment. Biomarkers associated with dementias have been identified and can be categorized into 2 main categories: (1) chemical analytes measured within the cerebrospinal fluid (CSF) and (2) brain imaging (**Table 3**). In patients with AD, several biomarkers have been identified.[29,30] Within the CSF, these biomarkers include a decrease in CSF $A\beta_{1-42}$ and $A\beta_{1-40}$ peptides, and an increase in tau protein, specifically as total tau and phosphorylated tau. $A\beta_{1-42}$ is the predominant form of Aβ found in amyloid plaques, whereas $A\beta_{1-40}$ is much less abundant. Within the brain, these biomarkers include brain atrophy, ventricular enlargement, white matter hyperintensities (WMHs), lobar microhemorrhages, glucose hypometabolism, reduction in cerebral blood flow and oxygenation, and the abnormal accumulation of proteins or protein fragments (ie, Aβ or tau) (see **Table 3**).

Some of these biomarkers reflect the general process of neurodegeneration, such as brain atrophy or glucose hypometabolism observed across many

Table 3
Biomarkers of Alzheimer disease and other dementias

	AD	Other Dementias
CSF	**Imaging**	**Imaging**
• ↓ CSF Aβ$_{1-42}$[a] • ↓ CSF Aβ$_{1-40}$ • ↑ CSF total tau (t-tau)[b] • ↑ CSF phosphorylated tau (p-tau)[b]	Structural: • Brain atrophy • Ventricular enlargement • WMHs • Lobar microhemorrhages Functional: • Glucose hypometabolism • Reduction in cerebral blood flow and oxygenation	Changes observed in these biomarkers in other degenerative dementias, but in patterns specific to each disease or dementia

	Molecular:
	• Abnormal accumulation of proteins:
	  ○ Aβ
	  ○ Tau (experimental)
		Abnormal accumulation of other proteins (experimental):
		• Tau, TDP-43, FUS (FTLD)
		• α-synuclein (Lewy bodies, DLB)
		• Prions (CJD)

Abbreviations: CJD, Creutzfeldt-Jakob disease; FUS, fused in sarcoma; TDP-43, transactive response-DNA-binding protein of 43 kDa.
[a] Aβ$_{1-42}$ is the predominant form of Aβ found in amyloid plaque, whereas Aβ$_{1-40}$ is a much less abundant in amyloid plaque.
[b] CSF t-tau and p-tau are increased in patients with AD. However, CSF concentrations of t-tau or p-tau are not elevated in patients with other tauopathies, including FTLD.

degenerative dementias, although in a pattern that varies according to the symptoms observed and specific to the dementia diagnosed. Other biomarkers seem to be more specific to a certain disease and can involve abnormal accumulations of specific proteins described as proteinopathies or differential expression of a single protein, such as the tau protein described as tauopathies.[31] Therefore, in AD are found the abnormal accumulation of Aβ and tau proteins; in FTLD, the accumulation of 3 different proteins (tau, transactive response-DNA-binding protein of 43 kDa [TDP-43], or fused in sarcoma [FUS] protein); in DLB, the accumulation of α-synuclein (Lewy bodies); and in Creutzfeldt-Jakob disease, the accumulation of prions. Although these proteinopathies are characteristic features of specific degenerative dementias, there is evidence for shared proteinopathies with some individuals demonstrating evidence for both AD and DLB or AD and FTLD, at autopsy. Diagnostic imaging tools are available to assess the structural, functional, and molecular imaging of the brain, focusing on many of these biomarkers relevant to AD and other dementias.

STRUCTURAL IMAGING
Structural Imaging in the Assessment of Cognitive Impairment

Many types of neurologic insult can have cognitive consequence. This article focuses on neurodegeneration (primary and secondary). As with many other neurologic symptoms, cognitive decline is evaluated early with structural neuroimaging (MRI and computed tomography [CT]). With the ever-increasing versatility and resolution of MRI, the role of CT in dementia has become secondary. CT is now typically used as a substitute when MRI is contraindicated (eg, the presence of metal in the body or claustrophobia). MRI is often part of the initial evaluation because it can provide a detailed definition of neuroanatomy that can be helpful for guiding diagnosis.

The most common cause of cognitive decline in the elderly (65 years and older) is neurodegeneration. The primary evidence of neurodegeneration on structural imaging is cerebral atrophy, which can be difficult to interpret visually in the clinical setting. Most clinicians are more familiar with imaging findings of secondary causes of cognitive decline, such as stroke, tumor, and demyelinating disease. Therefore, the primary role for structural imaging is to rule out these causes. However, with improvement in the image resolution, MRI evidence for neurodegeneration has been shown to be reliable for clinical interpretation.[32] This section presents a systematic approach using MRI to help determine the cause of cognitive decline in the elderly. Because AD is by far the most common neurodegenerative cause of cognitive decline, most validated MRI biomarkers are for AD. Less validated MRI biomarkers for non-AD dementias are also presented.

MRI uses strong magnetic fields, radio waves, and field gradients to generate images. Adjustment of these and other related parameters can produce images focused on different tissues with varying water or fat content. Clinically useful MRI sequences include T1-weighted (T1W), T2-weighted fluid-attenuated inversion recovery (T2-FLAIR), diffusion-weighted imaging (DWI), and gradient-recalled echo (GRE). Each of these sequences defines specific tissue characteristics. Together they provide evidence of atrophy and ventriculomegaly (T1W) and vascular injury (T2-FLAIR, T2 fast spin echo, DWI, GRE, and susceptibility weighted [SWI]), which is helpful for making a diagnosis.

Cerebral atrophy

Evaluation begins with the assessment of global cerebral volume in comparison with ventricular size. Although nonspecific, global cerebral atrophy with corresponding sulcal widening is predictive of further cognitive decline. Focal atrophy corresponds to the distribution of the underlying pathologic condition. In AD, atrophy follows the distribution of tauopathy in the form of NFT deposits (**Fig. 1**).[33,34] In particular, medial temporal atrophy (MTA) correlates well with cognitive decline and NFT accumulation. Studies have shown that the scale for MTA (Scheltens scale), measured on coronal T1W images, has approximately 80% to 85% sensitivity and specificity, respectively, for AD.[35] MTA also has approximately 73% sensitivity and approximately 81% specificity for predicting whether patients with amnestic MCI will convert to dementia.[35,36] Although not diagnostic by itself, in combination with positive CSF biomarkers (low amyloid-β and high tau), MTA has 94% positive predictive value for the conversion from MCI to AD.[37]

In clinical practice, the Scheltens scale can be useful in communicating the severity of MTA and providing the basis for calling pathologic MTA (adapted from A. Micheau, MD, Imaios, and Radiology Assistant, http://www.radiologyassistant.nl/en/p43dbf6d16f98d/dementia-role-of-mri.html). It is a 5-point scale, based on measurements of the choroid fissure, the temporal horn of lateral ventricle, and the hippocampal formation on coronal view (**Fig. 2A**). It is scored from 0 to 4, with higher numbers indicating worse atrophy. At stage 1, there is slight widening of the choroid fissure, at stage 2 there is also widening of temporal horn and decrease in the height of hippocampus, and at stages 3 and 4 the temporal horn appears larger than the hippocampus (see **Fig. 2**). The scoring is age-dependent, with pathologic atrophy defined as greater than or equal to 2 out of 4 in ages 75 years and younger and greater than or equal to 3 out of 4 in ages 75 years and older.

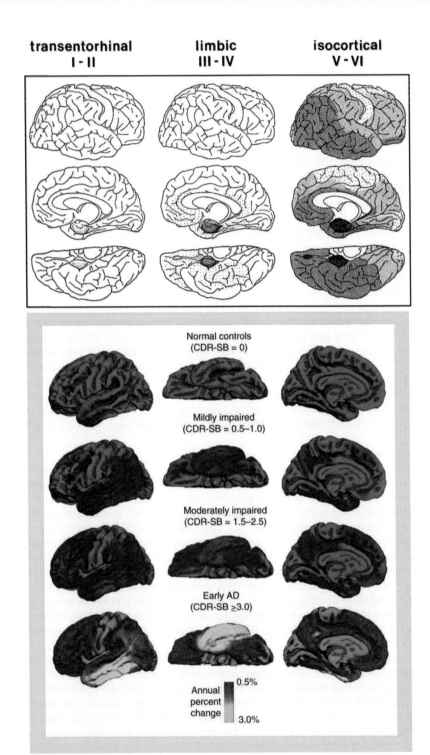

Fig. 1. Cortical atrophy corresponds to NFT deposition. Shown is the annual atrophy rates as a function of degree of clinical impairment as assessed with baseline Clinical Dementia Rating - Sum of Boxes (CDR-SB) score. (*Data from* Braak H, Braak E. Neuropathological staging of Alzheimer-related changes. Acta Neuropathol 1991;82(4):239–59; McEvoy LK, Brewer JB. Quantitative structural MRI for early detection of Alzheimer's disease. Expert Rev Neurother 2010;10(11):1675–88.)

A

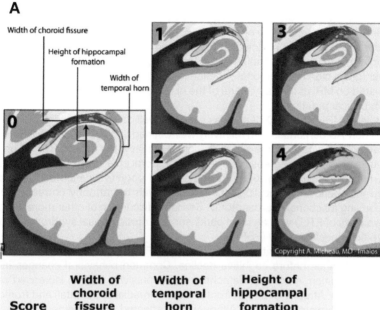

Score	Width of choroid fissure	Width of temporal horn	Height of hippocampal formation
0	N	N	N
1	↑	N	N
2	↑↑	↑↑	↓
3	↑↑↑	↑↑↑	↓↓
4	↑↑↑	↑↑↑	↓↓↓

B

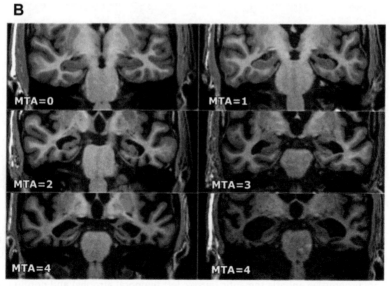

Fig. 2. Evaluation of MTA using Scheltens scale. (*A*) Visual assessment. (*B*) MRI of MTA (T1W coronal view). (*Adapted from* A. Micheau, MD, Imaios, and Radiology Assistant. Available at: http://www.radiologyassistant.nl/en/p43dbf6d16f98d/dementia-role-of-mri.html.)

Other than MTA, prominent posterior atrophy is prevalent, particularly among younger AD patients and more often in *APOE ε4* noncarriers. Atrophy of either the parietal lobe or the precuneus (including the posterior cingulate) may be the only finding in young-onset AD, and the finding of a normal hippocampus does not rule out AD.[32] However, given high interpersonal variation in gyral folding, lobar atrophy is often not appreciated on MRI at the early stage of the disease and, therefore, its evaluation less useful in clinical practice.

The role of MRI in non-AD dementias is not as well defined or validated. FTLD is a group of non-AD dementias with relatively well-defined findings on MRI. FTLD is characterized pathologically by the accumulation of primarily tau and/or TDP-43 proteins and involves in varying degrees the frontal or temporal pole, prefrontal cortex, insular cortex, and operculum (**Fig. 3**).[38] The patterns of cognitive deficit can be broadly grouped into behavioral and linguistic variants, with the atrophy corresponding to the underlying functional neuroanatomy. See later discussion of other more heterogeneous variants of FTLD with atypical parkinsonism, cortical basal syndrome, and progressive supranuclear palsy (PSP).

Behavioral variant (bv) frontotemporal dementia (FTD) is heralded by personality and behavioral changes before cognitive decline. Common behavioral changes include apathy, disinhibition, emotional detachment, compulsivity, and an increased preference for sweets. Atrophy of the prefrontal regions (medial and orbital) and frontotemporal poles is typically bilateral. Although the affected area affected corresponds functionally to behavioral changes, it is often difficult to appreciate this on MRI in the early stage of the disease. Metabolic scans (fluorodeoxyglucose [FDG] PET) have higher sensitivity and specificity for the diagnosis of the FTLDs.

Linguistic variants of FTLD, or primary progressive aphasias, have early changes in language functions, with proteinopathy (tau or TDP-43) in the left frontal and temporal

A Behavior Variant FTD   **B** Semantic Aphasia   Nonfluent Aphasia

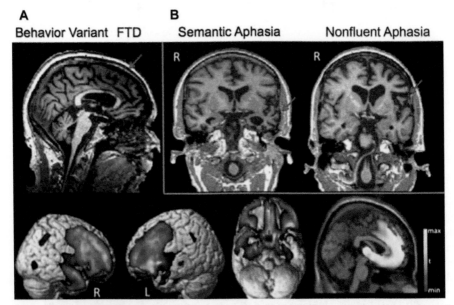

Fig. 3. FTLD: (*A*) behavioral variant frontotemporal dementia (*arrow*: frontal atrophy) and (*B*) primary progressive aphasia semantic (*arrow*: left temporal atrophy) and nonfluent (*arrow*: left frontal opercular atrophy) variants. (*From* Tartaglia MC, Rosen HJ, Miller BL. Neuroimaging in dementia. Neurotherapeutics. 2011;8(1):82–92; with permission.)

operculum and left temporal pole. Subtypes (nonfluent, semantic, and logopenic) have been characterized based on the language deficits. In nonfluent aphasia, impairment in speech production and grammar with telegraphic pattern of speech corresponds to atrophy in the left perisylvian regions, particularly the inferior frontal and insular cortices. In contrast, semantic aphasia is a fluent aphasia with loss of word meaning and conceptual knowledge, with atrophy in the left temporal lobe (see **Fig. 3**B). A rare variant with right temporal lobe atrophy can have prosopagnosia (deficit in face recognition) as the presenting symptom. The third subtype, logopenic aphasia, is most commonly associated with AD, with presenting deficits in word-search and phonological working memory (difficulty repeating complex sentences) and atrophy in the posterior temporal and inferior parietal cortices. In group comparisons, atrophy in these subtypes can be differentiated on MRI but FDG-PET has higher positive predictive value.[39]

With increasing availability of high-resolution MRI, assessment of global and hippocampal volumes with automated software has become reality in the clinical setting. However, its value over qualitative visual assessment is controversial and requires further validation.

Vascular injury

One of the most productive uses of structural neuroimaging is in defining vascular injury. MRI is able to visualize ischemic and hemorrhagic strokes as fast as clinician's can get the patients into the scanners. It provides information about perfusion and diffusion status related to ischemic lesions, hemosiderin deposition, and its evolution in hemorrhage. Although CT is not as versatile, it has remained the first-line imaging tool for stroke for its rapid acquisition and accuracy in assessing perfusion and vessel stenosis or occlusion for intervention. The ability to demonstrate acute changes on MRI and CT allows correlation of the location of the lesions with acute cognitive changes, such as the inferior frontal region with expressive aphasia. Furthermore, vascular injury can be asymptomatic and have a cumulative effect on cognition. This type of silent injury has also been characterized with MRI and CT, corresponding to pathologic states in the small vessels, such as arteriolosclerotic (hyaline and/or hyperplastic changes) vessel occlusion and wall rupture. Such vascular injury can trigger neurodegeneration and ultimately lead to VaD, typically with frontal subcortical deficits (eg, executive dysfunction, poor motivation, psychomotor slowing). This section is focused on imaging findings of small vessel disease associated with VaD, namely microinfarction and microhemorrhage.

Microinfarctions are best seen on T2-FLAIR and T2W MRI as WMHs and lacunes (**Fig. 4**A).[40–42] WMH (also known as leukoaraiosis) is considered chronic partial infarction from damages to small vessels. It is radiologically described as mild, moderate, and severe, with scattered, clustered, and confluent appearances, respectively. Scales (eg, Fazekas and Longstreth) are widely used in publication but not generally used in clinical practice. It is most commonly associated with psychomotor slowing, executive dysfunction, and memory retrieval deficits. Cognitive decline typically occurs at a threshold of approximately 25% white matter involvement. WMH is also a known risk factor for neurodegeneration and atrophy. Arteriopathy with striking WMH on MRI is traditionally known as Binswanger disease. An inherited form (NOTCH-3 gene mutation), known as cerebral autosomal dominant arteriopathy with subcortical infarcts and leukoencephalopathy (CADASIL), has characteristic U-fiber involvement in the temporal poles and the vertex (see **Fig. 4**A). In other small vessel arteriopathies (eg, Susac disease and systemic lupus erythematosus), MRI findings might be nonspecific but, with clinical correlation, they can be used to guide treatment.

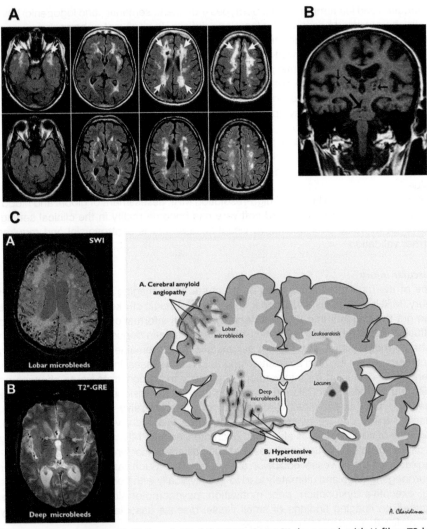

Fig. 4. SVD associated with VaD and AD. (*A*) WMH: CADASIL (*top row*) with U-fiber T2 hyperintensity in temporal poles and vertex (*white arrows*) and Binswanger disease (*bottom row*). (*B*) Lacunar infarcts in pons (*large arrow*), internal or external capsules, and bilateral thalami (*small arrows*). (*C*) Microhemorrhages from cerebral amyloid angiopathy in a lobar distribution (*a*) and from hypertension involving basal ganglia (*b*) (*arrows* highlight location of several microhemorrhages). SVD, small vessel disease. (*Data from* [*A*] and [*B*] Bastos Leite AJ, van der Flier WM, van Straaten EC. Infratentorial abnormalities in vascular dementia. Stroke 2006;37(1):105–10. and [*C*] *From* Charidimou A, Shakeshaft C, Werring DJ. Cerebral microbleeds on magnetic resonance imaging and anticoagulant-associated intracerebral hemorrhage risk. Front Neurol 2012;3:133.)

Lacunar infarcts result from occlusion of small perforating vessels in white matter and subcortical nuclei (see **Fig. 4**B). As with territorial stroke, DWI sequence has high sensitivity and specificity for acute lacunar infarcts. Chronic lesions are well visualized on T2-FLAIR and T2W images. Although they are typically not as extensive as WMH, lacunes in strategic locations can cause significant neurologic and cognitive symptoms. A syndrome with acute onset of dysarthria and hand incoordination (dysarthria-clumsy hand syndrome) was found to have significant association with lacunes in the internal capsule, pons, and corona radiate.[43] Lacunes in the thalamus and the posterior limb of the internal capsule can significantly affect information processing speed and executive function, respectively.[44] Accumulation of lacunar infarcts is associated with deficits in executive function, verbal fluency, and verbal memory.[45]

Like microinfarction, microhemorrhage can be asymptomatic at its onset and have a cumulative effect on cognition. Microhemorrhages are best visualized on GRE and SWI sequences as hypointensities (see **Fig. 4**C).[42] MRI evidence of microhemorrhages is associated with cognitive decline, independent of WMH or atrophy. Microhemorrhages can be categorized into hypertensive and amyloid types. Chronic hypertension is associated with hyaline and hyperplastic changes in the wall of small vessels, ensued by rupture. This type of microhemorrhage has a more central location, frequently involving the basal ganglia and other deep structures compared with the amyloid type (see **Fig. 4**C). Vessel wall weakening and rupture also occurs with intramural amyloid deposition, possibly associated with poor clearance of amyloid protein in AD. Excluding the rare hereditary types, cerebral amyloid angiopathy (CAA) is a disease of aging. The prevalence of CAA increases from about 2% at age 50 years to 74% by 90 years. One out of 5 AD patients has at least 1 microhemorrhage on MRI at the time of diagnosis. Different from hypertensive microhemorrhage, CAA commonly has a peripheral or lobar distribution, nearing the gray-white junction (see **Fig. 4**C). The finding of 3 more microhemorrhages in a lobar distribution is suggestive of the presence of CAA. The diagnosis of CAA in the elderly is suggestive of the simultaneous deposition of amyloid in the parenchyma and, therefore, AD.

Both microinfarcts and microhemorrhages of VaD are now known to increase the risk of AD, especially in the late onset form. *APOE ε4* positivity, a major genetic risk for late-onset AD, is associated with microinfarcts in the white matter. Without significant MTA, the presence of severe WMH is associated with an odds ratio of 1.6 for developing AD. It is estimated that 60% to 90% of AD patients have significant pathologic VaD. By clinical criteria, the overlapping disease, or mixed dementia, is probably underdiagnosed, with 1 mixed dementia for every 4 AD dementias.[46] New MRI techniques are being developed to detect earlier vascular pathologic states, such as decline in perfusion, blood-brain barrier breakdown, and arterial stiffening.

Degeneration of subcortical nuclei

Non-AD dementias with early degeneration of subcortical nuclei and structures (eg, substantia nigra, ventral tegmental area, and midbrain) typically present with symptoms in motor function as well as cognition. This group often presents with a normal-appearing MRI, at least in the early symptomatic stages. Some of the characteristic MRI findings in DLB, corticobasal degeneration (CBD), and PSP are presented.

The most common dementia in this group is DLB (intraneuronal proteinaceous inclusions containing alpha-synuclein and ubiquitin). Deposition of Lewy bodies in the limbic system and substantia nigra correlates with symptoms. A typical patient presents with some features of parkinsonism (eg, bilateral bradykinesia and shuffling gait), hallucinations (visual more than auditory), and fluctuating attention and alertness. Nonspecific mild global atrophy is common in early stages, with some predominance in the occipital lobe. Molecular (dopaminergic PET) and metabolic (FDG-PET) imaging can be performed in some cases to help identify the presence of pathologic Lewy bodies.

CBD is a tauopathy with asymmetrical deposition in the posterior frontal and parietal regions. Clinical features include impairment in executive function, language, and higher motor function (apraxia), often difficult to differentiate from other subtypes of FTLD at symptom onset. There is usually no specific MRI correlate. Asymmetrical frontoparietal atrophy may be present as the disease progresses but is not specific to CBD.

In PSP, the pathological tau deposits are found in subcortical and brainstem nuclei and the cerebellar dentate nucleus. Characteristic MRI findings include midbrain atrophy, divergence of the red nuclei, dilatation of the third ventricle, atrophy of the superior cerebellar peduncle, and frontal cortical atrophy. Atrophic changes in the midbrain have been called the Mickey Mouse sign on the axial view (**Fig. 5**A) and the hummingbird sign on the midsagittal view (**Fig. 5**B).[32]

Ventriculomegaly

Along with atrophy, ventriculomegaly is commonly seen on MRI and CT in the elderly. Ventriculomegaly can be seen as a result of atrophy (ex vacuo ventriculomegaly) but can also be an indication of chronic hydrocephalus, which is associated with the triad of gait disturbance, cognitive decline, and urinary incontinence. This syndrome is called normal pressure hydrocephalus (NPH), to be differentiated from other types with elevated intracranial pressure (ICP). It is caused by gradual reduction of CSF absorption at the arachnoid granulation, with measurable transient elevation of ICP in the initial stages. It is thought that alternative routes of CSF absorption through ependymal and perivascular space help keep ICP in the normal range. Though it can be associated with leptomeningeal fibrosis in the setting of subarachnoid hemorrhage, meningitis, or traumatic brain injury, idiopathic NPH is common.

In patients with a clinical history suggestive of NPH, the role of structural imaging is to demonstrate ventriculomegaly disproportional to cerebral atrophy (**Fig. 6**A).[47] Visual findings include bowing and thinning of the corpus callosum, and dilatation of the temporal horns, in the absence of sulcal widening. Measurement of frontal horn in coronal and axial views has been used to quantify the severity (see **Fig. 6**B, callosal

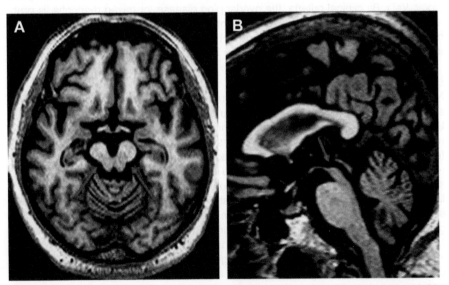

Fig. 5. Midbrain atrophy in PSP: thinning of midbrain on axial view. (*A*) Mickey Mouse sign (*red arrows*) and (*B*) sagittal view of hummingbird sign (*red arrow*). (*Data from* Barkhof F, Fox NC, Bastos-Leite AJ, et al. Neuroimaging in dementia. New York: Springer, 2011.)

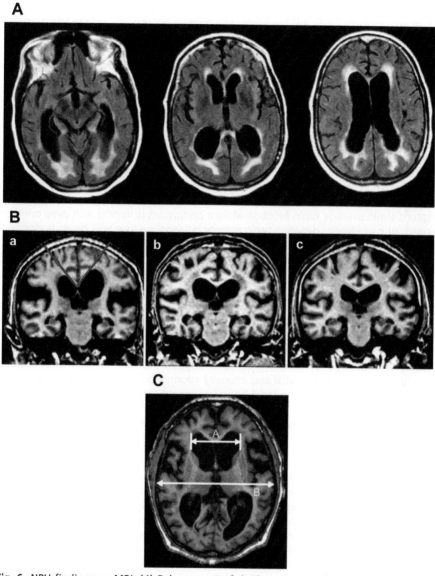

Fig. 6. NPH findings on MRI. (*A*) Enlargement of the lateral ventricles with minimal sulcal widening, and periventricular transependymal flow (T2-FLAIR) (http://casemed.case.edu/clerkships/neurology/Web%20Neurorad/nph01.htm). (*B*) Narrowing of callosal angle (CA) on T1W coronal view (at the posterior commissure perpendicular to the anteroposterior commissure plane). (*a*) CA of 69° in NPH (*red*), (*b*) CA of 102° in AD (not indicated), and (*c*) CA of 112° normal control (*green*). (*C*) Ratio of maximal frontal horns (*double arrow,* A) over maximal width of the inner skull (*double arrow,* B) greater than 0.3 indicates ventriculomegaly (Evans index). (*Adapted from* Ishii K, Kanda T, Harada A, et al. Clinical impact of the callosal angle in the diagnosis of idiopathic normal pressure hydrocephalus. Eur Radiol 2008;18(11):2678–83; with permission.)

angle; and **Fig. 6**C, Evans ratio). It is uncertain if these measurements add to overall visual assessment. T2-FLAIR hyperintensity homogeneously around the lateral ventricles indicating transependymal flow can be seen (see **Fig. 6**A). Recent application of dynamic MRI sequences (eg, phase-contrast and arterial spin labeling) to NPH might someday provide a more accurate diagnosis and better understanding of the pathophysiology.

FUNCTIONAL IMAGING

Functional imaging focuses on an underlying physiologic process and includes brain imaging by PET, and single-photon emission CT (SPECT). These brain imaging scanners use tracers to identify functional biomarkers or molecules of interest within the brain. Common physiologic targets of functional imaging include glucose metabolism, blood perfusion, oxygen use, or the loss of specific neurons. Functional imaging can capture static average brain function while a participant is resting with eyes open or closed, or can identify dynamic brain activity in response to a task being performed during image acquisition (ie, cognitive tasks associated with memory or language, or sensory or motor activities).

PET

PET imaging facilitates the detection of subtle changes in brain physiology. PET uses positron emitters to label target physiologic or pathologic brain processes. Positrons are positively charged unstable particles that interact with electrons while traveling through brain tissue. This interaction produces photons. These coincident tissue interactions are detected by sensitive detector rings in the PET scanner that make it possible to identify both spatial and intensity information. Various types of positron-emitting nuclei can be used to label tracers to identify physiologic targets of interest in vivo. The most common are ^{15}O, ^{11}C, and ^{18}F, with ^{18}F being the most widely used in clinical practice, mostly because its longer half-life makes it a more practical molecular isotope.

Fluorodeoxyglucose PET

Neurons use glucose as their primary energy source and, therefore, tracking glucose utilization within the brain provides a method to detect the general level of neuronal activity. PET imaging with a glucose analog, ^{18}F FDG, has been used to identify subtle changes in metabolic glucose utilization in the brain. After intravenous injection, FDG is phosphorylated and incorporated into cells. The amount of regional FDG uptake then provides a spatial and intensity representation of cerebral metabolic rate for glucose (CMRgl). In the resting state, FDG uptake is driven mostly by basal neuronal activity. In general, basal state FDG-PET imaging represents underlying neuronal integrity, with decreased function leading to regional reduction in glucose turnover.

In AD, patients show a characteristic pattern of glucose hypometabolism consisting of a reduced FDG-PET signal in temporal-parietal, posterior cingulate, and frontal cortices.[48] These brain regions are well known to be associated with cognitive function, such as memory and spatial orientation, and the pattern observed is consistent with the known pattern of AD.[49] In patients with postmortem evidence of AD, Minoshima and colleagues[50] reported the presence of hypometabolic changes within the temporal-parietal, posterior cingulate, and frontal cortices in prior FDG-PET scans. Hoffman and colleagues[51] reported that temporal-parietal hypometabolism was the typical abnormality observed in patients with pathologically verified AD. The decline in glucose utilization as evidenced by FDG-PET imaging in patients with AD has been shown to be progressive, to correlate with dementia severity, and to predict an AD diagnosis at autopsy.[52–55]

In MCI, glucose hypometabolism occurs in patterns similar to those with AD but to a lesser degree.[48] Cross-sectional studies have consistently demonstrated that FDG-PET imaging and the resulting hypometabolic patterns can reliably differentiate groups of MCI patients from healthy controls, and from patients with AD dementia.[56–60] Several studies have identified a predictive value of FDG-PET as a biomarker for the future development of AD.[55,57,58,60–66] All these studies were able to identify typical hypometabolic changes in FDG-PET baseline examinations of MCI patients, associated with later conversion to AD dementia, whereas stable subjects showed fewer or no abnormalities. Several studies demonstrated higher accuracy of FDG-PET for prediction of AD dementia in MCI patients relative to neuropsychological examination.[55,64]

FDG-PET has also been evaluated in populations of patients who are presymptomatic but at heightened risk for the development of AD. Early-onset familial AD (FAD) is associated with autosomal-dominant inheritance of mutations in the presenilin and amyloid precursor protein genes.[67,68] Regional glucose hypometabolism on FDG-PET has been associated with asymptomatic FAD gene carriers, in a pattern consistent with the typical AD PET pattern but with the relative absence of structural brain atrophy.[69] Compared with the more common late-onset sporadic AD (LOAD), cases of FAD with autosomal-dominant inheritance represent only a small percentage of all AD cases and have a very different clinical onset and course.[70]

The ε4 allele of apolipoprotein E (*APOE* ε4) is currently the most potent known genetic risk factor for LOAD.[71,72] Several studies have been able to demonstrate hypometabolic abnormalities in cognitively impaired individuals at increased risk for AD, including carriers of the *APOE* ε4 allele and those with family histories of AD. For example, compared with age- and education matched noncarriers (ages 50–65 years), Reiman and colleagues showed reduced glucose metabolism in ε4 homozygotes in the same brain regions as that observed in patients with probable AD.[73] These same authors later demonstrated that even relatively young (20–39 years) ε4 homozygotes had abnormally low rates of glucose metabolism bilaterally in the posterior cingulate, parietal, temporal, and prefrontal cortex, and that the ε4-gene dose is correlated with lower glucose metabolism in each of these brain regions.[74,75] Furthermore, in several studies, decline of glucose metabolism over time in AD-typical regions has been demonstrated in cognitively healthy ε4 carriers.[76,77] Recent studies have also shown hypometabolic changes in subjects with maternal history of AD who are at higher risk for dementia, suggesting additional genetic or environmental risks for LOAD.[78,79]

Other dementias show patterns of glucose hypometabolism that distinguish them from normal controls and AD patients. In FTLD, the typical pattern of hypometabolism includes a combination of frontal or temporal predominant reductions in CMRgl.[80] Early in the course of the disease, the pattern observed will often show relative sparing of the parietal lobes, which can help to distinguish FTLD and its associated variants from AD.[81,82] Adding FDG-PET to clinical diagnostic criteria can significantly increase the accuracy of diagnosis. In one study involving 6 dementia experts who were asked to provide a diagnostic decision for 45 subjects with pathologically confirmed AD (n = 31) or FTD (n = 14), the addition of FDG-PET data to clinical summaries was superior to clinical assessment and resulted in the best measures of inter-rater reliability (mean kappa = 0.78) and diagnostic accuracy (89.6%).[82]

There have been relatively few investigations of DLB with functional imaging. Consistent with structural findings, the overall pattern of glucose hypometabolism is similar to that observed in AD including significant metabolic reductions involving parietotemporal, poster cingulate, and frontal association cortices.[50,83,84] However, decreased glucose utilization is also seen in the primary visual and the occipital association cortices in patients diagnosed with DLB, consistent with the clinical presentation of DLB.[50,83,84] This pattern of hypometabolism is consistent with a finding of diffuse cortical Lewy bodies on autopsy.[85]

FDG-PET scanning is approved for clinical use. Recent recommendations from the European Federation of Neurological Societies (EFNS) include use of FDG-PET in patients in whom there is diagnostic doubt in clinical dementia presentation.[86] In the United States, Medicare has specific National Coverage Determinations for use of FDG-PET as a diagnostic test for dementia and neurodegenerative diseases (Medicare Manual Section Number 220.6.13). Medicare generally covers FDG-PET scans for the differential diagnosis of FTLD and AD, and is considered reasonable and necessary in patients with a recent diagnosis of dementia and documented cognitive decline of at least 6 months who meet diagnostic criteria for both AD and FTD. Coverage varies from state to state, with no guarantee that the cost of the imaging procedure will be approved or covered by a patient's private insurance carrier.

Single-photon emission computed tomography

SPECT imaging uses gamma photon-emitting radioisotopes attached to biologically relevant molecules that have been injected intravenously and distributed throughout the body. As gamma-emitting molecules are dispersed in the body, they are attenuated as they pass through different types of tissue. This attenuation is assumed to be homogenous throughout the brain. A gamma camera is used to detect the photon signal, and collimators funnel photon activity to the camera as they are emitted in defined directions, allowing for the detection of spatial patterns. The gamma camera rotates around the patient, generating 2-dimensional (2D) images projected from various angles. Three-dimensional reconstruction of these 2D images facilitates the modeling of biologically meaningful physiologic processes, such as blood flow and receptor-binding capacity. SPECT is commonly used to measure regional cerebral blood flow but also dopaminergic transporter loss in the striatum and cardiac uptake of metaiodobenzylguanidine (MIBG).

In AD, SPECT shows decreased cerebral perfusion in bilateral temporal-parietal lobes and in the frontal lobes, which often occurs in the later stages of dementia.[87,88] The primary sensorimotor strips and basal ganglia typically do not show decreased cerebral perfusion. These findings are similar to pattern of glucose hypometabolism seen with FDG-PET imaging. In MCI, SPECT also reveals consistent patterns of cerebral hypoperfusion, although to a lesser degree than that seen in AD, and SPECT has shown some predictive value for AD.[89–91]

Other dementias also show regions of hypoperfusion on SPECT scanning that are similar to the pattern of hypometabolism seen with FDG-PET imaging. FTLD patients show an expected pattern of frontal and anterior temporal lobe hypoperfusion.[92,93] McNeill and colleagues[92] found that frontal blood flow had a sensitivity of 80% and specificity of 65% in distinguishing AD from FTD. DLB patients show expected patterns of cerebral hypoperfusion similar to that observed in AD but relatively more blood flow reduction in the visual cortex.[94,95] However, modest sensitivity and specificity of 65% and 87%, respectively, suggest limited usefulness of HMPAO SPECT to distinguish AD from DLB.[95]

SPECT imaging has also been used to identify loss of dopamine transporters in the striatum of patients with DLB. Previous studies have demonstrated nigrostriatal degeneration and subsequent loss of dopamine transporters within the striatum that is significantly more severe in DLB than in AD.[96] Nigrostriatal dopaminergic neurons can be visualized *in vivo* using the SPECT ligand ^{123}I-Fluoropropyl-2-beta-carbome-thoxy-3-beta(4-iodophenyl)nortropane (^{123}I-FP-CIT), which binds to the dopamine transporter. Studies have demonstrated IFP-CIT SPECT imaging (DaTscan) to have an overall accuracy of around 86%, with a sensitivity of 78% and specificity of 90% for distinguishing DLB from other dementias (primarily AD),[97] and 78% sensitivity and 94% specificity for distinguishing it from AD.[98]

Cardiac uptake of MIBG is also reduced in DLB patients compared with normal controls and AD.[99] MIBG SPECT is thought to be a measure of cardiac sympathetic denervation in DLB patients. MIBG cardiac imaging has shown sensitivities of 95% to 100%, and specificity of 87% to 100% for distinguishing DLB from AD and normal controls.[99–101] This association seems related to clinical symptoms of orthostatic hypotension.[102]

Dopamine imaging has been included as a "suggestive feature" in the International Consensus criteria for diagnosis of DLB.[97] Dopaminergic SPECT is also now recommended, with strong evidence for clinical evaluations to distinguish AD from DLB by the EFNS.[86]

MOLECULAR IMAGING

Molecular imaging focuses on visualizing cellular function and molecular processes in living humans, tissues, or organisms, and includes brain imaging by PET. As described previously for functional imaging, brain imaging scanners use tracers to identify molecular biomarkers or molecules of interest within the brain. Common molecular targets of molecular imaging include abnormal accumulation of specific proteins, such as $A\beta$ peptide, and most recently tau protein.

Amyloid Imaging by PET

The presence of $A\beta$ neuritic plaques is a hallmark finding of AD at autopsy.[12] The abnormal accumulation of amyloid oligomers, precursors to amyloid fibrils and amyloid deposits, is thought to be central to the pathogenesis of AD.[103] Biomarkers of increased brain amyloidosis in AD include decreased CSF levels of $A\beta_{1-42}$ or increased radiolabeled amyloid PET tracer binding within the brain.[29,30] Several amyloid PET tracers have been developed to measure fibrillary $A\beta$ in the living human brain.[104,105] The Pittsburgh compound B (PiB), C11-(2-[4-methyl-amino phenyl]-1,3-benzothiazol-6-ol) (^{11}C), was the first amyloid PET tracer to be described and has been the most extensively studied.[106] A direct correlation has been observed between $A\beta$ amyloid plaques and in vivo (^{11}C)PiB binding, demonstrating specificity of PiB PET for detecting pathologic $A\beta$ within brain regions known to be affected in AD.[107–110] However, the short half-life of the ^{11}C isotope (20 minutes) has minimized the commercial use of (^{11}C)PiB. Therefore, development of other amyloid PET tracers such as ^{18}F-ligands with a longer half-life ($\sim$2 hours) was critical for enabling possible commercial development and broad patient access.

Several ^{18}F-labeled $A\beta$ PET tracers have been developed, including [18]F39-F-PiB (flutemetamol),[111] [18]FAV-45 (florbetapir),[112,113] ^{18}F-AV-1 or ^{18}F-BAY94-9172 (florbetaben),[114] and ^{18}F-AZD4694 or NAV4694.[115–117] Three of these amyloid-binding ligands are currently approved by the Food and Drug Administration (FDA): (1) florbetapir (Amyvid, Eli Lilly), (2) florbetaben (Neuracq, Piramal), and (3) flutemetamol (Vizamyl, GE). Florbetapir was the first ^{18}F amyloid-binding ligand to be approved by the FDA in 2012. Original studies demonstrated that florbetapir PET imaging was correlated with the presence and density of β-amyloid at autopsy.[113,118] The sensitivity and specificity of florbetapir PET imaging for detection of moderate to frequent amyloid plaques was 92% and 100%, respectively, in individuals who had an autopsy within 2 years of PET imaging, and 96% and 100%, respectively, for those who had an autopsy within 1 year.[118] Similar associations between amyloid burden estimated by use of PET imaging and histopathological amyloid levels have also been reported for florbetaben at autopsy[119,120] and for flutemetamol after cortical biopsy.[111,121]

Morris and colleagues[122] performed a meta-analysis assessing the diagnostic accuracy of florbetaben, florbetapir, and flutemetamol in AD. They systematically reviewed articles published between 1990 and 2014 and identified 9 studies that met several criteria, including patients with a diagnosis of AD and a control group; analysis of more than 10 subjects; investigation of the diagnostic accuracy of florbetapir, florbetaben, or flutemetamol PET uptake compared with clinical diagnosis or histopathology; and publication of the full paper in a peer-reviewed scientific journal. The results from their meta-analysis showed that pooled sensitivity and specificity values were high for all 3 tracers; the sensitivity for all subgroups ranged from 89% to 97%, whereas for specificity the values ranged more widely, from 63% to 93%. The values for sensitivity and specificity were similar for both visual and quantitative analyses and, overall, the sensitivity was higher than specificity for all subgroups. All tracers performed better when discriminating between subjects with AD and healthy controls. No marked differences were noted in the diagnostic accuracy of the 3 Aβ PET radiotracers. Moreover, the sensitivity and specificity for both the quantitative and visual analysis of the ^{18}F-labeled tracers (combined) was generally comparable to those of other imaging or biomarker techniques used to diagnose AD.

In contrast, there is currently insufficient evidence to support the use of amyloid PET tracers as a biomarker to distinguish FTLD from AD, or to distinguish DLB from AD.[123] However, amyloid PET imaging may assist physicians in the differential diagnosis of neurodegenerative disorders by including or excluding the presence of pathologic Aβ. Among a clinical cohort of participants with probable AD, MCI, or older healthy controls, 80.9%, 40.0%, and 20.7%, respectively, met cortical florbetapir standardized uptake value ratio (SUVR) criteria (≥1.17) for levels of amyloid associated with AD and 85.3%, 46.6%, and 28.1%, respectively, met SUVR criteria (>1.08) for the presence of any identifiable Aβ.[124] Thus while 81% of participants with probable AD demonstrated significant levels of florbetapir PET binding, nearly 50% of subjects who were clinically diagnosed with MCI due to AD were negative on amyloid PET scans, and approximately 30% of cognitively normal elderly individuals present with positive amyloid PET scans. Indeed, amyloid PET imaging studies report that a certain percentage of patients clinically diagnosed with AD dementia do not show evidence of significant Aβ accumulation within their brains (two recent studies: 20–25% were amyloid PET negative),[125,126] corroborating earlier data demonstrating that up to 30% of patients with clinically diagnosed AD lack evidence of AD pathology at autopsy.[26]

These findings emphasize the difficulty of an accurate clinical diagnosis in the absence of a pathologic biomarker and the potential utility of such biomarkers in facilitating the differential diagnostic process for dementia. A negative amyloid brain scan is inconsistent with a diagnosis of AD, suggesting that a different pathophysiological process is likely the cause for the patient's cognitive complaints or dementia. A positive amyloid brain scan is more complicated to interpret because a positive scan may indicate that a patient is at risk for AD and lies somewhere along the prodromal-MCI-AD dementia continuum. However, other diseases and dementias can also show increased amyloid binding within the brain. Also, as noted, even healthy individuals can show increased amyloid binding and still be cognitively normal, indicating a risk for impending cognitive decline.[127,128]

What is the appropriate role of amyloid PET imaging in the differential diagnosis of dementia? Morris and colleagues[122] highlighted some of the recent changes that have occurred in the diagnostic guidelines for AD, especially in regard to biomarkers and amyloid PET imaging:

- In 2011, the National Institute on Aging Alzheimer's Association workgroups on diagnostic guidelines for AD recommended updated criteria for the diagnosis of AD. None of these revisions include the use of biomarker tests in the routine diagnostic process for AD. The authors concluded that the core criteria provide sufficient diagnostic accuracy and that more research is required regarding standardization and availability of the tests.[20]
- In 2012, the EFNS proposed guidelines on the use of neuroimaging in the diagnosis of dementia.[129] The guidelines do not include the use of amyloid imaging in routine clinical setting. It was concluded that amyloid scans may find clinical utility in patients with MCI, in patients with atypical symptoms, and for differentiating between AD and FTLD.
- In 2013, the Amyloid Imaging Task Force in association with the Society of Nuclear Medicine and Molecular imaging and the Alzheimer's Association developed a set of specific appropriate use criteria (AUC) to identify patients and clinical circumstances in which amyloid PET could be used.[130,131] Out of a list of 10 situations, 3 situations were considered an appropriate use of the technique and 7 were not (**Box 1**). Ordering amyloid imaging was suggested to be done only by dementia specialists instead of in the primary care setting.
- In 2014, the International Working Group (IWG) for New Research Criteria for the Diagnosis of Alzheimer's Disease proposed updated guidelines for the diagnosis of typical AD,[132] updating their original 2007 criteria.[133] In addition to clinical criteria, these revised criteria include *in vivo* evidence of AD pathology, requiring one of the following: 1) CSF biomarker tests (low amyloid β_{1-42} together with high T-tau or P-tau), 2) amyloid PET imaging (high retention of amyloid tracer), or 3) genetic tests.[133]

Box 1
Appropriate use criteria for amyloid PET imaging

Amyloid imaging is appropriate in the following situations:

1. Persistent or progressive unexplained MCI

2. Patients satisfying core clinical criteria for possible AD because of unclear clinical presentation, either an atypical clinical course or an etiologically mixed presentation

3. Patients with progressive dementia and atypically early age of onset (usually defined as ≤65 years in age)

Amyloid imaging is inappropriate in the following situations:

1. Patients with core clinical criteria for probable AD with typical age of onset

2. To determine dementia severity

3. Based solely on a positive family history of dementia or presence of APOE ε4

4. Patients with a cognitive complaint that is unconfirmed on clinical examination

5. In lieu of genotyping for suspected autosomal mutation carriers

6. In asymptomatic individuals

7. Nonmedical use (eg, legal, insurance coverage, or employment screening).

Amyloid PET is not currently reimbursed by US Centers for Medicare and Medicaid Services (CMS), limiting the availability of this imaging modality for routine clinical use.[105,123] Coverage with evidence development is planned to provide for reimbursement for amyloid-PET as part of clinical research studies and is currently being assessed in a community-based longitudinal imaging program, the Imaging Dementia–Evidence for Amyloid Scanning (IDEAS) study. The IDEAS study is designed to determine the clinical usefulness and value in diagnosing AD and other dementias in Medicare patients meeting AUC (ClinicalTrials.gov: NCT02420756). This process may provide outcomes data needed for CMS to reconsider the coverage decision for amyloid-PET.

Use of amyloid PET in the clinic

Even though amyloid imaging represents the most recent advance in the ability to detect amyloid burden in vivo within the brain of a living human who present with cognitive complaint, to date, amyloid PET imaging is not commonly used in clinical practice. Is there evidence that inclusion of amyloid PET imaging can significantly influence the diagnosis and management of patients undergoing evaluation for memory deficits?

A number of studies have begun to report that incorporation of amyloid PET imaging in addition to routine assessment in patients with cognitive impairment can have a significant effect on diagnosis, diagnostic confidence, and drug treatment. Grundman and colleagues[134] assessed the potential value of incorporating amyloid PET imaging in diagnostic plans for evaluation and management of 229 subjects with progressive cognitive decline and an uncertain diagnosis. In their study, a provisional diagnosis was given, diagnostic confidence estimated, and a plan for diagnostic evaluation and management was created both before and immediately following receipt of the florbetapir ^{18}F PET results. Results revealed that, after amyloid PET imaging, physicians changed their diagnosis for 54.6% (125 out of 229) of the subjects. Diagnostic confidence increased by an average of 21.6% and 86.9% of the cases had a least 1 change in their management plan. Cholinesterase inhibitor or memantine use increased by 17.7% among amyloid positive cases and decreased by 23.3% among those with amyloid negative scans. In addition, planned brain structural imaging decreased by 24.4% and planned neuropsychological testing decreased by 32.8%. The investigators concluded that amyloid PET imaging altered physician diagnostic thinking, intended testing, and management plans in patients undergoing evaluation for cognitive decline. Similar findings highlighting the potential value of information from amyloid PET imaging have now been reported across a variety of different studies and with different amyloid PET tracers including florbetpir,[135–137] flutemetamol,[138] and florbetaben[139] and even for vignettes reporting "positive," "negative," or no β-amyloid imaging information for hypothetical patients with symptoms of unexplained mild cognitive impairment, possible AD, or young-onset dementia.[140]

Tau Imaging by PET

The role of tau protein in the pathophysiology of AD and in other tauopathies, such as FTLD, has been based primarily on data from postmortem autopsies.[12,141,142] FTLD involves 3 different histologies: (1) abnormal accumulation of microtubule-associated protein tau (FTLD-tau, 45% cases); (2) RNA-binding and DNA-binding protein, TDP-43 (FTLD-TDP, 50% cases); and (3) FUS protein (FTLD-FUS, 5%).[142]

Only recently have PET tracers become available that allow in vivo detection of tau protein within the human brain. At least 7 pathologic tau PET tracers have been developed and used in clinical studies.[143] ^{18}F-AV-1451 ([18]FT807) is a PET tracer for the in vivo detection of pathologic tau in AD and has been recently confirmed by neuropathology.[144] This PET tracer is currently in phase 2 development as a diagnostic PET tracer for in vivo imaging of pathologic tau in patients with AD and related neurodegenerative diseases.[143] Several studies have reported early clinical findings with several of these tau PET tracers.[145–150] Using multimodal imaging techniques to assess the relationship among clinical symptoms, in vivo pathologic tau, amyloid distribution, and glucose hypometabolism, several studies have now shown that pathologic tau is more closely linked to the pattern of glucose hypometabolism and development of clinical symptoms than amyloid deposition.[148–150]

Similar to the accumulation of Aβ peptide, increases in tau PET binding is also observed in healthy controls with aging.[151] Whereas older age was related to increased retention of the PET tracer in regions of the medial temporal lobe (predicting worse episodic memory performance), increased detection of pathologic tau in other isocortical regions required the presence of β-amyloid and was associated with decline in global cognition.

Tau PET imaging is the most recent advance in molecular brain imaging. At present, a role of tau PET imaging has not been defined within the AD diagnostic schemes.

Use of Biomarker Combinations for Understanding Disease Progress

Jack and colleagues[152] have proposed amyloid/tau/neurodegeneration (A/T/N) as an unbiased descriptive classification scheme for AD biomarkers. The investigators argue that there are gaps with regard to the current use of biomarkers in AD and propose the A/T/N scheme to address 4 key issues: (1) include tau PET imaging, (2) make no assumption about temporal ordering of biomarkers or their putative causal relationship, (3) do not specify disease or syndromic labels so that the classification scheme is applicable across all clinical diagnostic states, and (4) include all individuals in any population regardless of the mix of biomarker findings. In their scheme, referred to as A/T/N system, 7 major AD biomarkers are divided into 3 binary categories based on the nature of the pathophysiology that each measures: A refers to the value of a Aβ biomarker (ie, amyloid PET or CSF Ab42); T, the value of a tau biomarker (ie, CSF phospho-tau or tau PET); and N, biomarkers of neurodegeneration or neuronal injury (ie, ^{18}F-fluorodeoxyglucose–PET, structural MRI, or CSF total tau). Each biomarker category is rated as positive or negative, resulting in individual scores such as A1/T1/N2. This scheme is argued to have potential value in categorizing patients according to accuracy of AD diagnosis and likelihood of clinical progression. This has potential value for clinical diagnostic accuracy, disease categorization, prognostication, and design of treatment trials targeting specific disease states.

SUMMARY

Currently, only the use of structural imaging is standard of care in clinical practice, with newer imaging techniques offering great promise to aid in diagnostic accuracy and benefit patient management. Brain imaging in AD, MCI, and in other dementias will continue to evolve, reflecting improvements in imaging techniques, signal detection, and the development of new tracers to track various biomarkers of interest in vivo. Continued scientific discovery should provide greater understanding of the pathophysiology of degenerative brain diseases, especially in regard to understanding the changes occurring within the brain of individuals who are asymptomatic but in the early stages of what is thought to be prodromal or preclinical dementia. It is hoped that this knowledge will continue to inform clinical practice in the use of brain imaging as a whole and, specifically, with respect to newer imaging modalities of amyloid and tau PET imaging.

REFERENCES

1. American Psychiatric Association. Diagnostic and statistical manual of mental disorders. 5th edition. Arlington (VA): American Psychiatric Publishing; 2013.
2. Ross GW, Bowen JD. The diagnosis and differential diagnosis of dementia. Med Clin North Am 2002;86(3):455–76.
3. Kelley RE, Minagar A. Memory complaints and dementia. Prim Care 2004;31(1): 129–48.
4. Barker WW, Luis CA, Kashuba A, et al. Relative frequencies of Alzheimer disease, Lewy body, vascular and frontotemporal dementia, and hippocampal sclerosis in the State of Florida Brain Bank. Alzheimer Dis Assoc Disord 2002; 16(4):203–12.
5. O'Brien JT, Holmes C, Jones M, et al. Clinical practice with anti-dementia drugs: A revised (third) consensus statement from the British Association for Psychopharmacology. J Psychopharmacol 2017;31(2):147–68.
6. Jellinger KA, Attems J. Neuropathological evaluation of mixed dementia. J Neurol Sci 2007;257(1–2):80–7.
7. Schneider JA, Arvanitakis Z, Bang W, Bennett DA. Mixed brain pathologies account for most dementia cases in community-dwelling older persons. Neurology 2007;69(24):2197–204.
8. Schneider JA, Arvanitakis Z, Leurgans SE, Bennett DA. The neuropathology of probable Alzheimer disease and mild cognitive impairment. Ann Neurol 2009; 66(2):200–8.
9. Viswanathan A, Rocca WA, Tzourio C. Vascular risk factors and dementia: how to move forward? Neurology 2009;72(4):368–74.
10. Alzheimer's Association. 2016 Alzheimer's disease facts and figures. Alzheimers Dement 2016;12(4):459–509.
11. Gorno-Tempini ML, Hillis AE, Weintraub S, et al. Classification of primary progressive aphasia and its variants. Neurology 2011;76(11):1006–14.
12. Hyman BT, Phelps CH, Beach TG, et al. National Institute on Aging-Alzheimer's Association guidelines for the neuropathologic assessment of Alzheimer's disease. Alzheimers Dement 2012;8(1):1–13.
13. Villemagne VL, Burnham S, Bourgeat P, et al. Amyloid β deposition, neurodegeneration, and cognitive decline in sporadic Alzheimer's disease: a prospective cohort study. Lancet Neurol 2013;12(4):357–67.
14. Reiman EM, Quiroz YT, Fleisher AS, et al. Brain imaging and fluid biomarker analysis in young adults at genetic risk for autosomal dominant Alzheimer's disease in the presenilin 1 E280A kindred: a case-control study. Lancet Neurol 2012;11(12):1048–56.
15. Bateman RJ, Xiong C, Benzinger TL, et al. Clinical and biomarker changes in dominantly inherited Alzheimer's disease. N Engl J Med 2012;367(9):795–804.
16. Petersen RC, Doody R, Kurz A, et al. Current concepts in mild cognitive impairment. Arch Neurol 2001;58(12):1985–92.
17. Mistridis P, Krumm S, Monsch AU, et al. The 12 years preceding mild cognitive impairment due to Alzheimer's disease: the temporal emergence of cognitive decline. J Alzheimers Dis 2015;48(4):1095–107.
18. Mufson EJ, Ikonomovic MD, Counts SE, et al. Molecular and cellular pathophysiology of preclinical Alzheimer's disease. Behav Brain Res 2016;311:54–69.

19. Jack CR Jr, Albert MS, Knopman DS, et al. Introduction to the recommendations from the National Institute on Aging-Alzheimer's Association workgroups on diagnostic guidelines for Alzheimer's disease. Alzheimers Dement 2011;7(3): 257–62.

20. McKhann GM, Knopman DS, Chertkow H, et al. The diagnosis of dementia due to Alzheimer's disease: recommendations from the National Institute on Aging-Alzheimer's Association workgroups on diagnostic guidelines for Alzheimer's disease. Alzheimers Dement 2011;7(3):263–9.

21. Albert MS, DeKosky ST, Dickson D, et al. The diagnosis of mild cognitive impairment due to Alzheimer's disease: recommendations from the National Institute on Aging-Alzheimer's Association workgroups on diagnostic guidelines for Alzheimer's disease. Alzheimers Dement 2011;7(3):270–9.

22. Sperling RA, Aisen PS, Beckett LA, et al. Toward defining the preclinical stages of Alzheimer's disease: recommendations from the National Institute on Aging-Alzheimer's Association workgroups on diagnostic guidelines for Alzheimer's disease. Alzheimers Dement 2011;7(3):280–92.

23. Flanagan EP, Duffy JR, Whitwell JL, et al. Mixed Tau and TDP-43 pathology in a patient with unclassifiable primary progressive aphasia. Neurocase 2016;22(1): 55–9.

24. Wicklund MR, Duffy JR, Strand EA, et al. Quantitative application of the primary progressive aphasia consensus criteria. Neurology 2014;82(13):1119–26.

25. Knopman DS, DeKosky ST, Cummings JL, et al. Practice parameter: diagnosis of dementia (an evidence-based review). Report of the Quality Standards Subcommittee of the American Academy of Neurology. Neurology 2001;56(9): 1143–53.

26. Beach TG, Monsell SE, Phillips LE, et al. Accuracy of the clinical diagnosis of Alzheimer disease at National Institute on Aging Alzheimer Disease Centers, 2005-2010. J Neuropathol Exp Neurol 2012;71(4):266–73.

27. Silverman DH, Gambhir SS, Huang HW, et al. Evaluating early dementia with and without assessment of regional cerebral metabolism by PET: a comparison of predicted costs and benefits. J Nucl Med 2002;43(2):253–66.

28. Zamrini E, De Santi S, Tolar M. Imaging is superior to cognitive testing for early diagnosis of Alzheimer's disease. Neurobiol Aging 2004;25(5):685–91.

29. Thal LJ, Kantarci K, Reiman EM, et al. The role of biomarkers in clinical trials for Alzheimer disease. Alzheimer Dis Assoc Disord 2006;20(1):6–15.

30. Hampel H, Bürger K, Teipel SJ, et al. Core candidate neurochemical and imaging biomarkers of Alzheimer's disease. Alzheimers Dement 2008;4(1):38–48.

31. Kovacs GG. Molecular pathological classification of neurodegenerative diseases: turning towards precision medicine. Int J Mol Sci 2016;17(2):189.

32. Barkhof F, Fox NC, Bastos-Leite AJ, et al. Neuroimaging in Dementia. Berlin Heidelberg: Springer; 2011. Chapter 5.

33. Braak H, Braak E. Neuropathological staging of Alzheimer-related changes. Acta Neuropathol 1991;82(4):239–59.

34. McEvoy LK, Brewer JB. Quantitative structural MRI for early detection of Alzheimer's disease. Expert Rev Neurother 2010;10(11):1675–88.

35. Frisoni GB, Fox NC, Jack CR, et al. The clinical use of structural Mrl in Alzheimer disease. Nat Rev Neurol 2010;6:67–77.

36. Yuan Y, Gu ZX, Wei WS. Fluorodeoxyglucose-positron-emission tomography, single-photon emission tomography, and structural MR imaging for prediction of rapid conversion to Alzheimer disease in patients with mild cognitive impairment: a meta-analysis. AJNR Am J Neuroradiol 2009;30(2):404–10.

37. Bouwman FH, Schoonenboom SNM, van der Flier WM, et al. CSF biomarkers and medial temporal lobe atrophy predict dementia in mild cognitive impairment. Neurobiol Aging 2007;28(7):1070–4.

38. Tartaglia MC, Rosen HJ, Miller BL. Neuroimaging in dementia. Neurotherapeutics 2011;8(1):82–92.

39. Silverman DHS. Brain 18 F-FDG PET in the diagnosis of neurodegenerative dementias: comparison with perfusion SPECT and with clinical evaluations lacking nuclear imaging. J Nucl Med 2004;45(4):594–607.

40. Auer DP, Pütz B, Gössl C, et al. Differential lesion patterns in CADASIL and sporadic subcortical arteriosclerotic encephalopathy: MR imaging study with statistical parametric group comparison. Radiology 2001;218(2):443–51.

41. Bastos Leite AJ, van der Flier WM, van Straaten ECW, et al. Infratentorial abnormalities in vascular dementia. Stroke 2006;37(1):105–10.

42. Charidimou A, Shakeshaft C, Werring DJ. Cerebral microbleeds on magnetic resonance imaging and anticoagulant-associated intracerebral hemorrhage risk. Front Neurol 2012;3:133.

43. Arboix A, Bell Y, García-Eroles L, et al. Clinical study of 35 patients with dysarthria-clumsy hand syndrome. J Neurol Neurosurg Psychiatry 2004;75(2):231–4.

44. Benjamin P, Lawrence AJ, Lambert C, et al. Strategic lacunes and their relationship to cognitive impairment in cerebral small vessel disease. Neuroimage Clin 2014;4:828–37.

45. Blanco-Rojas L, Arboix A, Canovas D, et al. Cognitive profile in patients with a first-ever lacunar infarct with and without silent lacunes: a comparative study. BMC Neurol 2013;13:203.

46. Lopez OL, Kuller LH, Fitzpatrick A, et al. Evaluation of dementia in the cardiovascular health cognition study. Neuroepidemiology 2003;22(1):1–12.

47. Ishii K, Kanda T, Harada A, et al. Clinical impact of the callosal angle in the diagnosis of idiopathic normal pressure hydrocephalus. Eur Radiol 2008;18(11): 2678–83.

48. Langbaum JB, Chen K, Lee W, et al. Categorical and correlational analyses of baseline fluorodeoxyglucose positron emission tomography images from the Alzheimer's Disease Neuroimaging Initiative (ADNI). Neuroimage 2009;45(4): 1107–16.

49. Braak H, Braak E. Evolution of the neuropathology of Alzheimer's disease. Acta Neurol Scand Suppl 1996;165:3–12.

50. Minoshima S, Foster NL, Sima AA, et al. Alzheimer's disease versus dementia with Lewy bodies: cerebral metabolic distinction with autopsy confirmation. Ann Neurol 2001;50:358–65.

51. Hoffman JM, Welsh-Bohmer KA, Hanson M, et al. FDG PET imaging in patients with pathologically verified dementia. J Nucl Med 2000;41:1920–8.

52. Matthews B, Siemers ER, Mozley PD. Imaging-based measures of disease progression in clinical trials of disease-modifying drugs for Alzheimer disease. Am J Geriatr Psychiatry 2003;11(2):146–59.

53. Alexander GE, Chen K, Pietrini P, et al. Longitudinal PET evaluation of cerebral metabolic decline in dementia: a potential outcome measure in Alzheimer's disease treatment studies. Am J Psychiatry 2002;159(5):738–45.

54. Kawano M, Ichimiya A, Ogomori K, et al. Relationship between both IQ and Mini-Mental State Examination and the regional cerebral glucose metabolism in clinically diagnosed Alzheimer's disease: a PET study. Dement Geriatr Cogn Disord 2001;12(2):171–6.

55. Silverman DH, Small GW, Chang CY, et al. Positron emission tomography in evaluation of dementia: Regional brain metabolism and long-term outcome. JAMA 2001;286(17):2120–7.

56. Minoshima S, Giordani B, Berent S, et al. Metabolic reduction in the posterior cingulate cortex in very early Alzheimer's disease. Ann Neurol 1997;42:85–94.

57. Drzezga A, Lautenschlager N, Siebner H, et al. Cerebral metabolic changes accompanying conversion of mild cognitive impairment into Alzheimer's disease: a PET follow-up study. Eur J Nucl Med Mol Imaging 2003;30:1104–13.

58. Drzezga A, Grimmer T, Riemenschneider M, et al. Prediction of individual clinical outcome in MCI by means of genetic assessment and (18)F-FDG PET. J Nucl Med 2005;46(10):1625–32.

59. Del Sole A, Clerici F, Chiti A, et al. Individual cerebral metabolic deficits in Alzheimer's disease and amnestic mild cognitive impairment: an FDG PET study. Eur J Nucl Med Mol Imaging 2008;35:1357–66.

60. Nobili F, Salmaso D, Morbelli S, et al. Principal component analysis of FDG PET in amnestic MCI. Eur J Nucl Med Mol Imaging 2008;35:2191–202.

61. Herholz K, Nordberg A, Salmon E, et al. Impairment of neocortical metabolism predicts progression in Alzheimer's disease. Dement Geriatr Cogn Disord 1999; 10:494–504.

62. Arnaiz E, Jelic V, Almkvist O, et al. Impaired cerebral glucose metabolism and cognitive functioning predict deterioration in mild cognitive impairment. Neuroreport 2001;12:851–5.

63. Chetelat G, Desgranges B, De La Sayette V, et al. Mild cognitive impairment: can FDG-PET predict who is to rapidly convert to Alzheimer's disease? Neurology 2003;60:1374–7.

64. Mosconi L, Perani D, Sorbi S, et al. MCI conversion to dementia and the APOE genotype: a prediction study with FDG-PET. Neurology 2004;63(12):2332–40.

65. Hunt A, Schonknecht P, Henze M, et al. Reduced cerebral glucose metabolism in patients at risk for Alzheimer's disease. Psychiatry Res 2007;155:147–54.

66. Landau SM, Harvey D, Madison CM, et al. Associations between cognitive, functional, and FDG-PET measures of decline in AD and MCI. Neurobiol Aging 2011;32(7):1207–18.

67. Goate AM. Molecular genetics of Alzheimer's disease. Geriatrics 1997;52: S9–12.

68. Ermak G, Davies KJ. Gene expression in Alzheimer's disease. Drugs Today (Barc) 2002;38:509–16.

69. Mosconi L, Sorbi S, de Leon MJ, et al. Hypometabolism exceeds atrophy in presymptomatic early-onset familial Alzheimer's disease. J Nucl Med 2006;47: 1778–86.

70. Sorbi S, Forleo P, Tedde A, et al. Genetic risk factors in familial Alzheimer's disease. Mech Ageing Dev 2001;122(16):1951–60.

71. Corder EH, Saunders AM, Strittmatter WJ, et al. Gene dose of apolipoprotein E type 4 allele and the risk of Alzheimer's disease in late onset families. Science 1993;261:921–3.

72. Farrer L, Cupples L, Haines J, et al. Effects of age, sex, and ethnicity on the association between apolipoprotein E genotype and Alzheimer disease. J Am Med Assoc 1997;278:1349–56.

73. Reiman EM, Caselli RJ, Yun LS, et al. Preclinical evidence of Alzheimer's disease in persons homozygous for the epsilon 4 allele for apolipoprotein E. N Engl J Med 1996;334:752–8.

74. Reiman EM, Chen K, Alexander GE, et al. Functional brain abnormalities in young adults at genetic risk for late-onset Alzheimer's dementia. Proc Natl Acad Sci U S A 2004;101:284–9.

75. Reiman EM, Chen K, Alexander GE, et al. Correlations between apolipoprotein E epsilon4 gene dose and brain-imaging measurements of regional hypometabolism. Proc Natl Acad Sci U S A 2005;102:8299–302.

76. Small GW, Ercoli LM, Silverman DH, et al. Cerebral metabolic and cognitive decline in persons at genetic risk for Alzheimer's disease. Proc Natl Acad Sci U S A 2000;97:6037–42.

77. Reiman EM, Caselli RJ, Chen K, et al. Declining brain activity in cognitively normal apolipoprotein E epsilon 4 heterozygotes: a foundation for using positron emission tomography to efficiently test treatments to prevent Alzheimer's disease. Proc Natl Acad Sci U S A 2001;98:3334–9.

78. Mosconi L, Brys M, Switalski R, et al. Maternal family history of Alzheimer's disease predisposes to reduced brain glucose metabolism. Proc Natl Acad Sci U S A 2007;104:19067–72.

79. Mosconi L, Mistur R, Switalski R, et al. Declining brain glucose metabolism in normal individuals with a maternal history of Alzheimer disease. Neurology 2009a;72:513–20.

80. Ishii K, Sakamoto S, Sasaki M, et al. Cerebral glucose metabolism in patients with frontotemporal dementia. J Nucl Med 1998;39:1875–8.

81. Ishii K. Clinical application of positron emission tomography for diagnosis of dementia. Ann Nucl Med 2002;16:515–25.

82. Foster NL, Heidebrink JL, Clark CM, et al. FDG-PET improves accuracy in distinguishing frontotemporal dementia and Alzheimer's disease. Brain 2007; 130(Pt 10):2616–35.

83. Gilman S, Koeppe RA, Little R, et al. Differentiation of Alzheimer's disease from dementia with Lewy bodies utilizing positron emission tomography with [18F]fluorodeoxyglucose and neuropsychological testing. Exp Neurol 2005;191(Suppl 1):S95–103.

84. Albin RL, Minoshima S, D'Amato CJ, et al. Fluoro-deoxyglucose positron emission tomography in diffuse Lewy body disease. Neurology 1996;47:462–6.

85. Mirzaei S, Knoll P, Koehn H, et al. Assessment of diffuse Lewy body disease by 2-[18F]fluoro-2-deoxy-D-glucose positron emission tomography (FDG PET). BMC Nucl Med 2003;3(1):1.

86. Hort J, O'Brien JT, Gainotti G, et al. EFNS guidelines for the diagnosis and management of Alzheimer's disease. Eur J Neurol 2010;17:1236–48.

87. Song IU, Chung YA, Chung SW, et al. Early diagnosis of Alzheimer's disease and Parkinson's disease associated with dementia using cerebral perfusion SPECT. Dement Geriatr Cogn Disord 2014;37(5–6):276–85.

88. Pakrasi S, O'Brien JT. Emission tomography in dementia. Nucl Med Commun 2005;26:189–96.

89. Johnson KA, Jones K, Holman BL, et al. Preclinical prediction of Alzheimer's disease using SPECT. Neurology 1998;50:1563–71.

90. Huang C, Wahlund LO, Svensson L, et al. Cingulate cortex hypoperfusion predicts Alzheimer's disease in mild cognitive impairment. BMC Neurol 2002;2:9.

91. Staffen W, Schonauer U, Zauner H, et al. Brain perfusion SPECT in patients with mild cognitive impairment and Alzheimer's disease: comparison of a semiquantitative and a visual evaluation. J Neural Transm 2006;113:195–203.

92. McNeill R, Sare GM, Manoharan M, et al. Accuracy of single-photon emission computed tomography in differentiating frontotemporal dementia from Alzheimer's disease. J Neurol Neurosurg Psychiatry 2007;78:350–5.
93. Archer HA, Smailagic N, John C, et al. Regional cerebral blood flow single photon emission computed tomography for detection of Frontotemporal dementia in people with suspected dementia. Cochrane Database Syst Rev 2015;(6):CD010896.
94. Donnemiller E, Heilmann J, Wenning GK, et al. Brain perfusion scintigraphy with 99mTc-HMPAO or 99mTc-ECD and 123I-beta-CIT single-photon emission tomography in dementia of the Alzheimer-type and diffuse Lewy body disease. Eur J Nucl Med 1997;24:320–5.
95. Lobotesis K, Fenwick JD, Phipps A, et al. Occipital hypoperfusion on SPECT in dementia with Lewy bodies but not AD. Neurology 2001;56:643–9.
96. Piggott MA, Marshall EF, Thomas N, et al. Striatal dopaminergic markers in dementia with Lewy bodies, Alzheimer's and Parkinson's diseases: rostrocaudal distribution. Brain 1999;122(Pt 8):1449–68.
97. McKeith I, O'Brien J, Walker Z, et al. Sensitivity and specificity of dopamine transporter imaging with 123I-FP-CIT SPECT in dementia with Lewy bodies: a phase III, multicentre study. Lancet Neurol 2007;6:305–13.
98. O'Brien JT, Colloby S, Fenwick J, et al. Dopamine transporter loss visualized with FP-CIT SPECT in the differential diagnosis of dementia with Lewy bodies. Arch Neurol 2004;61:919–25.
99. Hanyu H, Shimizu S, Hirao K, et al. The role of 123I-metaiodobenzylguanidine myocardial scintigraphy in the diagnosis of Lewy body disease in patients with dementia in a memory clinic. Dement Geriatr Cogn Disord 2006;22:379–84.
100. Hanyu H, Shimizu S, Hirao K, et al. Comparative value of brain perfusion SPECT and [(123)I]MIBG myocardial scintigraphy in distinguishing between dementia with Lewy bodies and Alzheimer's disease. Eur J Nucl Med Mol Imaging 2006;33:248–53.
101. Yoshita M, Taki J, Yokoyama K, et al. Value of 123I-MIBG radioactivity in the differential diagnosis of DLB from AD. Neurology 2006;66:1850–4.
102. Kobayashi S, Tateno M, Morii H, et al. Decreased cardiac MIBG uptake, its correlation with clinical symptoms in dementia with Lewy bodies. Psychiatry Res 2009;174:76–80.
103. Salahuddin P, Fatima MT, Abdelhameed AS, et al. Structure of amyloid oligomers and their mechanisms of toxicities: targeting amyloid oligomers using novel therapeutic approaches. Eur J Med Chem 2016;114:41–58.
104. Zeng F, Goodman MM. Fluorine-18 radiolabeled heterocycles as PET tracers for imaging β-amyloid plaques in Alzheimer's disease. Curr Top Med Chem 2013; 13(8):909–19.
105. Anand K, Sabbagh M. Amyloid Imaging: poised for Integration into Medical Practice. Neurotherapeutics 2017;14(1):54–61.
106. Klunk WE, Engler H, Nordberg A, et al. Imaging brain amyloid in Alzheimer's disease with Pittsburgh Compound-B. Ann Neurol 2004;55(3):306–19.
107. Bacskai BJ, Frosch MP, Freeman SH, et al. Molecular imaging with Pittsburgh compound B confirmed at autopsy: a case report. Arch Neurol 2007;64:431–4.
108. Ikonomovic MD, Klunk WE, Abrahamson EE, et al. Post-mortem correlates of in vivo PiB-PET amyloid imaging in a typical case of Alzheimer's disease. Brain 2008;131:1630–45.
109. Kadir A, Marutle A, Gonzalez D, et al. Positron emission tomography imaging and clinical progression in relation to molecular pathology in the first Pittsburgh

Compound B positron emission tomography patient with Alzheimer's disease. Brain 2011;134(Pt 1):301–17.

110. Sojkova J, Driscoll I, Iacono D, et al. In vivo fibrillar beta-amyloid detected using [11C]PiB positron emission tomography and neuropathologic assessment in older adults. Arch Neurol 2011;68:232–40.

111. Wolk DA, Grachev ID, Buckley C, et al. Association between in vivo fluorine 18-labeled flutemetamol amyloid positron emission tomography imaging and in vivo cerebral cortical histopathology. Arch Neurol 2011;68(11):1398–403.

112. Wong DF, Rosenberg PB, Zhou Y, et al. In vivo imaging of amyloid deposition in Alzheimer disease using the radioligand 18F-AV-45 (florbetapir [corrected] F 18). J Nucl Med 2010;51(6):913–20.

113. Clark CM, Schneider JA, Bedell BJ, et al. Use of florbetapir-PET for imaging beta-amyloid pathology. JAMA 2011;305(3):275–83.

114. Rowe CC, Ackerman U, Browne W, et al. Imaging of amyloid beta in Alzheimer's disease with 18F-BAY94-9172, a novel PET tracer: proof of mechanism. Lancet Neurol 2008;7:129–35.

115. Cselenyi Z, Jonhagen ME, Forsberg A, et al. Clinical validation of 18F-AZD4694, an amyloid-beta-specific PET radioligand. J Nucl Med 2012;53:415–24.

116. Jureus A, Swahn BM, Sandell J, et al. Characterization of AZD4694, a novel fluorinated Abeta plaque neuroimaging PET radioligand. J Neurochem 2010;114: 784–94.

117. Rowe CC, Pejoska S, Mulligan RS, et al. Head-to-head comparison of 11C-PiB and 18F-AZD4694 (NAV4694) for β-amyloid imaging in aging and dementia. J Nucl Med 2013;54(6):880–6.

118. Clark CM, Pontecorvo MJ, Beach TG, et al. Cerebral PET with florbetapir compared with neuropathology at autopsy for detection of neuritic amyloid-beta plaques: a prospective cohort study. Lancet Neurol 2012;11:669–78.

119. Sabri O, Seibyl J, Rowe C, et al. Beta-amyloid imaging with florbetaben. Clin Transl Imaging 2015;3:13–26.

120. Sabri O, Sabbagh MN, Seibyl J, et al. Florbetaben PET imaging to detect amyloid beta plaques in Alzheimer's disease: phase 3 study. Alzheimers Dement 2015;11(8):964–74.

121. Rinne JO, Wong DF, Wolk DA, et al. [(18)F]Flutemetamol PET imaging and cortical biopsy histopathology for fibrillary amyloid B detection in living subjects with normal pressure hydrocephalus: pooled analysis of four studies. Acta Neuropathol 2012;124(6):833–45.

122. Morris E, Chalkidou A, Hammers A, et al. Diagnostic accuracy of (18)F amyloid PET tracers for the diagnosis of Alzheimer's disease: a systematic review and meta-analysis. Eur J Nucl Med Mol Imaging 2016;43(2):374–85.

123. McConathy J, Sheline YI. Imaging biomarkers associated with cognitive decline: a review. Biol Psychiatry 2015;77(8):685–92.

124. Fleisher AS, Chen K, Liu X, et al. Using positron emission tomography and florbetapir F18 to image cortical amyloid in patients with mild cognitive impairment or dementia due to Alzheimer disease. Arch Neurol 2011;68(11):1404–11.

125. Degenhardt EK, Witte MM, Case MG, et al. Florbetapir F18 PET Amyloid neuroimaging and characteristics in patients with mild and moderate Alzheimer Dementia. Psychosomatics 2016;57(2):208–16.

126. Sabbagh MN, Schäuble B, Anand K, et al. Histopathology and florbetaben PET in patients incorrectly diagnosed with Alzheimer's disease. J Alzheimers Dis 2017;56(2):441–6.

127. Doraiswamy PM, Sperling RA, Coleman RE, et al. Amyloid-B assessed by florbetapir F18 PET and 18-month cognitive decline: a multicenter study. Neurology 2012;79(16):1636–44.

128. Doraiswamy PM, Sperling RA, Johnson K, et al. Florbetapir F 18 amyloid PET and 36-month cognitive decline: a prospective multicenter study. Mol Psychiatry 2014;19(9):1044–51.

129. Filippi M, Agosta F, Barkhof F, et al. EFNS task force: the use of neuroimaging in the diagnosis of dementia. Eur J Neurol 2012;19(12):e131–40, 1487–501.

130. Johnson KA, Minoshima S, Bohnen NI, et al. Appropriate use criteria for amyloid PET: a report of the Amyloid Imaging Task Force, the Society of Nuclear Medicine and Molecular Imaging, and the Alzheimer's Association. Alzheimers Dement 2013;9(1):e1–16.

131. Johnson KA, Minoshima S, Bohnen NI, et al. Update on appropriate use criteria for amyloid PET imaging: dementia experts, mild cognitive impairment, and education. Amyloid Imaging Task Force of the Alzheimer's Association and Society for Nuclear Medicine and Molecular Imaging. Alzheimers Dement 2013;9(4): e106–9.

132. Dubois B, Feldman HH, Jacova C, et al. Advancing research diagnostic criteria for Alzheimer's disease: the IWG-2 criteria. Lancet Neurol 2014;13(6):614–29.

133. Dubois B, Feldman HH, Jacova C, et al. Research criteria for the diagnosis of Alzheimer's disease: revising the NINCDS-ADRDA criteria. Lancet Neurol 2007;6(8):734–46.

134. Grundman M, Pontecorvo MJ, Salloway SP, et al. Potential impact of amyloid imaging on diagnosis and intended management in patients with progressive cognitive decline. Alzheimer Dis Assoc Disord 2013;27(1):4–15.

135. Zannas AS, Doraiswamy PM, Shpanskaya KS, et al. Impact of 18F-florbetapir PET imaging of B-amyloid neuritic plaque density on clinical decision-making. Neurocase 2014;20(4):466–73.

136. Boccardi M, Altomare D, Ferrari C, et al. Assessment of the incremental diagnostic value of florbetapir F 18 imaging in patients with cognitive impairment: the incremental diagnostic value of amyloid PET With [18F]-florbetapir (INDIA-FBP) study. JAMA Neurol 2016;73(12):1417–24.

137. Mitsis EM, Bender HA, Kostakoglu L, et al. A consecutive case series experience with [18F] florbetapir PET imaging in an urban dementia center: impact on quality of life, decision making, and disposition. Mol Neurodegener 2014;9: 10.

138. Zwan MD, Bouwman FH, Konijnenberg E, et al. Diagnostic impact of [18F]flutemetamol PET in early-onset dementia. Alzheimers Res Ther 2017;9(1):2.

139. Schipke CG, Peters O, Heuser I, et al. Impact of beta-amyloid-specific florbetaben PET imaging on confidence in early diagnosis of Alzheimer's disease. Dement Geriatr Cogn Disord 2012;33(6):416–22.

140. Zhong Y, Karlawish J, Johnson MK, et al. The potential value of β-amyloid imaging for the diagnosis and management of dementia: a survey of clinicians. Alzheimer Dis Assoc Disord 2017;31(1):27–33.

141. Khanna MR, Kovalevich J, Lee VM, et al. Therapeutic strategies for the treatment of tauopathies: hopes and challenges. Alzheimers Dement 2016;12(10): 1051–65.

142. Mann DM, Snowden JS. Frontotemporal lobar degeneration: Pathogenesis, pathology and pathways to phenotype. Brain Pathol 2017. http://dx.doi.org/10. 1111/bpa.12486.

143. James OG, Doraiswamy PM, Borges-Neto S. PET imaging of tau pathology in Alzheimer's disease and tauopathies. Front Neurol 2015;6:1–4.
144. Marquié M, Normandin MD, Vanderburg CR, et al. Validating novel tau positron emission tomography tracer [F-18]-AV-1451 (T807) on postmortem brain tissue. Ann Neurol 2015;78(5):787–800.
145. Maruyama M, Shimada H, Suhara T, et al. Imaging of tau pathology in a tauopathy mouse model and in Alzheimer patients compared to normal controls. Neuron 2013;79(6):1094–108.
146. Chien DT, Bahri S, Szardenings AK, et al. Early clinical PET imaging results with the novel PHF-tau radioligand [F-18]-T807. J Alzheimers Dis 2013;34(2):457–68.
147. Chien DT, Szardenings AK, Bahri S, et al. Early clinical PET imaging results with the novel PHF-tau radioligand [F18]-T808. J Alzheimers Dis 2014;38(1):171–84.
148. Ossenkoppele R, Schonhaut DR, Baker SL, et al. Tau, amyloid, and hypometabolism in a patient with posterior cortical atrophy. Ann Neurol 2015;77(2):338–42.
149. Ossenkoppele R, Schonhaut DR, Schöll M, et al. Tau PET patterns mirror clinical and neuroanatomical variability in Alzheimer's disease. Brain 2016;139(Pt 5): 1551–67.
150. Dronse J, Fliessbach K, Bischof GN, et al. In vivo patterns of tau pathology, amyloid-β burden, and neuronal dysfunction in clinical variants of Alzheimer's disease. J Alzheimers Dis 2017;55(2):465–71.
151. Schöll M, Lockhart SN, Schonhaut DR, et al. PET Imaging of Tau Deposition in the Aging Human Brain. Neuron 2016;89(5):971–82.
152. Jack CR Jr, Bennett DA, Blennow K, et al. A/T/N: An unbiased descriptive classification scheme for Alzheimer disease biomarkers. Neurology 2016;87(5): 539–47.

Early-Onset Alzheimer Disease

Mario F. Mendez, MD, PhD[a,b,*]

KEYWORDS

- Dementia • Alzheimer disease • Early-onset dementia • Young-onset dementia
- Logopenic variant primary progressive aphasia • Progressive cortical atrophy

KEY POINTS

- Early-onset Alzheimer disease (EOAD) is not just late-onset AD (LOAD) at a younger age; there are substantial differences between these 2 categories of AD.
- Compared with LOAD, EOAD has greater neocortical pathology, particularly in the parietal cortex, greater tau compared with amyloid burden, and less hippocampal disease.
- Fifty percent or more of patients with EOAD have nonamnestic, phenotypic variants, including logopenic variant primary progressive aphasia, posterior cortical atrophy, progressive ideomotor apraxia, behavioral/dysexecutive AD, corticobasal syndrome, and others. These may be conceptualized as "Type 2 AD."
- Compared with LOAD, the phenotypic variants of EOAD preferentially involve alternate, fronto-parietal neural networks rather than the posterior default mode network.
- The management of EOAD differs from LOAD in the emphasis on targeted cognitive interventions and age-appropriate psychosocial support.

INTRODUCTION

Alzheimer disease (AD) originally meant a disorder of early-onset (EOAD; <65 years of age) and did not include older patients with "senile dementia." In fact, the first patient reported with the neuropathology of AD, Auguste Deter (1850–1906), appeared to have the onset of symptoms in her late 40s, before being diagnosed with dementia at age 51.[1] Her symptoms included memory loss, confusion, language impairment, and unpredictable, agitated, aggressive, and paranoid behavior, and, on autopsy, she had what we now

Disclosure Statement: The author has nothing to disclose. The author has no commercial or financial conflicts of interest.
Funding Source (author PI): NIA R01AG050967; NIA R01AG034499.
[a] Behavioral Neurology Program, David Geffen School of Medicine at UCLA, 300 Westwood Plaza, Suite B-200, Box 956975, Los Angeles, CA 90095, USA; [b] Neurobehavior Unit, VA Greater Los Angeles Healthcare System, 11301 Wilshire Boulevard, Building 206, Los Angeles, CA 90073, USA
* Neurobehavior Unit, VA Greater Los Angeles Healthcare System, 11301 Wilshire Boulevard, Building 206, Los Angeles, CA 90073.
E-mail address: mfmendez@mednet.ucla.edu

recognize as the characteristic neuropathological markers of AD, extracellular amyloid-positive neuritic plaques and intracellular tau-positive neurofibrillary tangles (NFTs). With the observation of similar neuropathology associated with cognitive decline in all age groups, investigators subsequently broadened the diagnosis of AD to include the much more common late-onset AD (LOAD).[2] In recent years, the main focus of interest and research has been on LOAD; however, like Auguste Deter, patients with EOAD remain an important and impactful subgroup of patients with this disorder.

EOAD is the most common early-onset neurodegenerative dementia. The few epidemiologic studies on EOAD indicate that the vast majority are nonfamilial, making up approximately 4% to 6% of all AD,[3] with an annual incidence rate of approximately 6.3 per 100,000[4] and a prevalence rate of approximately 24.2 per 100,000 in the 45-year to 64-year age group,[5] or between 220,000 and 640,000 Americans.[6] These incidence and prevalence rates of EOAD rise exponentially as patients approach age 65.[7] Unfortunately, EOAD is often atypical and missed, resulting in an approximately 1.6-year average delay in diagnosis compared with older patients.[8] Yet, from 1999 to 2010, mortality reports show that EOAD accounted for a large number of premature deaths among US adults aged 40 to 64, with many years of potential life lost, as well as losses in productivity.[9]

EARLY-ONSET ALZHEIMER DISEASE VERSUS LATE-ONSET ALZHEIMER DISEASE

EOAD is not just LOAD occurring at an arbitrarily younger age cutoff; EOAD differs from LOAD in many respects (**Box 1**). EOAD differs from LOAD in the greater extent of evaluation required for diagnosis,[10] the increased impact of dementia risk factors, such as lower cardiovascular fitness and cognitive fitness,[11] and the potentially increased consequence of traumatic brain injury the lower the age of onset of dementia.[12] There are psychosocial problems specific to early-onset dementia,[13–17] such as the effects of unexpected loss of independence, grief with a sense of an "out-of-step" decline in midlife, difficulty juggling ongoing responsibilities, and relatively preserved insight with associated depression and anxiety. Given that autosomal dominant familial AD tends to be of early onset, there are subgroups of EOAD with higher rates of neurologic symptoms than LOAD and a greater risk for the development of AD among relatives.[18,19] In contrast, compared with LOAD, patients with EOAD have decreased overall comorbidities, such as diabetes, obesity, and circulatory disorders.[18]

Patients with EOAD differ, on average, from patients with LOAD on a number of clinical, neuropsychological, neuroimaging, and neuropathological variables. Several studies indicate that these early-onset patients have a more aggressive clinical course.[20–24] EOAD, compared with LOAD, presents less commonly with memory deficits and more frequently as focal cortical or phenotypic variants (described later in this article).[25] Overall, patients with EOAD, compared with comparably impaired patients with LOAD, have better memory recognition scores and semantic memory,[26] but they tend to have worse attention, executive functions, ideomotor praxis, and visuospatial skills.[25,26] On MRI, EOAD shows greater neocortical atrophy, particularly in the parietal cortex, with less atrophy in the mesial temporal lobe (MTL).[27,28] MRI shows larger sulcal widths in the temporoparietal cortex among patients with EOAD with preserved hippocampal volumes relative to LOAD.[29] Resting state fluorodeoxyglucose (FDG)-PET shows greater parietal hypometabolism, worse on the left in one study,[30] in EOAD compared with greater bilateral temporal hypometabolism in LOAD.[15] FDG-PET also suggests dysfunction in brain metabolic activity, especially in the salience network among patients with EOAD with behavioral disturbances.[31] Neuropathologically, both EOAD and LOAD have temporoparietal-precuneus atrophy, but

> **Box 1**
> **Early-onset Alzheimer disease**
>
> *Reported Differences in Comparison with the More Common Late-Onset Disorder*
> - Greater delay to diagnosis
> - Lower cardiovascular fitness in early adulthood
> - Lower cognitive reserve in early adulthood
> - Lower incidence of diabetes, obesity, circulatory disorders
> - Higher prevalence of traumatic brain injury (TBI), with evidence that TBI lowers age of onset of dementia
> - Greater psychosocial problems
>   - Unexpected loss of independence
>   - Grief, severe and feeling the dementia is "out-of-step" with age
>   - Difficulty juggling active responsibilities (job and family)
> - More insight and depression
> - Lower frequency of the *APOE ε4* allele among the phenotypic variants
> - Subset with familial Alzheimer disease, neurologic symptoms, and/or increased family risk
> - Somewhat more aggressive course
> - Increased occurrence of nonamnestic, focal variants or phenotypes with early posterior neocortical involvement
> - Relatively greater deficits in attention, executive functions, praxis, and visuospatial functions
> - Greater neocortical atrophy in parietal areas and temporoparietal junction sulcal width on neuroimaging
> - Greater parietal versus temporal hypometabolism
> - Less hippocampal and mesial temporal lobe disease and hippocampal volume loss compared with late-onset Alzheimer disease
> - Greater white matter changes, especially in posterior association areas and fronto-parietal networks
> - Decreased central hubs, nodal connections, and rich club networks
> - Decreased involvement of mesial temporal-posterior cingulate network of default mode network (DMN)
> - Greater involvement of non-DMN neural networks, including central executive, language, working memory, and visuospatial networks
> - Higher burden of neurofibrillary tangles and neuritic plaques, especially in posterior neocortex
> - Greater tau/neurofibrillary tangle load per stage of dementia and per gray matter atrophy

patients with EOAD have higher burdens of neuritic plaques and NFTs in these regions, and, to a lesser extent, frontal cortex, than patients with LOAD.[25]

EOAD, regardless of clinical variant, has an early and prominent pattern of white matter (WM) damage that is more severe in posterior areas.[32] Diffusion tensor imaging (DTI) measures in EOAD demonstrate more damage to WM pathways in both deep long-range limbic and association fibers and superficially located short-range association fibers in the frontal, temporal, and parietal lobes associated with fronto-parietal dysfunction.[33,34] Compared with LOAD, the WM involvement in patients with EOAD is particularly greater in posterior WM (posterior cingulate and parietal regions) and main anterior-posterior pathways with less mesial temporal involvement.[14,34,35] Moreover, WM damage in EOAD is more widely distributed than would be predicted by the extent of gray matter (GM) atrophy.[35] Using graph theory analysis of DTI, EOAD appears to target the nodal connectivity of the brain, mainly affecting the rich club network in the superior frontal regions, precuneus, posterior cingulate, and insula with differential disruption of the major central hubs that transfer information between brain regions.[36]

Variant Early-Onset Alzheimer Disease Phenotypes (or "Type 2 Alzheimer Disease")

One of the most important aspects of EOAD is its common presentation as a number of nonamnestic, variant phenotypes, potentially justifying their grouping under the label "Type 2" AD. These variants represent the young tail of the normally distributed age of AD onset curve (**Fig. 1**). About 22% to 64% of EOAD are nonamnestic variant phenotypes, which differ from typical amnestic AD (either EOAD or LOAD) not only in nonmemory presentations,[21,25,37–41] but also in the decreased prevalence of the apolipoprotein E (*APOE*) ε4 allele,[23,40] and early posterior cortical NFTs with relative hippocampal sparing.[42]

The variant phenotypes of EOAD constitute a number of syndromes (**Table 1**).[37,43,44] The most common may be a language-impaired phenotype known as logopenic progressive aphasia.[14,38,45] Investigators report a "posterior cortical atrophy" (PCA) variant with visuospatial deficits.[46,47] Others suggest that a biparietal phenotype with progressive ideomotor apraxia (PIA) and visuospatial and other deficits is a common form of EOAD.[43] The literature stresses the occurrence of a behavioral/dysexecutive variant, sometimes referred to as "frontal variant AD."[37,48] In addition, patients with corticobasal syndrome, characterized by progressive limb apraxia and motor changes, have AD in up to 25% at autopsy,[49] indicating another manifestation of variant EOAD which greatly overlaps with PIA. These phenotypes are clinical syndromes that appear to overlap with one another, while differing in basic respects from typical amnestic AD.[50,51]

Neuroimaging studies indicate differences among the EOAD variants (further discussed below). In general, the typical amnestic patients with EOAD have more hippocampal atrophy; whereas, the variant phenotypes of EOAD with language presentations have more left parietal atrophy, and the variant phenotypes of EOAD with visuospatial presentations have more right parietal-occipital changes. Typical

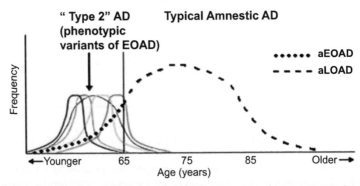

Fig. 1. Type 2 AD (variant phenotypes of EOAD) versus typical amnestic AD (aEOAD and aLOAD). The nonamnestic variant phenotypes (logopenic variant PPA, PCA, and other proposed variants) tend to occur in the early-onset age range and are depicted as colored lines. (*Adapted from* van der Flier WM, Pijnenburg YA, Fox NC, Scheltens P. Early-onset versus late-onset Alzheimer's disease: the case of the missing APOE epsilon4 allele. Lancet Neurol 2011;10(3):280–8.)

Table 1
Alternative classifications for variant phenotypes of EOAD

Brain Regions	Koedam et al,[43] 2010 (N = 87)	Alladi et al,[38] 2007 (N = 34)	Stopford et al,[37] 2008[a] (N = 17)
Left parietal	Apraxia/visuospatial (37.5%)	Corticobasal syndrome (17.5%)	Praxis (23.5%)
Left parietal, left temporo-occipital	Language (28.1%), aphasia-apraxia-agnosia (25%)	Language (56%): nonfluent (35%), semantic (6%), mixed (15%)	Language (23.5%)
Dorsolateral frontal	Dysexecutive (6.3%)	Non-AD: FTD (6%)	Dysexecutive (41.2%)
Right parietal, right temporo-occipital	Posterior cortical atrophy (3.1%)	Posterior cortical atrophy (20.5%)	Perceptuo-spatial (11.8%)

Abbreviations: AD, Alzheimer disease; EOAD, early-onset AD; FTD, frontotemporal dementia.
[a] With this exception, the dysexecutive phenotype may be less common in EOAD, versus late-onset AD.
Data from Refs.[37,148–153]

amnestic AD has WM damage in the genu and splenium of the corpus callosum and the parahippocampal tract bilaterally[35]; whereas, the variant phenotypes of EOAD have extensive degeneration of major anterior-posterior connecting fiber bundles and of commissural frontal lobe tracts, implying deafferentation within fronto-parietal cortical networks.[52]

Functional MRI (fMRI) studies suggest that EOAD is driven by early involvement of fronto-parietal networks (central executive and salience networks; language, working memory, and higher visual networks) rather than the decreased posterior default mode network (DMN) and MTL-hippocampal connectivity of typical amnestic AD.[53–66] In typical AD, functional connectivity shows enhanced effective connectivity within frontally based executive and salience networks, even before the detection of any WM changes.[3,67,68] In contrast, fMRI in EOAD demonstrates decreased fronto-parietal connectivity.[43,44,69–72]

Logopenic Variant Primary Progressive Aphasia

A major EOAD phenotypic variant is the progressive decline in language known as logopenic variant primary progressive aphasia (lvPPA). Patients with this syndrome present with word-finding difficulty, decreased sentence repetition, and abnormalities in echoic memory, with impairments in their phonological buffer (ie, limitations in the number of spoken words that they can keep in working memory). Clinicians must distinguish these patients from nonfluent and semantic forms of primary progressive aphasia (PPA), which are typically due to frontotemporal lobar degenerations. The presence of some degree of difficulty in episodic memory and visuospatial skills helps distinguish lvPPA from other PPAs. In addition, a history of dyslexia is common among patients with lvPPA,[73–75] suggesting a preexisting vulnerability in language networks. In one study, 25% of patients with lvPPA had self or informant reports of delay in spelling or reading.[74]

The clinical criteria for lvPPA are as follows (**Box 2**)[45]: an insidious onset and progression of (1) impaired single-word retrieval in spontaneous speech and naming (anomia); (2) impaired repetition of sentences and phrases; and (3) at least 3 of the following also must be present: speech (phonologic) errors, spared single-word comprehension and object knowledge, spared motor speech, and/or (4) absence of frank agrammatism.

Box 2
Characteristics of logopenic variant primary progressive aphasia (lvPPA)

- An insidious onset and progressive disorder of language
- Word-finding difficulty with frequent word-finding pauses, may have circumlocutions
- Decreased word retrieval with phonological paraphasias (errors)
- Disproportionately decreased repetition of sentences ("hallmark finding")
- Decreased comprehension for long (not complex) sentences but not for words
- Preserved grammar and articulation (motor speech)
- Other evidence of decreased phonologic store (eg, decreased digit or word span)
- Word-length effect but decreased phonological similarity effect
- Left posterior temporal/inferior parietal dysfunction on neuroimaging

---

Although some patients may have frontotemporal lobar degeneration or other pathologies, the clinical syndrome of lvPPA usually results from AD with focal involvement of temporoparietal language areas in the left hemisphere. Neuroimaging shows atrophy, decreased metabolism, and decreased WM in the left temporoparietal junction.[76] Patients with lvPPA usually have positive AD biomarkers, including amyloid-PET positive scans[77] and decreased Aβ42/elevated tau levels in the cerebrospinal fluid (CSF).[78] DTI analysis of lvPPA reveals bilateral but predominantly left-sided alterations in frontal origin pathways, such as superior and inferior longitudinal fasciculi and the uncinate fasciculus, as well as the parietotemporal junction (**Fig. 2**).[50,69,79] Compared with typical AD, those with lvPPA have reduced connectivity in the left posterior superior temporal region and temporal language network, the inferior parietal and prefrontal regions and fronto-parietal networks, and the left working memory networks,[66,71,80] and less involvement of the ventral DMN associated with episodic memory impairment.[66]

There is a pathophysiological explanation for this syndrome's impairments. In lvPPA, disease in the left inferior parietal lobule and superior and middle temporal gyri disturbs the phonological loop of verbal working memory (phonological short-term memory or store that holds phonological traces for brief periods),[66,81] resulting in deficits in digit, letter, and word span and an absent phonological similarity effect.[82]

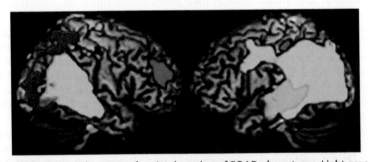

Fig. 2. Voxel-based morphometry of parietal overlap of EOAD phenotypes. Light green represents overlap of all EOAD variants. Blue, Type 2 AD-PCA; Green, Type 2 AD-lvPPA; Red, Other EOAD. (*From* Migliaccio R, Agosta F, Rascovsky K, et al. Clinical syndromes associated with posterior atrophy: early age at onset AD spectrum. Neurology 2009;73(19):1571–8; with permission.)

Posterior Cortical Atrophy

Many patients with EOAD present with a progressive decline in visuospatial skills, known as PCA or "Benson disease" after D. Frank Benson, who described the syndrome in 1988.[83] Patients with this syndrome present with complex visual symptoms, including alexia, apperceptive visual agnosia, Balint syndrome (simultanagnosia, optic ataxia, oculomotor apraxia) and difficulty with visuospatial localization, Gerstmann syndrome, and a possible left visual field deficit with disproportionate impairments on tests of visual constructions (**Box 3**). PCA is most commonly a visual variant of AD, but may result from dementia with Lewy bodies, Creutzfeldt-Jakob (Heidenheim variant), or other lesions or disorders involving the posterior visual cortex. Patients with PCA have better verbal fluency and somewhat less impaired episodic memory than typical AD,[84] and they differ from many dementias in having relatively preserved insight into their illness and a tendency to depression. Some investigators suggest that PCA is a focal Alzheimer neurodegeneration of the occipital, occipitoparietal, and occipitotemporal cortex,[85,86] and that there may be prior learning disabilities and a preexisting vulnerability in the cortical visual systems.[75]

The clinical criteria for PCA are as follows (**Box 4**)[46,47]: an insidious onset and progression of the following: (1) visual complaints with intact primary visual functions, except for possible visual field deficits; (2) evidence of predominant complex visual disorder (oculomotor apraxia, optic ataxia, dressing apraxia, environmental disorientation, abnormal antisaccades, neglect, constructional difficulty, simultanagnosia, visual agnosia, prosopagnosia); (3) proportionally less impaired deficits in memory and verbal fluency.

Neuroimaging shows predominant areas of atrophy, hypoperfusion, and hypometabolism from primary visual cortex through dorsal visual association cortex and posterior regions of the temporal lobes. On DTI, there may be predominate right-sided WM changes in superior and inferior longitudinal fasciculi, inferior fronto-occipital fasciculus, and right fronto-parietal pathways (see **Fig. 2**).[14,87] These areas and WM tracts impact on midlevel cortical visual processing, resulting in abnormal perceptual integration and organization, and difficulty with figure-ground discrimination and global-local precedence. Many patients have difficulty finding things in their spatial environment, left more than right visual field constriction, and elements of Balint

---

Box 3
Complex visual disorders among patients with posterior cortical atrophy (approximate order of frequency)

- Alexia (>oral difficulty)
- Balint (whole or partial), especially optic ataxia
- Visual object agnosia
- Environmental disorientation
- Dressing apraxia/other spatial
- Prosopagnosia (apperceptive)
- Color perception problems
- Hemispatial neglect or visual field constriction on the left

Adapted from Mendez MF, Ghajarania M, Perryman KM. Posterior cortical atrophy: clinical characteristics and differences compared to Alzheimer's disease. Dement Geriatr Cogn Disord 2002;14(1):33–40.

Box 4
Developing criteria for posterior cortical atrophy

- Clinical features:
  Insidious onset and gradual progression
  Prominent early disturbances of visual and/or other posterior cognitive symptoms/signs

- Cognitive features:
  At least 3 of the following must be early or presenting features: visuospatial difficulty, elements of Balint syndrome, visual object agnosia, visuoconstructional difficulty, environmental disorientation, dressing apraxia, alexia, elements of Gerstmann syndrome, ideomotor apraxia, apperceptive prosopagnosia, visual field deficit
  All of following must be evident: relative sparing of anterograde memory, speech and verbal language, executive functions, and behavior and personality

- Neuroimaging:
  Predominant occipito-parietal or occipito-temporal changes

- Exclusion criteria:
  Lesions or disorders of the brain that could cause similar symptoms and findings

Consortium developing criteria under the leadership of Sebastian Crutch, MD.
Data from Crutch SJ, Schott JM, Rabinovici GD, et al. Shining a light on posterior cortical atrophy. Alzheimers Dement 2012;9(4):463–465.

---

syndrome, especially optic ataxia with "magnetic misreaching" toward the point of fixation when reaching for items in their peripheral fields.[88]

Other Variants

Other than for lvPPA and PCA, there is no consensus on the number of EOAD variants or on their classification. Two addition EOAD variants are worth noting. One is a PIA variant, which overlaps with corticobasal syndrome from AD as well as with lvPPA and PCA. This variant results from focal left parietal neuropathology and manifests as difficulty performing learned limb movements on command and to imitation. It is often accompanied by Gerstmann syndrome with acalculia, alexia with agraphia, and problems with visual constructions. Another variant is "behavioral/dysexecutive AD," also described as "frontal variant AD."[48] This variant can present with apathy, and half can meet clinical criteria for behavioral variant frontotemporal dementia (bvFTD). However, persons with behavioral/executive variant EOAD tend to perform worse on memory tests than those with bvFTD and can show marked atrophy in bilateral temporoparietal regions with milder atrophy in frontal cortex.[48]

The recent literature suggests that the variant phenotypes of EOAD could be related to each other, potentially comprising a "Type 2" AD that differs in its neurocognitive-neural network profile from typical amnestic AD.[25,41,50,51] Clinically, they all relatively spare memory, and pathologically, they may all have hippocampal sparing with greater posterior cortical NFTs.[42] There is additionally specific involvement of left hemisphere language areas in lvPPA[78,89] and the visual neocortex in PCA.[90,91] Neuroimaging data also suggest posterior neocortical rather than mesotemporal cortical overlap of these phenotypes.[76,92,93]

Cerebrospinal Fluid and Amyloid PET Biomarkers in Early-Onset Alzheimer Disease

Similar to typical LOAD, amyloid β42 (Aβ) peptide levels are decreased and total tau and phospho-tau levels are increased in the cerebrospinal fluid (CSF) in EOAD and its variants.[94] Some studies suggest phenotypic variations in these CSF biomarkers, particularly lower tau levels in PCA,[52,95,96] but this is not confirmed across studies and with neuropathology. Where EOAD differs from LOAD is the better correspondence of lower Aβ levels, rather than increased tau levels, with GM atrophy.[94] One possible explanation for this difference is the decreased release of tau into the ventricular space in EOAD in light of the neurodegeneration occurring farther from the ventricular surface (eg, in the neocortex rather than medial temporal lobe).

Amyloid PET is especially useful in the differentiation of EOAD from other dementias of early onset. The prevalence of amyloid positivity decreases in AD from age 50 to 90, particularly among apolipoprotein E (APOE) ε4 noncarriers, and increasing with age in non-AD dementias.[97] This suggests an increased utility of amyloid PET among those with dementia onset of less than 65 years of age. Amyloid positivity by PET is almost always associated with low CSF Aβ in symptomatic AD, and amyloid PET positivity is a better predictor of clinical diagnosis.[98]

Genetics

Genetic changes are becoming increasingly important in the analysis and understanding of EOAD.[99] There is growing awareness of polymorphisms and genetic mutations that increase susceptibility for EOAD. The identification of determinant AD genes in this population overall, however, is rare. Despite an autosomal dominant history in approximately 14.2% of persons with EOAD, only approximately 1.6% of the total EOAD population carries a presenilin 1 (*PSEN1*), presenilin 2 (*PSEN2*), or amyloid precursor protein (APP) gene that conveys an autosomal dominant inheritance for AD.[100] These 3 pathogenic mutations, which lead to aberrant cleavage or aggregation of the APP, result in the more typical amnestic AD but can have distinctive features such as spastic paraparesis, early myoclonus, seizures, dysarthria, pseudobulbar affect, more extensive amyloid angiopathy, and atypical amyloid plaque morphology and distribution.[101] Nevertheless, there may be a need to screen patients with EOAD for these mutations. Investigators report a *PSEN1* mutation in an analysis of a specimen from Auguste Deter, Alzheimer's original patient,[102] and some PSEN1 mutations, such as A79 V, can be variable and sometimes mild with ages of onset ranging from 53 to 84.[103] One study found 3 PSEN1 and 1 PSEN2 in 4 (1.5%) of 264 patients with EOAD, but no effect of having a positive family history of LOAD.[104] Another whole-exome sequencing of 23 German patients with EOAD revealed 3 with potential pathogenic *PSEN2* variants.[105] Finally, on screening 451 patients with sporadic EOAD for known causative mutations of the APP gene, investigators found 4 heterozygous for *A713T, V717I, V717G*.[106]

There is a polygenic risk for AD from a number of susceptibility genes, but none increases risk as much as does the presence of the APOE ε4 allele. *APOE* is a regulator of lipoprotein metabolism that binds soluble Aβ and influences its clearance and aggregation. The presence of ε4 alleles accelerates Aβ deposition; 1 allele increases AD risk 3-fold, and 2 alleles increase AD risk 12-fold. For typical amnestic AD, the presence of an ε4 allele decreases the age of onset (but, paradoxically, within EOAD it occurs within the older range[107]); whereas, ε3 alleles tend to be found in variant phenotypes of EOAD, and ε2 alleles decrease the risk or delay AD. Other rare variants that increase risk for EOAD occur in genes including *SORL1* (sortilin-related receptor, L [DLR class]), a neuronal *APOE* receptor that plays a protective role against the secretion of Aβ[108]; the *ABCA7* (ATP binding cassette subfamily A member 7), which was present in 6.6% of patients with EOAD compared with only 2.0% of controls[109]; and coding variants such as *PLD3* (phospholipase D Family Member 3), which catalyzes the hydrolysis of membrane phospholipid, and *TREM2* (Triggering Receptor Expressed On Myeloid Cells 2), a receptor on microglia that stimulates phagocytosis and suppresses inflammation.[99]

Neuropathology

The neuropathology of EOAD resembles that of LOAD in the presence of neuritic plaques and NFTs, but differs in several respects. First, there is a greater likelihood of hippocampal sparing and more involvement of neocortex, particularly parietal and occipitoparietal, but also, to a lesser extent, frontal.[42] Second, despite early Aβ deposition, the clinicopathological manifestations are driven more by tau than by Aβ, with a relatively greater tau burden in EOAD than in LOAD. For example, in lvPPA the regional tau deposition in the left inferior parietal lobule is more closely linked to hypometabolism than amyloid density,[110] and in PCA the best correspondence with clinical symptoms is with the tau burden.[111] Although unclear, it is possible that EOAD variants could result from differences in the "strains" of soluble Aβ or oligomeric Aβ. Third, EOAD variants also may depend on greater WM involvement and selective vulnerability of long, projection neurons, which connect higher association cortex.[74]

Neural Networks

The human brain is organized as separate networks, and there is growing evidence that AD targets and spreads along network pathways with different networks being involved in different clinicopathological forms of AD.[95,112–116] Progressive changes and disconnection in neural networks are present before symptom onset in AD and before neuronal loss and regional atrophy.[117–120] All forms of AD may begin with Aβ deposition in the precuneus and related areas years before clinical symptoms, and this amyloid deposition has a permissive effect on tau and NFT spread.[121–123] The network degeneration hypothesis postulates that Aβ promotes the spread of pathologic forms of tau trans-synaptically along networks, which, in typical amnestic AD follows the "Braak and Braak progression" from the MTL-entorhinal-hippocampus to limbic and then neocortical regions probably along the DMN.[124–129] EOAD variant phenotypes reflect differences from typical amnestic AD in probable trans-synaptic spread along alternate fronto-parietal neural networks, such as the central executive network.[124,130,131] In sum, the literature suggests that Type 2 EOAD proceeds to earlier and more prominent NFTs in the posterior neocortex compared with LOAD, and involves alternate, vulnerable neural networks rather than the DMN.[27,34,37,71,76,89,132–146]

Management

Management is similar to that for LOAD but with emphasis on targeting the specific cognitive areas involved and more age-appropriate psychosocial support and education. Targeting cognition includes speech therapy for language impairment, interventions for the partially sighted for PCA, and occupational therapy for ideomotor apraxia. There must be greater psychosocial support for these patients, who are often in a highly productive time of their life, maintaining jobs and careers and supporting families. Clinicians can help these patients and their families by providing information, education, and resources on these frequently poorly understood manifestations of AD. Clinicians also must take care to provide services, such as support groups, that are specifically for those with young-onset dementia, rather than the elderly. Often the best support groups and programs are even more specifically targeted to the EOAD phenotype. For example, groups of lvPPA caregivers may discuss methods to improve communication, and groups of PCA caregivers may discuss methods to improve visual functioning in the home. As for medications, nonmemory symptoms may not significantly respond to acetylcholinesterase inhibitors or memantine, but, considering their safety, these interventions are worth trying in these patients. Finally, in the absence of disease-modifying interventions, patients and families usually appreciate the opportunity to participate in clinical drug trials.

SUMMARY

EOAD, with onset in individuals younger than 65 years, while overshadowed by the more common LOAD, differs significantly from LOAD. EOAD comprises approximately 5% of AD and is associated with delays in diagnosis, distress and confusion over symptoms, an aggressive or problematic course, and age-related psychosocial needs. One source of confusion is that a substantial percentage of EOADs are phenotypic variants ("Type 2 AD") that differ from the usual memory-disordered presentation of typical AD. These variants include lvPPA, PCA, PIA, and corticobasal syndrome from AD, and behavioral/dysexecutive AD. In addition, there is a small percentage (1.5%–5.0%) of persons with EOAD in whom the disease is inherited as an autosomal dominant trait due to identifiable gene mutations.

Patients with EOAD overall have greater parietal atrophy, more WM disturbances, and less hippocampal volume loss, compared with those with LOAD. The phenotypic variants have atrophy and WM changes in corresponding cognitive areas of the brain. On neuropathology, patients with EOAD overall have disproportionate regional amyloid and tau accumulation in the posterior neocortex. Abnormal tau drives this neocortical pathology with greater posterior cortical NFTs per GM atrophy compared with typical AD. The focal neocortical burden of NFTs is greater in left hemisphere language areas in lvPPA and in visual neocortex in PCA. The variants tended to hippocampal sparing compared with typical AD, and, in more advanced stages, the pattern of atrophy converged across the variants.[147]

Neural network differences characterize EOAD and the different phenotypes. Compared with LOAD, the phenotypic variants of EOAD involve alternate, frontoparietal and syndrome-specific neural networks rather than the posterior DMN, as in typical AD. Language networks are affected in lvPPA, visual networks in PCA, and the posterior cingulate cortex-hippocampal circuit in amnestic EOAD and LOAD. In Type 2 AD there may be primary spread along alternate neural networks rather than from mesiotemporal entorhinal cortex along the DMN as in more typical amnestic AD.

These scientific advancements in our understanding of EOAD and its variants is only a first step in advancing our management of this disorder, which is particularly devastating because of its onset in middle life. Currently, the management is similar to that for LOAD with the addition of targeting interventions for specific cognitive impairments, the provision of education on the disease, and psychosocial support aimed at the unique patient and caregiver problems due to EOAD. The advancements in our understanding of the neurobiology of EOAD holds great promise for the development of therapeutic interventions specifically targeted to the initiation, spread, and expression of the neuropathology of this disease.

REFERENCES

1. Maurer K, Volk S, Gerbaldo H. Auguste D and Alzheimer's disease. Lancet 1997;349(9064):1546–9.
2. Terry RD, Davies P. Dementia of the Alzheimer type. Annu Rev Neurosci 1980;3: 77–95.
3. Zhu XC, Tan L, Wang HF, et al. Rate of early onset Alzheimer's disease: a systematic review and meta-analysis. Ann Translational Med 2015;3(3):38.
4. Bickel H, Burger K, Hampel H, et al. Presenile dementia in memory clinics–incidence rates and clinical features. Nervenarzt 2006;77(9):1079–85 [in German].

5. Renvoize E, Hanson M, Dale M. Prevalence and causes of young onset dementia in an English health district. Int J Geriatr Psychiatry 2011;26(1):106–7.

6. Alzheimer's A. Early-onset dementia: a national challenge, a future crisis. Washington, DC: Alzheimer's Association; 2006.

7. Lambert MA, Bickel H, Prince M, et al. Estimating the burden of early onset dementia; systematic review of disease prevalence. Eur J Neurol 2014;21(4): 563–9.

8. van Vliet D, de Vugt ME, Bakker C, et al. Time to diagnosis in young-onset dementia as compared with late-onset dementia. Psychol Med 2013;43(2):423–32.

9. Moschetti K, Barragan N, Basurto-Davila R, et al. Mortality and productivity losses from Alzheimer disease among US adults aged 40 to 64 years, 1999 to 2010. Alzheimer Dis Assoc Disord 2015;29(2):165–8.

10. Eriksson H, Fereshtehnejad SM, Falahati F, et al. Differences in routine clinical practice between early and late onset Alzheimer's disease. J Alzheimers Dis 2014;41(2):411–9.

11. Nyberg J, Aberg MA, Schioler L, et al. Cardiovascular and cognitive fitness at age 18 and risk of early-onset dementia. Brain 2014;137(Pt 5):1514–23.

12. Mendez MF, Paholpak P, Lin A, et al. Prevalence of traumatic brain injury in early versus late-onset Alzheimer's disease. J Alzheimers Dis 2015;47(4):985–93.

13. Clemerson G, Walsh S, Isaac C. Towards living well with young onset dementia: an exploration of coping from the perspective of those diagnosed. Dementia (London) 2013;13(4):451–66.

14. Migliaccio R, Agosta F, Toba MN, et al. Brain networks in posterior cortical atrophy: a single case tractography study and literature review. Cortex 2012;48(10): 1298–309.

15. Kaiser NC, Melrose RJ, Liu C, et al. Neuropsychological and neuroimaging markers in early versus late-onset Alzheimer's disease. Am J Alzheimers Dis Other Demen 2012;27(7):520–9.

16. Ducharme F, Kergoat MJ, Antoine P, et al. The unique experience of spouses in early-onset dementia. Am J Alzheimers Dis Other Demen 2013;28(6):634–41.

17. Rosness TA, Barca ML, Engedal K. Occurrence of depression and its correlates in early onset dementia patients. Int J Geriatr Psychiatry 2010;25(7):704–11.

18. Gerritsen AA, Bakker C, Verhey FR, et al. Prevalence of comorbidity in patients with young-onset Alzheimer disease compared with late-onset: a comparative cohort study. J Am Med Dir Assoc 2016;17(4):318–23.

19. Jarvik L, LaRue A, Blacker D, et al. Children of persons with Alzheimer disease: what does the future hold? Alzheimer Dis Assoc Disord 2008;22(1):6–20.

20. Koedam EL, Pijnenburg YA, Deeg DJ, et al. Early-onset dementia is associated with higher mortality. Dement Geriatr Cogn Disord 2008;26(2):147–52.

21. Schott JM, Ridha BH, Crutch SJ, et al. Apolipoprotein e genotype modifies the phenotype of Alzheimer disease. Arch Neurol 2006;63(1):155–6.

22. Panegyres PK, Chen HY. Differences between early and late onset Alzheimer's disease. Am J Neurodegenerative Dis 2013;2(4):6.

23. Smits LL, Pijnenburg YA, van der Vlies AE, et al. Early onset APOE E4-negative Alzheimer's disease patients show faster cognitive decline on non-memory domains. Eur Neuropsychopharmacol 2015;25(7):1010–7.

24. Stanley K, Walker Z. Do patients with young onset Alzheimer's disease deteriorate faster than those with late onset Alzheimer's disease? A review of the literature. Int psychogeriatr 2014;26(12):1945–53.

25. Palasi A, Gutierrez-Iglesias B, Alegret M, et al. Differentiated clinical presentation of early and late-onset Alzheimer's disease: is 65 years of age providing a reliable threshold? J Neurol 2015;262(5):1238–46.
26. Joubert S, Gour N, Guedj E, et al. Early-onset and late-onset Alzheimer's disease are associated with distinct patterns of memory impairment. Cortex 2016;74:217–32.
27. Cho H, Jeon S, Kang SJ, et al. Longitudinal changes of cortical thickness in early- versus late-onset Alzheimer's disease. Neurobiol Aging 2013;34(7): 1921.e09–15.
28. Migliaccio R, Agosta F, Possin KL, et al. Mapping the progression of atrophy in early- and late-onset Alzheimer's disease. J Alzheimers Dis 2015;46(2):351–64.
29. Hamelin L, Bertoux M, Bottlaender M, et al. Sulcal morphology as a new imaging marker for the diagnosis of early onset Alzheimer's disease. Neurobiol Aging 2015;36(11):2932–9.
30. Chiaravalloti A, Koch G, Toniolo S, et al. Comparison between early-onset and late-onset Alzheimer's disease patients with amnestic presentation: CSF and (18)F-FDG PET study. Dement Geriatr Cogn Disord 2016;6(1):108–19.
31. Ballarini T, Iaccarino L, Magnani G, et al. Neuropsychiatric subsyndromes and brain metabolic network dysfunctions in early onset Alzheimer's disease. Hum Brain Mapp 2016;37(12):4234–47.
32. Daianu M, Mendez MF, Baboyan VG, et al. An advanced white matter tract analysis in frontotemporal dementia and early-onset Alzheimer's disease. Brain Imaging Behav 2015;10(4):1038–53.
33. Kim MJ, Seo SW, Kim ST, et al. Diffusion tensor changes according to age at onset and apolipoprotein E genotype in Alzheimer disease. Alzheimer Dis Assoc Disord 2016;30(4):297–304.
34. Canu E, Agosta F, Spinelli EG, et al. White matter microstructural damage in Alzheimer's disease at different ages of onset. Neurobiol Aging 2013;34(10): 2331–40.
35. Caso F, Agosta F, Mattavelli D, et al. White matter degeneration in atypical Alzheimer disease. Radiology 2015;277(1):162–72.
36. Daianu M, Jahanshad N, Mendez MF, et al. Communication of brain network core connections altered in behavioral variant frontotemporal dementia but possibly preserved in early-onset Alzheimer's disease. Proc SPIE Int Soc Opt Eng 2015;9413 [pii: 941322].
37. Stopford CL, Snowden JS, Thompson JC, et al. Variability in cognitive presentation of Alzheimer's disease. Cortex 2008;44(2):185–95.
38. Alladi S, Xuereb J, Bak T, et al. Focal cortical presentations of Alzheimer's disease. Brain 2007;130(Pt 10):2636–45.
39. Davidson Y, Gibbons L, Pritchard A, et al. Apolipoprotein E epsilon4 allele frequency and age at onset of Alzheimer's disease. Dement Geriatr Cogn Disord 2007;23(1):60–6.
40. van der Flier WM, Pijnenburg YA, Fox NC, et al. Early-onset versus late-onset Alzheimer's disease: the case of the missing APOE epsilon4 allele. Lancet Neurol 2011;10(3):280–8.
41. Park HK, Choi SH, Park SA, et al. Cognitive profiles and neuropsychiatric symptoms in Korean early-onset Alzheimer's disease patients: a CREDOS study. J Alzheimers Dis 2015;44(2):661–73.
42. Murray ME, Graff-Radford NR, Ross OA, et al. Neuropathologically defined subtypes of Alzheimer's disease with distinct clinical characteristics: a retrospective study. Lancet Neurol 2011;10(9):785–96.

43. Koedam EL, Lauffer V, van der Vlies AE, et al. Early-versus late-onset Alzheimer's disease: more than age alone. J Alzheimers Dis 2010;19(4):1401–8.

44. Smits LL, Pijnenburg YA, Koedam EL, et al. Early onset Alzheimer's disease is associated with a distinct neuropsychological profile. J Alzheimers Dis 2012; 30(1):101–8.

45. Gorno-Tempini ML, Hillis AE, Weintraub S, et al. Classification of primary progressive aphasia and its variants. Neurology 2011;76(11):1006–14.

46. Tsai PH, Teng E, Liu C, et al. Posterior cortical atrophy: evidence for discrete syndromes of early-onset Alzheimer's disease. Am J Alzheimers Dis Other Demen 2011;26(5):413–8.

47. Mendez MF, Ghajarania M, Perryman KM. Posterior cortical atrophy: clinical characteristics and differences compared to Alzheimer's disease. Dement Geriatr Cogn Disord 2002;14(1):33–40.

48. Ossenkoppele R, Pijnenburg YA, Perry DC, et al. The behavioural/dysexecutive variant of Alzheimer's disease: clinical, neuroimaging and pathological features. Brain 2015;138(Pt 9):2732–49.

49. Lee SE, Rabinovici GD, Mayo MC, et al. Clinicopathological correlations in corticobasal degeneration. Ann Neurol 2011;70(2):327–40.

50. Magnin E, Sylvestre G, Lenoir F, et al. Logopenic syndrome in posterior cortical atrophy. J Neurol 2013;260(2):528–33.

51. Ahmed S, de Jager CA, Haigh AM, et al. Logopenic aphasia in Alzheimer's disease: clinical variant or clinical feature? J Neurol Neurosurg Psychiatr 2012; 83(11):1056–62.

52. Cerami C, Crespi C, Della Rosa PA, et al. Brain changes within the visuo-spatial attentional network in posterior cortical atrophy. J Alzheimers Dis 2014;43(2): 385–95.

53. Gour N, Felician O, Didic M, et al. Functional connectivity changes differ in early and late-onset Alzheimer's disease. Hum Brain Mapp 2014;35(7):2978–94.

54. Laforce R Jr, Tosun D, Ghosh P, et al. Parallel ICA of FDG-PET and PiB-PET in three conditions with underlying Alzheimer's pathology. Neuroimage Clin 2014;4:508–16.

55. Lehmann M, Madison CM, Ghosh PM, et al. Intrinsic connectivity networks in healthy subjects explain clinical variability in Alzheimer's disease. Proc Natl Acad Sci U S A 2013;110(28):11606–11.

56. Blautzik J, Keeser D, Berman A, et al. Long-term test-retest reliability of resting-state networks in healthy elderly subjects and with amnestic mild cognitive impairment patients. J Alzheimers Dis 2013;34(3):741–54.

57. Dennis EL, Thompson PM. Functional brain connectivity using fMRI in aging and Alzheimer's disease. Neuropsychol Rev 2014;24(1):49–62.

58. Sorg C, Riedl V, Perneczky R, et al. Impact of Alzheimer's disease on the functional connectivity of spontaneous brain activity. Curr Alzheimer Res 2009;6(6): 541–53.

59. Krajcovicova L, Mikl M, Marecek R, et al. Disturbed default mode network connectivity patterns in Alzheimer's disease associated with visual processing. J Alzheimers Dis 2014;41(4):1229–38.

60. Hampel H. Amyloid-beta and cognition in aging and Alzheimer's disease: molecular and neurophysiological mechanisms. J Alzheimers Dis 2013; 33(Suppl 1):S79–86.

61. Sperling R. Potential of functional MRI as a biomarker in early Alzheimer's disease. Neurobiol Aging 2011;32(Suppl 1):S37–43.

62. Agosta F, Pievani M, Geroldi C, et al. Resting state fMRI in Alzheimer's disease: beyond the default mode network. Neurobiol Aging 2012;33(8):1564–78.
63. de Haan W, van der Flier WM, Koene T, et al. Disrupted modular brain dynamics reflect cognitive dysfunction in Alzheimer's disease. Neuroimage 2012;59(4): 3085–93.
64. Das SR, Pluta J, Mancuso L, et al. Increased functional connectivity within medial temporal lobe in mild cognitive impairment. Hippocampus 2013; 23(1):1–6.
65. Lehmann M, Madison C, Ghosh PM, et al. Loss of functional connectivity is greater outside the default mode network in nonfamilial early-onset Alzheimer's disease variants. Neurobiol Aging 2015;36(10):2678–86.
66. Whitwell JL, Jones DT, Duffy JR, et al. Working memory and language network dysfunctions in logopenic aphasia: a task-free fMRI comparison with Alzheimer's dementia. Neurobiol Aging 2015;36(3):1245–52.
67. Neufang S, Akhrif A, Riedl V, et al. Disconnection of frontal and parietal areas contributes to impaired attention in very early Alzheimer's disease. J Alzheimers Dis 2011;25(2):309–21.
68. Balthazar ML, Pereira FR, Lopes TM, et al. Neuropsychiatric symptoms in Alzheimer's disease are related to functional connectivity alterations in the salience network. Hum Brain Mapp 2014;35(4):1237–46.
69. Mahoney CJ, Malone IB, Ridgway GR, et al. White matter tract signatures of the progressive aphasias. Neurobiol Aging 2013;34(6):1687–99.
70. Seeley WW, Menon V, Schatzberg AF, et al. Dissociable intrinsic connectivity networks for salience processing and executive control. J Neurosci 2007; 27(9):2349–56.
71. Frisoni GB, Pievani M, Testa C, et al. The topography of grey matter involvement in early and late onset Alzheimer's disease. Brain 2007;130(Pt 3):720–30.
72. Kalpouzos G, Eustache F, de la Sayette V, et al. Working memory and FDG-PET dissociate early and late onset Alzheimer disease patients. J Neurol 2005; 252(5):548–58.
73. Rogalski E, Johnson N, Weintraub S, et al. Increased frequency of learning disability in patients with primary progressive aphasia and their first-degree relatives. Arch Neurol 2008;65(2):244–8.
74. Miller ZA, Mandelli ML, Rankin KP, et al. Handedness and language learning disability differentially distribute in progressive aphasia variants. Brain 2013; 136(Pt 11):3461–73.
75. Seifan A, Assuras S, Huey ED, et al. Childhood learning disabilities and atypical dementia: a retrospective chart review. PLoS One 2015;10(6):e0129919.
76. Migliaccio R, Agosta F, Rascovsky K, et al. Clinical syndromes associated with posterior atrophy: early age at onset AD spectrum. Neurology 2009;73(19): 1571–8.
77. Rabinovici GD, Jagust WJ, Furst AJ, et al. Abeta amyloid and glucose metabolism in three variants of primary progressive aphasia. Ann Neurol 2008; 64(4):388–401.
78. Mesulam M, Wicklund A, Johnson N, et al. Alzheimer and frontotemporal pathology in subsets of primary progressive aphasia. Ann Neurol 2008;63(6):709–19.
79. Galantucci S, Tartaglia MC, Wilson SM, et al. White matter damage in primary progressive aphasias: a diffusion tensor tractography study. Brain 2011; 134(Pt 10):3011–29.
80. Leyton CE, Piguet O, Savage S, et al. The neural basis of logopenic progressive aphasia. J Alzheimers Dis 2012;32(4):1051–9.

81. Baldo JV, Katseff S, Dronkers NF. Brain regions underlying repetition and auditory-verbal short-term memory deficits in aphasia: evidence from voxel-based lesion symptom mapping. Aphasiology 2012;26(3–4):338–54.

82. Meyer AM, Snider SF, Campbell RE, et al. Phonological short-term memory in logopenic variant primary progressive aphasia and mild Alzheimer's disease. Cortex 2015;71:183–9.

83. Benson DF, Davis RJ, Snyder BD. Posterior cortical atrophy. Arch Neurol 1988; 45(7):789–93.

84. Ahmed S, Baker I, Husain M, et al. Memory impairment at initial clinical presentation in posterior cortical atrophy. J Alzheimers Dis 2016;52(4):1245–50.

85. Crutch SJ, Schott JM, Rabinovici GD, et al. Shining a light on posterior cortical atrophy. Alzheimers Dement 2012;9(4):463–5.

86. Tang-Wai DF, Graff-Radford NR. Looking into posterior cortical atrophy: providing insight into Alzheimer disease. Neurology 2011;76(21):1778–9.

87. Migliaccio R, Agosta F, Scola E, et al. Ventral and dorsal visual streams in posterior cortical atrophy: A DT MRI study. Neurobiol Aging 2012;33(11):2572–84.

88. Meek BP, Shelton P, Marotta JJ. Posterior cortical atrophy: visuomotor deficits in reaching and grasping. Front Hum Neurosci 2013;7:294.

89. Gefen T, Gasho K, Rademaker A, et al. Clinically concordant variations of Alzheimer pathology in aphasic versus amnestic dementia. Brain 2012; 135(Pt 5):1554–65.

90. Tang-Wai DF, Graff-Radford NR, Boeve BF, et al. Clinical, genetic, and neuropathologic characteristics of posterior cortical atrophy. Neurology 2004;63(7): 1168–74.

91. Carrasquillo MM, Khan QU, Murray ME, et al. Late-onset Alzheimer disease genetic variants in posterior cortical atrophy and posterior AD. Neurology 2014; 82(16):1455–62.

92. Ridgway GR, Lehmann M, Barnes J, et al. Early-onset Alzheimer disease clinical variants: multivariate analyses of cortical thickness. Neurology 2012; 79(1):80–4.

93. Lehmann M, Koedam EL, Barnes J, et al. Posterior cerebral atrophy in the absence of medial temporal lobe atrophy in pathologically-confirmed Alzheimer's disease. Neurobiol Aging 2012;33(3):627.e1–12.

94. Ossenkoppele R, Mattsson N, Teunissen CE, et al. Cerebrospinal fluid biomarkers and cerebral atrophy in distinct clinical variants of probable Alzheimer's disease. Neurobiol Aging 2015;36(8):2340–7.

95. Teng E, Yamasaki TR, Tran M, et al. Cerebrospinal fluid biomarkers in clinical subtypes of early-onset Alzheimer's disease. Dement Geriatr Cogn Disord 2014;37(5–6):307–14.

96. Molinuevo JL, Blennow K, Dubois B, et al. The clinical use of cerebrospinal fluid biomarker testing for Alzheimer's disease diagnosis: a consensus paper from the Alzheimer's Biomarkers Standardization Initiative. Alzheimers Dement 2014;10(6):808–17.

97. Ossenkoppele R, Jansen WJ, Rabinovici GD, et al. Prevalence of amyloid PET positivity in dementia syndromes: a meta-analysis. JAMA 2015;313(19): 1939–49.

98. Fagan AM. What does it mean to be 'amyloid-positive'? Brain 2015;138(Pt 3): 514–6.

99. Karch CM, Goate AM. Alzheimer's disease risk genes and mechanisms of disease pathogenesis. Biol Psychiatry 2015;77(1):43–51.

100. Jarmolowicz AI, Chen HY, Panegyres PK. The patterns of inheritance in early-onset dementia: Alzheimer's disease and frontotemporal dementia. Am J Alzheimers Dis Other Demen 2015;30(3):299–306.

101. Joshi A, Ringman JM, Lee AS, et al. Comparison of clinical characteristics between familial and non-familial early onset Alzheimer's disease. J Neurol 2012; 259(10):2182–8.

102. Muller U, Winter P, Graeber MB. A presenilin 1 mutation in the first case of Alzheimer's disease. Lancet Neurol 2013;12(2):129–30.

103. Ringman JM. Are late-onset autosomal dominant and sporadic Alzheimer disease "Separate but Equal"? JAMA Neurol 2016;73(9):1060–1.

104. Nicolas G, Wallon D, Charbonnier C, et al. Screening of dementia genes by whole-exome sequencing in early-onset Alzheimer disease: input and lessons. Eur J Hum Genet 2016;24(5):710–6.

105. Blauwendraat C, Wilke C, Jansen IE, et al. Pilot whole-exome sequencing of a German early-onset Alzheimer's disease cohort reveals a substantial frequency of PSEN2 variants. Neurobiol Aging 2016;37:208.e11–7.

106. Barber IS, Garcia-Cardenas JM, Sakdapanichkul C, et al. Screening exons 16 and 17 of the amyloid precursor protein gene in sporadic early-onset Alzheimer's disease. Neurobiol Aging 2016;39:220.e1–7.

107. De Luca V, Orfei MD, Gaudenzi S, et al. Inverse effect of the APOE epsilon4 allele in late- and early-onset Alzheimer's disease. Eur Arch Psychiatry Clin Neurosci 2015;266(7):599–606.

108. Nicolas G, Charbonnier C, Wallon D, et al. SORL1 rare variants: a major risk factor for familial early-onset Alzheimer's disease. Mol Psychiatry 2016;21(6): 831–6.

109. Le Guennec K, Nicolas G, Quenez O, et al. ABCA7 rare variants and Alzheimer disease risk. Neurology 2016;86(23):2134–7.

110. Pascual B, Masdeu JC. Tau, amyloid, and hypometabolism in the logopenic variant of primary progressive aphasia. Neurology 2016;86(5):487–8.

111. Ossenkoppele R, Schonhaut DR, Baker SL, et al. Tau, amyloid, and hypometabolism in a patient with posterior cortical atrophy. Ann Neurol 2015;77(2):338–42.

112. Seppala TT, Nerg O, Koivisto AM, et al. CSF biomarkers for Alzheimer disease correlate with cortical brain biopsy findings. Neurology 2012;78(20):1568–75.

113. Dai Z, He Y. Disrupted structural and functional brain connectomes in mild cognitive impairment and Alzheimer's disease. Neurosci Bull 2014;30(2): 217–32.

114. Bokde AL, Ewers M, Hampel H. Assessing neuronal networks: understanding Alzheimer's disease. Prog Neurobiol 2009;89(2):125–33.

115. Sun Y, Yin Q, Fang R, et al. Disrupted functional brain connectivity and its association to structural connectivity in amnestic mild cognitive impairment and Alzheimer's disease. PLoS One 2014;9(5):e96505.

116. Pineda-Pardo JA, Garces P, Lopez ME, et al. White matter damage disorganizes brain functional networks in amnestic mild cognitive impairment. Brain Connect 2014;4(5):312–22.

117. Savioz A, Leuba G, Vallet PG, et al. Contribution of neural networks to Alzheimer disease's progression. Brain Res Bull 2009;80(4–5):309–14.

118. Brier MR, Thomas JB, Fagan AM, et al. Functional connectivity and graph theory in preclinical Alzheimer's disease. Neurobiol Aging 2014;35(4):757–68.

119. D'Amelio M, Rossini PM. Brain excitability and connectivity of neuronal assemblies in Alzheimer's disease: from animal models to human findings. Prog Neurobiol 2012;99(1):42–60.

120. Jacobs HI, Radua J, Luckmann HC, et al. Meta-analysis of functional network alterations in Alzheimer's disease: toward a network biomarker. Neurosci Biobehav Rev 2013;37(5):753–65.
121. Mattsson N, Insel PS, Nosheny R, et al. Emerging beta-amyloid pathology and accelerated cortical atrophy. JAMA Neurol 2014;71(6):725–34.
122. Jack CR Jr, Knopman DS, Jagust WJ, et al. Hypothetical model of dynamic biomarkers of the Alzheimer's pathological cascade. Lancet Neurol 2010;9(1): 119–28.
123. Sperling RA, Aisen PS, Beckett LA, et al. Toward defining the preclinical stages of Alzheimer's disease: recommendations from the National Institute on Aging-Alzheimer's Association workgroups on diagnostic guidelines for Alzheimer's disease. Alzheimers Dement 2011;7(3):280–92.
124. Braak H, Braak E. Neuropathological stageing of Alzheimer-related changes. Acta Neuropathol 1991;82(4):239–59.
125. Buerger K, Ewers M, Pirttila T, et al. CSF phosphorylated tau protein correlates with neocortical neurofibrillary pathology in Alzheimer's disease. Brain 2006; 129(Pt 11):3035–41.
126. Spreng RN, Turner GR. Structural covariance of the default network in healthy and pathological aging. J Neurosci 2013;33(38):15226–34.
127. Spires-Jones TL, Hyman BT. The intersection of amyloid beta and tau at synapses in Alzheimer's disease. Neuron 2014;82(4):756–71.
128. Jack CR Jr, Wiste HJ, Knopman DS, et al. Rates of beta-amyloid accumulation are independent of hippocampal neurodegeneration. Neurology 2014;82(18): 1605–12.
129. Jack CR Jr, Knopman DS, Jagust WJ, et al. Tracking pathophysiological processes in Alzheimer's disease: an updated hypothetical model of dynamic biomarkers. Lancet Neurol 2013;12(2):207–16.
130. Jack CR Jr, Holtzman DM. Biomarker modeling of Alzheimer's disease. Neuron 2013;80(6):1347–58.
131. de Calignon A, Polydoro M, Suarez-Calvet M, et al. Propagation of tau pathology in a model of early Alzheimer's disease. Neuron 2012;73(4):685–97.
132. Tang-Wai D, Mapstone M. What are we seeing? Is posterior cortical atrophy just Alzheimer disease? Neurology 2006;66(3):300–1.
133. Davidson YS, Raby S, Foulds PG, et al. TDP-43 pathological changes in early onset familial and sporadic Alzheimer's disease, late onset Alzheimer's disease and Down's syndrome: association with age, hippocampal sclerosis and clinical phenotype. Acta Neuropathol 2011;122(6):703–13.
134. Malkani RG, Dickson DW, Simuni T. Hippocampal-sparing Alzheimer's disease presenting as corticobasal syndrome. Parkinsonism Relat Disord 2011;18(5): 683–5.
135. Ossenkoppele R, Zwan MD, Tolboom N, et al. Amyloid burden and metabolic function in early-onset Alzheimer's disease: parietal lobe involvement. Brain 2012;135(Pt 7):2115–25.
136. Shibuya Y, Kawakatsu S, Hayashi H, et al. Comparison of entorhinal cortex atrophy between early-onset and late-onset Alzheimer's disease using the VSRAD, a specific and sensitive voxel-based morphometry. Int J Geriatr Psychiatry 2013; 28(4):372–6.
137. Ishii K, Kawachi T, Sasaki H, et al. Voxel-based morphometric comparison between early- and late-onset mild Alzheimer's disease and assessment of diagnostic performance of z score images. AJNR Am J Neuroradiol 2005;26(2): 333–40.

138. Rabinovici GD, Furst AJ, Alkalay A, et al. Increased metabolic vulnerability in early-onset Alzheimer's disease is not related to amyloid burden. Brain 2010; 133(Pt 2):512–28.
139. Shiino A, Watanabe T, Maeda K, et al. Four subgroups of Alzheimer's disease based on patterns of atrophy using VBM and a unique pattern for early onset disease. Neuroimage 2006;33(1):17–26.
140. Kim EJ, Cho SS, Jeong Y, et al. Glucose metabolism in early onset versus late onset Alzheimer's disease: an SPM analysis of 120 patients. Brain 2005; 128(Pt 8):1790–801.
141. Sakamoto S, Ishii K, Sasaki M, et al. Differences in cerebral metabolic impairment between early and late onset types of Alzheimer's disease. J Neurol Sci 2002;200(1–2):27–32.
142. Mielke R, Herholz K, Grond M, et al. Differences of regional cerebral glucose metabolism between presenile and senile dementia of Alzheimer type. Neurobiol Aging 1992;13(1):93–8.
143. Karas G, Scheltens P, Rombouts S, et al. Precuneus atrophy in early-onset Alzheimer's disease: a morphometric structural MRI study. Neuroradiology 2007;49(12):967–76.
144. Whitwell JL, Jack CR Jr, Przybelski SA, et al. Temporoparietal atrophy: a marker of AD pathology independent of clinical diagnosis. Neurobiol Aging 2011;32(9): 1531–41.
145. Moller C, Vrenken H, Jiskoot L, et al. Different patterns of gray matter atrophy in early- and late-onset Alzheimer's disease. Neurobiol Aging 2013;34(8):2014–22.
146. Marshall GA, Fairbanks LA, Tekin S, et al. Early-onset Alzheimer's disease is associated with greater pathologic burden. J Geriatr Psychiatry Neurol 2007; 20(1):29–33.
147. Ossenkoppele R, Cohn-Sheehy BI, La Joie R, et al. Atrophy patterns in early clinical stages across distinct phenotypes of Alzheimer's disease. Hum Brain Mapp 2015;36(11):4421–37.
148. Mendez MF, Lee AS, Joshi A, et al. Nonamnestic presentations of early-onset Alzheimer's disease. Am J Alzheimers Dis Other Demen 2012;27(6):413–20.
149. Snowden JS, Stopford CL, Julien CL, et al. Cognitive phenotypes in Alzheimer's disease and genetic risk. Cortex 2007;43(7):835–45.
150. Binetti G, Magni E, Padovani A, et al. Executive dysfunction in early Alzheimer's disease. J Neurol Neurosurg Psychiatr 1996;60(1):91–3.
151. Johnson JK, Head E, Kim R, et al. Clinical and pathological evidence for a frontal variant of Alzheimer disease. Arch Neurol 1999;56(10):1233–9.
152. Swanberg MM, Tractenberg RE, Mohs R, et al. Executive dysfunction in Alzheimer disease. Arch Neurol 2004;61(4):556–60.
153. Woodward M, Jacova C, Black SE, et al. Differentiating the frontal variant of Alzheimer's disease. Int J Geriatr Psychiatry 2010;25(7):732–8.

Late-Onset Alzheimer Disease

Aimee L. Pierce, MD[a],*, Szofia S. Bullain, MD[b], Claudia H. Kawas, MD[c]

KEYWORDS

- Late-onset • Alzheimer disease • Dementia • Oldest-old • Pathology

KEY POINTS

- There is an urgent societal need for interventions to delay or treat Alzheimer disease (AD), particularly in the oldest-old, which represent the fastest growing segment of society.
- Rates of dementia continue to increase as people age into their 9th and 10th decades.
- Dementia in the oldest-old is often due to mixed pathologies, including amyloid plaques and neurofibrillary tangles of AD, as well as microinfarcts, hippocampal sclerosis, and more rarely Lewy Bodies.
- The typical presentation of AD in the oldest-old is short-term memory impairment gradually progressing to involve other domains of cognition (language, visuospatial, and executive dysfunction) and leading to functional impairment.
- It is challenging to diagnose dementia in the oldest-old due to reduced societal and familial expectations of function, medical comorbidities, and difficulty performing cognitive testing due to visual or hearing impairment, fatigue, and physical disability.

OVERVIEW

The oldest-old, people 85 years and older, are the fastest growing segment of society, and neurologists must be prepared to diagnose and treat dementia in this age group. The prevalence and risk of dementia in this group is high and continues to rise with advancing age. Increasingly, we have come to recognize that the oldest-old are a

Disclosure Statement: The authors have nothing to disclose and no commercial or financial conflicts of interest.
Funding Source: Supported by grants from the National Institutes of Health (R01AG21055, P50AG16573).
[a] Department of Neurology and Institute for Memory Impairments and Neurological Disorders, University of California, Irvine, 1100 Medical Plaza Drive, Irvine, CA 92697, USA; [b] Department of Neurology and Institute for Memory Impairments and Neurological Disorders, University of California, Irvine, 1515 Hewitt Hall, Irvine, CA 92697, USA; [c] Departments of Neurology, Neurobiology & Behavior, Epidemiology, and Institute for Memory Impairments and Neurological Disorders, University of California, Irvine, 1121 Gillespie, Irvine, CA 92697, USA
* Corresponding author.
E-mail address: piercea@uci.edu

unique population with unique risk factors for Alzheimer disease (AD) and dementia. AD remains the most common cause of dementia in the oldest-old, but mixed pathologies are often present and contribute to cognitive impairment. The typical presentation of clinical AD in the oldest-old often begins with the gradual onset of short-term memory impairment, then progresses to involve other domains of cognition, such as language, visuospatial, and executive function, ultimately leading to functional impairment. It can be challenging to diagnose dementia in the oldest-old due to lack of an informant for the many oldest-old who live alone, reduced functional expectations, difficulty performing and interpreting cognitive testing in this age group, and presence of positive amyloid biomarkers in many cognitively healthy elderly persons. Treatment of AD dementia in the oldest-old is extrapolated from younger elderly persons, because the oldest-old have generally been excluded from treatment trials. There is no treatment that can slow or reverse the progression of AD dementia, although acetylcholinesterase inhibitors and memantine can provide modest cognitive and functional benefits. Treating medical and psychiatric comorbidities and ensuring adequate home care and social support are critical. There is an urgent need for interventions to prevent or delay AD dementia in the oldest-old, for the benefit of individuals at risk, their families, and society.

EPIDEMIOLOGY

Our oldest citizens are the fastest growing segment of societies worldwide. In 2010, there were approximately 5.6 million people age 85 and older in the United States. This number is projected to quadruple by midcentury.[1] However, living long does not necessarily mean living well, as the oldest-old have the highest rates of incident and prevalent dementia and AD in the population.[2]

Fig. 1 shows the estimated total number of people age 85 and older[1] and the projected number of oldest-old with prevalent AD dementia[3] in the United States from

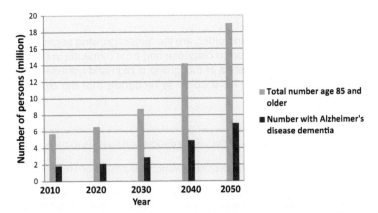

Fig. 1. Predicted number of oldest-old total and with dementia in the United States. The predicted total number of oldest-old and the predicted number of oldest-old with AD dementia in the United States 2010 to 2050 based on the national population projections data by the US Census Bureau and AD prevalence estimates by Hebert and colleagues. (*Data from* National Population Projections (Based on Census 2000). Table 12. Projections of the population by age and sex for the United States: 2010 to 2050 2008. Available at: http://www.census.gov/population/www/projections/summarytables.html. Accessed February 29, 2012; and Hebert LE, Weuve J, Scherr PA, et al. Alzheimer disease in the United States (2010–2050) estimated using the 2010 census. Neurology 2013;80:1778–83.)

2010 to 2050. In 2010, approximately 32% of the oldest-old had AD dementia, affecting approximately 1.8 million people. This number is predicted to increase to approximately 7 million (36.6%) oldest-old individuals with AD dementia by 2050. Based on the growth of the Baby Boomer generation, by midcentury 50% of all AD dementia cases will be in the oldest-old.[3]

The incidence of AD is also the highest among the oldest-old. In 2016, the estimated annual incidence of AD in people age 85 and older was approximately 37 new cases per 1000 persons, which is almost triple the incidence rate of 13 new cases per 1000 persons among people age 75 to 84. The higher incidence rate of all-cause dementia, including AD dementia, in the oldest-old has also been demonstrated by a number of different epidemiologic studies from around the globe, as shown in **Fig. 2**. Similarly, the mortality rate from AD is also highest among the oldest-old. Although the AD attributable death rate is estimated at 172 per 100,000 persons in people aged 75 to 84 years, this rate jumps to 930 per 100,000 persons in people aged 85 and older in the United States.[4]

RISK FACTORS

Studying risk and protective factors for AD in the oldest-old is particularly challenging, as the proportion of underlying mixed pathologies increases with age.[2] Subsequently,

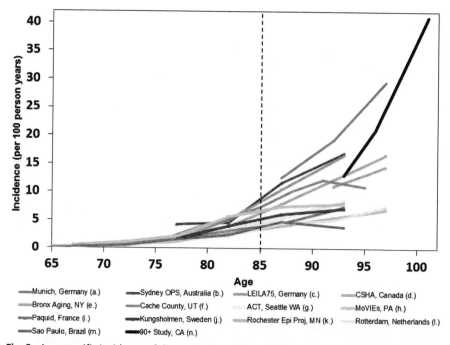

Fig. 2. Age-specific incidence of dementia in studies with oldest-old subjects. [a] Fichter MM, Eur Arch Psychiatry Clin Neurosci, 1996; [b] Waite LM, Int J Geriatr Psychiatry, 2001; [c] Riedel-Heller SG, Br J Psychiatry, 2001; [d] Canadian Study of Health and Aging, Neurology, 2000; [e] Hall CB, Neurology, 2005; [f] Miech RA, Neurology, 2002; [g] Kukull WA, Arch Neurol, 2002; [h] Ganguli M, Neurology, 2000; [i] Letenneur L, Int J Epidemiol, 1994; [j] Fratiglioni L, Neurology, 1997; [k] Edland SD, Arch Neurol, 2002; [l] Ruitenberg A, Neurobiol Aging, 2001; [m] Nitrini R, Alzheimer Dis Assoc Disord, 2004; and [n] Corrada MM, Ann Neurol, 2010. (*Courtesy of* Dr Maria M. Corrada.)

many studies have focused on identifying risk and protective factors for all-cause dementia in this age group. Nevertheless, it is evident that the constellation of risk and protective factors for all-cause dementia and AD change in the oldest-old. Among all risk factors, age remains the strongest risk factor for dementia and AD in the oldest-old.[5] Low levels of education, low levels of physical activity, and poor physical performance have also been associated with an increased risk of late-age dementia.[2,6] However, many of the traditional risk factors lose their effect or have the opposite effect on the risk of developing AD. In particular, Apolipoprotein E ε4 allele (APOE*E4), a strong genetic risk factor for AD dementia in younger elderly,[7] has been shown to have little effect on the risk of dementia in the oldest-old.[2,5,7] On the other hand, although the presence of elevated blood pressure increases the risk of dementia and AD in younger elderly, its effect after age 85 appears to be protective for dementia.[5,8] The mechanism of the observed protective effect of hypertension in the oldest-old is still under investigation, although one hypothesis is that it is related to protection from cerebral hypoperfusion that develops as an aging-associated phenomenon.[2,5] Moreover, data from the Oregon Brain Aging Study showed that good or optimal health (ie, having had no history of major medical, neurologic, or psychiatric illnesses; vitamin deficiencies; major surgeries; head trauma; or substance abuse) at age 85 and older was associated with delayed onset of AD, although the lifetime risk of the disease remained the same as in the general population.[9]

PATHOLOGY

The neuropathological signature of AD dementia is the presence of amyloid plaques and neurofibrillary tangles. The prevalence of AD plaques and tangles in the brain increases with advancing age, and 60% to 70% of the oldest-old with clinical dementia have intermediate and high levels of AD pathology, defined by the National Institute of Aging (NIA)-Reagan criteria.[10] Although AD is the most frequently detected pathology, the hallmark of the neuropathology underlying dementia in the oldest-old is the presence of multiple pathologies. Most individuals with dementia have 2 or more pathologies at autopsy, including many forms of vascular disease (small and large cerebral infarctions, microinfarcts, cerebral amyloid angiopathy, atherosclerosis), hippocampal sclerosis, and to a lesser extent, Lewy bodies and changes of frontotemporal lobar degeneration. The frequency of multiple pathologies complicates making the etiologic diagnosis of the dementia in these patients. Further confounding the diagnostic process is the high frequency of AD pathology in individuals without dementia in this age range. In The 90+ Study, a population-based cohort study of aging and dementia in people aged 90 years and older, approximately 40% of individuals without dementia had intermediate and high levels of AD pathology. It is not known if this represents preclinical disease or resilience.

Fig. 3 shows the distribution of primary and secondary pathologies in individuals aged 90 and older with and without dementia. One of the most frequent "other pathologies" is hippocampal sclerosis. The prevalence of hippocampal sclerosis is strongly age-related and occurs in 20% to 30% of individuals with dementia who die when older than 85. However, we have no validated clinical criteria for the diagnosis of this disorder, and most of these patients are clinically diagnosed as AD, which they frequently also have at autopsy. Similarly, the presence of microinfarcts increases with age. Several investigators have noted a relationship between microinfarcts and dementia that is independent and as strong as the relationship of AD neurofibrillary tangles to dementia.[11,12] The greater the number of pathologies detected at autopsy, the greater the risk and the severity of dementia.[13] Although

Dementia
(N = 98)

No Dementia
(N = 85)

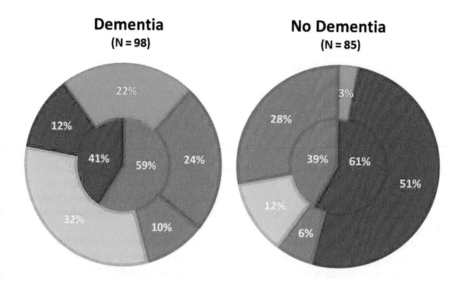

■ HS ■ AD Pathology ■ Other Pathologies ▨ Microinfarcts and Vascular ■ None

Fig. 3. Distribution of pathologic findings in participants aged 90 and older with and without dementia from *The 90+ Study*. The inner circles show the distribution of the primary pathology (AD or none). The outer circles depict the distribution of the secondary pathologies in relationship to the primary pathologies. AD: Intermediate/High level pathology by NIA-Reagan criteria; Vascular: Lacunar infarcts, large-vessel infarcts, white matter gliosis; Other: Lewy bodies, cerebral amyloid angiopathy, glioblastoma, cortical basal degeneration. (*Courtesy of* Mr Thomas Trieu.)

the number of neuropathologies at autopsy is related to risk and severity of dementia, not all pathologies are equal. **Fig. 4** shows the odds of having dementia in *The 90+ Study* in the presence of AD pathology alone, other types of pathology alone, and each in combination with one or more additional pathologies. Participants with

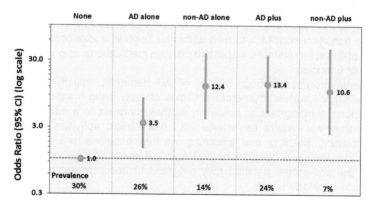

Type of Neuropathology

Fig. 4. Odds of dementia by type of neuropathology in *The 90+ Autopsy Study*. Analyses were done using logistic regression adjusting for age at death and sex (N = 183). CI, confidence interval. (*Data from* Kawas CH, Kim RC, Sonnen JA, et al. Multiple pathologies are common and related to dementia in the oldest-old: The 90+ Study. Neurology 2015;85:535–42.)

intermediate/high AD pathology alone were 3 times more likely to have dementia (odds ratio = 3.5), but those with single non-AD pathologies (mostly hippocampal sclerosis and microvascular ischemic disease) were 12 times more likely to have dementia (odds ratio = 12.4). When a second pathology was present, the likelihood of dementia increased fourfold in those with intermediate/high AD pathology but did not change in those with non-AD pathologies, suggesting that pathologies may interrelate in different ways.

CLINICAL FEATURES

The most typical clinical features of late-onset AD include the gradual onset of short-term memory impairment, which over the course of several years progresses to involve other aspects of cognition, including language impairment, executive dysfunction, and visuospatial impairment, and ultimately impacts the ability to perform activities of daily living.

Typical early symptoms of late-onset AD include forgetfulness, such as forgetting conversations, repeating statements and questions, and misplacing personal items. Long-term memory remains relatively preserved. In the early stages of AD, a patient may be aware of his or her short-term memory impairment and have preserved insight. Later symptoms may include word-finding difficulty, trouble with calculations, trouble with decision-making, and getting lost in familiar surroundings.

Often the earliest stage of symptoms may be subjective cognitive impairment, wherein patients may notice declines in memory, yet they are still testing normally on bedside cognitive testing and neuropsychological testing, and they remain able to perform all of their activities of daily living. The next stage may be mild cognitive impairment (MCI), wherein a patient or informant has a cognitive complaint, which is detectable on testing, yet he or she is still able to compensate and perform daily activities. MCI may be classified as amnestic or nonamnestic (signifying if memory impairment is present) and single domain or multiple domain. The most typical presentation of AD begins with subjective cognitive impairment, then amnestic single-domain MCI, then amnestic multiple-domain MCI, then mild dementia. However, it is important to note that many patients may not pass through these stages in a stereotypical fashion. In a study of the oldest-old, incidence of dementia was 31.4% per year in persons with amnestic MCI compared with 8.4% per year in persons with normal cognition.[14] The transition from MCI to mild dementia involves a loss of independence in functional abilities, for example, inability to manage medications, appointments, transportation, or finances.

As patients progress through stages of AD dementia, initially they may only require assistance with instrumental activities of daily living (medication management, finances, transportation); however, as they progress to a moderate stage of dementia, they will require assistance with more basic activities of daily living, such as dressing, bathing, and grooming. As they progress to a severe stage of AD dementia, they will need to be fed and will eventually become incontinent. Finally, in the end-stage, patients may progress to become nonverbal, unable to swallow, and bedridden.

The psychiatric symptoms associated with AD are varied and can be distressing to the patient and caregiver. Early psychiatric symptoms, most typical in the MCI stage, may include apathy, depression, and anxiety. Later psychiatric symptoms may include paranoid delusions, disinhibition (childlike behavior), and agitation. Sleep disorders are also common in late-onset AD, including insomnia, hypersomnia, disrupted sleep, and Circadian rhythm dysregulation.

DIAGNOSIS

The diagnostic evaluation for AD in the oldest-old can be challenging due to the many factors that may influence a person's cognitive or functional abilities that are not due to underlying neuropathology. These may include sensory impairments (visual or hearing), physical disability, and reduced family and societal expectations for functional independence.

Of note, the prior set of guidelines for the diagnosis of AD, the National Institute of Neurological and Communicative Disorders and Stroke–Alzheimer's Disease and Related Disorders Association (NINCDS-ADRDA) Criteria from 1984[15] specified that the onset of deficits begins between the ages of 40 and 90. However, the current set of guidelines for the diagnosis of dementia due to AD from the NIA–Alzheimer's Association (NIA-AA) workgroup does not set an upper age bound for the onset of symptoms.[16] Core clinical criteria for probable AD dementia (NIA-AA) include (1) dementia, (2) insidious onset, (3) cognitive deficits by history and examination with amnestic or nonamnestic (language, visuospatial, or executive) presentation, and (4) exclusion of other neurodegenerative, neurologic, medical, or medication comorbidities.[16]

The diagnostic evaluation for late-onset AD begins with a careful history. In many cases, patients in the early stages of AD (subjective cognitive impairment or early MCI) may have preserved insight and notice concerning changes in their own memory; however, it is typical in the later stages of MCI or dementia for patients to lose their insight and awareness of their memory impairment. Thus, it is optimal to obtain history from both the patient and an informant, who is aware of the patient's cognitive performance and functional abilities. The informant is often someone living with the patient (a spouse, adult child, or other family member), or it may be a staff member in the patient's living facility. However, many older adults are now living alone: in the United States in 2010, 48% of adults older than 85 lived alone.[17] In this case, the informant may be an adult child, other family member, or friend who does not have detailed knowledge of the patient, which may limit the accuracy of the clinical history.

A careful review of the past medical history and current medications may assist in identifying causes of dementia other than AD. Polypharmacy is common in older adults, and many commonly prescribed medications, such as benzodiazepines, anticholinergics, and antihistamines, can cause cognitive impairment. Also, alcohol use and depression are often-overlooked contributors to cognitive impairment in the elderly.

A detailed physical and neurologic examination often will be normal if the dementia is due to AD, thus abnormal findings may point toward other causes or contributors to the dementia. For example, subtle focal neurologic findings, such as pronator drift or subtle unilateral weakness, spasticity, or hyperreflexia, may indicate prior silent stroke and thus a vascular contribution to cognitive impairment. Parkinsonian features, such as bradykinesia, shuffling gait, and rigidity, may indicate a Lewy body spectrum disorder.

Cognitive testing should be performed next, which may be bedside cognitive testing, such as the Mini-Mental State Examination (MMSE), Montreal Cognitive Assessment (MoCA), or other tests. If cognitive impairment is not identified on bedside cognitive testing, but the clinician has a high suspicion for cognitive impairment, neuropsychological testing may be appropriate. It is important to note that both bedside cognitive tests and neuropsychological tests have age-adjusted norms, and the cutoffs used in younger populations may be too strict when applied in the oldest-old. For example, in *The 90+ Study*, the mean MMSE score in adults older than 90 years without dementia was 26.1, with the 10th percentile score being 23.[18]

In addition, sensory and physical limitations, such as visual impairment, hearing impairment, fatigue, or pain, may impact performance on cognitive testing in the oldest-old.

Laboratory assessment is critical and should include complete blood count and comprehensive metabolic panel to evaluate for infection, anemia, electrolyte abnormalities, liver, or kidney dysfunction that may contribute to cognitive dysfunction. Hormone abnormalities and vitamin deficiencies also may contribute to cognitive dysfunction, thus it is recommended to check thyroid function tests and vitamin levels (B12, folic acid, B1, and D) because deficiencies are commonly found in this age group.

Brain imaging is important in the assessment, and MRI is the preferred measure. Common findings that may not aid in differential diagnosis may include cerebral atrophy and periventricular and subcortical white matter hyperintensities, both of which are age-associated and frequently present to a mild or moderate degree in elderly individuals with and without dementia. The underlying pathologic substrates of white matter hyperintensities are not yet completely defined, but may represent microvascular ischemic change or gliosis. In AD, common findings may include biparietal and bitemporal atrophy, particularly involving the hippocampus; however, the wide range of normal age-related atrophy overlaps with findings in AD.

The NIA-AA guidelines for the diagnosis of dementia due to AD do not advocate the use of biomarkers for routine diagnostic purposes[16]; however, the guidelines give leeway to clinicians for use when deemed appropriate, such as in complex cases or when more certain diagnosis would change management. These specific AD biomarkers may include cerebrospinal fluid amyloid-beta42, phosphorylated-tau, and total tau. Also available is brain PET imaging for amyloid plaques using tracers such as florbetapir, flutemetamol, and florbetaben. However, it is important to note that many of the oldest-old with normal cognition may have positive biomarkers for AD. The overall prevalence of "amyloid positivity" among the cognitively normal oldest-old population has been estimated to be more than 50%.[19] For very old individuals, the significance of amyloid biomarkers is uncertain. For example, it is not known if they will ultimately develop AD dementia with the passage of time, or if perhaps they are somewhat "resistant" to these pathologies. In any case, testing for these biomarkers in an elderly adult with normal cognition is not recommended. Even in an oldest-old patient with clinical AD, the tests may not be helpful, as the dementia may be due to a different or multiple pathologies, and the Alzheimer pathology may be a bystander. Thus, testing for AD biomarkers may be most helpful when results are negative, providing information that it is highly unlikely that dementia is due to underlying AD.

TREATMENT

Bearing in mind the complexity of contributing factors to clinical AD in the oldest-old, an important first step is addressing medical contributors to dementia if possible, such as the removal of offending medications (eg, benzodiazepines, anticholinergics, antihistamines), and adequate treatment of depression, anxiety, and sleep disorders.

In the oldest-old, there is frequently a vascular contribution to AD dementia, so treatment of vascular risk factors is important; however, it is unclear how aggressively to treat hypertension, diabetes, and hypercholesterolemia in the oldest-old. It is possible that maintaining cerebral perfusion is critical to cognitive performance, so blood pressure targets may be somewhat liberalized in late life. Additionally, the side effects of medications to treat vascular risk factors may be problematic in the oldest-old. These may include orthostatic hypotension and renal insufficiency among the blood pressure medications, hypoglycemia among the diabetic medications in frail elderly patients with inadequate caloric intake, muscle cramps and weakness among the statins, and risk of cerebral hemorrhage in elderly individuals on anticoagulants, a higher prevalence of cerebral amyloid angiopathy, and with high fall risk. Each patient is an individual, and management of vascular risk factors as prevention and treatment of dementia should be undertaken in partnership between the primary care physician (who may be a family physician, internist, or geriatrician) and the neurologist.

The medications that are approved by the Food and Drug Administration for the treatment of AD dementia include acetylcholinesterase inhibitors: donepezil (Aricept), rivastigmine (Exelon), and galantamine (Reminyl); and memantine (Namenda.) These medications improve cognitive and functional performance but do not reduce the risk of progression from MCI to dementia nor do they slow progression of dementia. Acetylcholinesterase inhibitors are approved for use in all stages of AD dementia, and memantine is approved for moderate and severe-stage AD dementia. The clinical trials that demonstrated efficacy of these medications enrolled patients with a mean age between 72 and 76 years.[20–23] In some of the studies, patients older than 85 were excluded. Thus, the use of these medications in the oldest-old is an extrapolation from younger populations. It is appropriate to use these AD medications in the oldest-old population with the realization that the oldest-old may be more susceptible to the expected side effects, such as nausea, vomiting, diarrhea, and bradycardia, due to expected changes in pharmacokinetics and pharmacodynamics associated with aging.[24] The familiar adage for medication use in the elderly applies to the use of AD medications: *"Start low and go slow."*

As with patients of any age with AD, it is the neurologist's responsibility to assess safety, including ensuring the patient has adequate supervision and is not suffering from abuse or neglect. Significant safety issues to address include wandering and driving. Several states in the United States mandate that physicians report patients with AD or dementia to the Department of Public Health or Department of Motor Vehicles. Even in states that do not mandate physician reporting, it is important to discuss driving with patients and their families, including the fact that patients with AD are at high risk of car accidents. It is helpful to refer patients and their families to social services agencies, including the local chapter of the Alzheimer's Association or other advocacy groups for family support and future care planning. It is also important to involve and document the patients' wishes about future care (including cardiopulmonary resuscitation, invasive medical care, and feeding tube placement) while they are still able to participate in such discussions. Wishes should be recorded in an Advanced Directive, and 42 states have POLST (Physician Orders for Life-Sustaining Treatment) laws in place that allow physicians to document patients' end-of-life decisions in a portable medical order. Finally, as a patient reaches the end of life and develops difficulty with ambulation or feeding, it is appropriate to involve palliative care and hospice.

SUMMARY

AD dementia in the oldest-old is challenging to study, diagnose, and treat, relating to the complexities of mixed pathologies, medical comorbidities, and the expected changes of normal aging in cognition, physical performance, and functional status. Diagnosis relies on identifying progressive cognitive impairment, typically amnestic, leading to functional impairment, and excluding other causes through history, medication list, laboratory studies, and often neuroimaging. Symptomatic medical treatment with acetylcholinesterase inhibitors and memantine and supportive care are the mainstays of treatment. Identifying an intervention that can prevent or slow AD progression regardless of age is of critical importance; however, there is a particular urgency for the oldest-old, who represent the fastest growing segment of our society, and are at highest risk of developing AD dementia. Due to the differences in risk factors and pathology of dementia in the oldest-old compared with the younger elderly population, it is possible that successful treatment paradigms may ultimately differ based on age. Future clinical trial designs should include the oldest-old, as efficacy and tolerability need to be defined in this group in which the medications will be used.

REFERENCES

1. National Population Projections (Based on Census 2000). Table 12. Projections of the population by age and sex for the United States: 2010 to 2050 2008. Available at: http://www.census.gov/population/www/projections/summarytables.html. Accessed February 29, 2012.
2. Gardner R, Valcour V, Yaffe K. Dementia in the oldest old: a multi-factorial and growing public health issue. Alzheimers Res Ther 2013;5:27.
3. Hebert LE, Weuve J, Scherr PA, et al. Alzheimer disease in the United States (2010-2050) estimated using the 2010 census. Neurology 2013;80:1778–83.
4. Alzheimer's Association. 2016 Alzheimer's disease facts and figures. Alzheimers Dement 2016;12(4):459–509.
5. Bullain SS, Corrada MM. Dementia in the oldest old. Continuum 2013;19:457–69.
6. Bullain SS, Corrada MM, Perry SM, et al. Sound body sound mind? Physical performance and the risk of dementia in the oldest-old: the 90+ Study. J Am Geriatr Soc 2016;64:1408–15.
7. Farrer LA, Cupples LA, Haines JL, et al. Effects of age, sex, and ethnicity on the association between apolipoprotein E genotype and Alzheimer disease. A meta-analysis. APOE and Alzheimer Disease Meta Analysis Consortium. JAMA 1997; 278:1349–56.
8. Euser SM, van Bemmel T, Schram MT, et al. The effect of age on the association between blood pressure and cognitive function later in life. J Am Geriatr Soc 2009;57:1232–7.
9. McNeal MG, Zareparsi S, Camicioli R, et al. Predictors of healthy brain aging. J Gerontol A Biol Sci Med Sci 2001;56:B294–301.
10. Consensus recommendations for the postmortem diagnosis of Alzheimer's disease. The National Institute on Aging, and Reagan Institute Working Group on Diagnostic Criteria for the Neuropathological Assessment of Alzheimer's Disease. Neurobiol Aging 1997;18:S1–2.
11. Corrada MM, Sonnen JA, Kim RC, et al. Microinfarcts are common and strongly related to dementia in the oldest-old: The 90+ study. Alzheimers Dement 2016; 12:900–8.
12. White L, Petrovitch H, Hardman J, et al. Cerebrovascular pathology and dementia in autopsied Honolulu-Asia Aging Study participants. Ann N Y Acad Sci 2002; 977:9–23.
13. Kawas CH, Kim RC, Sonnen JA, et al. Multiple pathologies are common and related to dementia in the oldest-old: the 90+ Study. Neurology 2015;85:535–42.
14. Peltz CB, Corrada MM, Berlau DJ, et al. Incidence of dementia in oldest-old with amnestic MCI and other cognitive impairments. Neurology 2011;77:1906–12.
15. McKhann G, Drachman D, Folstein M, et al. Clinical diagnosis of Alzheimer's disease: report of the NINCDS-ADRDA work group under the auspices of

Department of Health and Human Services Task Force on Alzheimer's disease. Neurology 1984;34:939–44.

16. McKhann GM, Knopman DS, Chertkow H, et al. The diagnosis of dementia due to Alzheimer's disease: recommendations from the National Institute on Aging-Alzheimer's Association workgroups on diagnostic guidelines for Alzheimer's disease. Alzheimers Dement 2011;7:263–9.

17. West LA, Cole S, Goodkind D, et al. 65+ in the United States: 2010. 2014. Available at: https://www.census.gov/content/dam/Census/library/publications/2014/demo/p23-212.pdf. Accessed July 25, 2016.

18. Whittle C, Corrada MM, Dick M, et al. Neuropsychological data in nondemented oldest old: the 90+ Study. J Clin Exp Neuropsychol 2007;29:290–9.

19. Lopez OL, Klunk WE, Mathis C, et al. Amyloid, neurodegeneration, and small vessel disease as predictors of dementia in the oldest-old. Neurology 2014;83: 1804–11.

20. Seltzer B, Zolnouni P, Nunez M, et al. Efficacy of donepezil in early-stage Alzheimer disease: a randomized placebo-controlled trial. Arch Neurol 2004; 61:1852–6.

21. Rosler M, Anand R, Cicin-Sain A, et al. Efficacy and safety of rivastigmine in patients with Alzheimer's disease: international randomised controlled trial. BMJ 1999;318:633–8.

22. Wilcock GK, Lilienfeld S, Gaens E. Efficacy and safety of galantamine in patients with mild to moderate Alzheimer's disease: multicentre randomised controlled trial. Galantamine International-1 Study Group. BMJ 2000;321:1445–9.

23. Reisberg B, Doody R, Stoffler A, et al. Memantine in moderate-to-severe Alzheimer's disease. N Engl J Med 2003;348:1333–41.

24. Corsonello A, Pedone C, Incalzi RA. Age-related pharmacokinetic and pharmacodynamic changes and related risk of adverse drug reactions. Curr Med Chem 2010;17:571–84.

Vascular Contributions to Cognitive Impairment in Late Life

Helena C. Chui, MD[a],*, Liliana Ramirez Gomez, MD[b]

KEYWORDS

- Vascular cognitive impairment • Vascular dementia • Diagnosis • Treatment
- Neuropathology • MRI • White matter hyperintensity • Silent brain infarct

KEY POINTS

- A multifactorial approach to cognitive impairment in late life (eg, vascular, neurodegenerative, and systemic factors) may be more appropriate than the traditional dichotomous classifications (eg, vascular cognitive impairment vs Alzheimer disease).
- Quantitative neuroimaging enables detection of silent brain infarcts and white matter changes before onset of clinical symptoms.
- Multimodal imaging (eg, structural MRI combined with diffusion tensor tractography) can show the anatomically distributed effects of discrete infarcts.
- Amyloid PET imaging helps to identify concomitant Alzheimer conditions in persons with vascular brain injury.
- Management of vascular risk factors remains a proven and practical approach to reducing acute and progressive cognitive impairment and dementia.

BACKGROUND

History

The perceived contribution of vascular factors to cognitive impairment has oscillated significantly during the last century. In the early 20th century, progressive loss of intellectual function in late life was ascribed to hardening of the arteries, or so-called arteriosclerotic dementia. Alzheimer disease (AD) was considered a rare early-onset dementia associated with neurofibrillary tangles and senile plaques. When Tomlinson and colleagues[1] observed profuse tangle and plaques in sporadic, late-onset,

Disclosure Statement: The authors have nothing to disclose. This work was supported by the National Institute on Aging 1P50-05142.
[a] Department of Neurology, University of Southern California, 1540 Alcazar Street, CHP215, Los Angeles, CA 90033, USA; [b] Department of Neurology, University of California San Francisco, 400 Parnassus Avenue, A871, San Francisco, CA 94143, USA
* Corresponding author.
E-mail address: Helena.Chui@med.usc.edu

http://dx.doi.org/10.1016/j.ncl.2017.01.007
0733-8619/17/© 2017 Elsevier Inc. All rights reserved.
neurologic.theclinics.com

dementia cases, AD, not arteriosclerosis, became the preeminent etiology. Abrupt-onset, stepwise decline in cognition caused by acute strokes constituted the conceptual basis for multi-infarct dementia. Slowly progressive dementia caused by severe arteriopathy and demyelination of subcortical white matter, or Binswanger syndrome, was considered rare. In the 1980s, the landscape shifted with the advent of structural imaging. Asymptomatic white matter hyperintensities (WMH) and silent brain infarcts (SBI) were discovered on brain MRI in 20% to 30% of nondemented, community-dwelling, elderly subjects.[2] The ability to detect early and subclinical vascular disease without overt dementia prompted an earlier designation, vascular cognitive impairment (VCI). In the 1990s, epidemiologic studies noted associations between stroke risk factors and cognitive impairment (absent history of symptomatic stroke) and led to the still-unproven notion that vascular factors might promote Alzheimer disease. More recently, the frequent co-occurrence of vascular and AD conditions (15% between ages 65 and 89; 30% after age 90 years), suggests that a multifactorial, rather than dichotomous, approach to diagnosis and treatment may better reflect the realities of progressive cognitive impairment in late life.

Concepts

VCI is a syndrome or phenotype, not a disease. At its simplest, VCI embodies the concept that cognitive impairment is caused by vascular brain injury (VBI). The pathways leading from risk factors to cerebrovascular disease (CVD) to VBI are widely heterogeneous. Common sporadic forms of CVD include atherosclerosis, arteriolo-sclerosis, and cerebral amyloid angiopathy (CAA); rare genetic forms of CVD include CADASIL (cerebral autosomal dominant arteriopathy subcortical infarcts and leukoencephalopathy), and CARASIL (cerebral autosomal recessive arteriopathy with subcortical infarcts and leukoencephalopathy).[3] VBI may result from ischemia and hemorrhage and toxic, inflammatory, and oxidative stress.[4] To prevent or mitigate VCI, efforts must be directed toward risk factors, such as hypertension, diabetes mellitus, dyslipidemia, and smoking.

G&E → VRF → CVD → VBI → VCI

Genetic & Environmental factors → vascular risk factors → cerebrovascular disease → vascular brain injury → vascular cognitive impairment

The likelihood that VBI contributes to cognitive impairment varies with the patient and nature of the vascular insult. Location within cognitive networks and number and size of lesions are important determinants of the type and severity of cognitive impairment. For executive function, networks of parallel, frontal-subcortical circuits were first described based on anatomic studies in nonhuman primates.[5] Recently, Jeon and colleagues[6] scrutinized these parallel prefrontal-caudate-thalamic circuits in humans using task-activated high field 7T functional MRI combined with diffusion tensor imaging (Fig. 1). For the higher level branching executive tasks, activations were found in the ventroanterior portion of the prefrontal cortex (PFC), the head of the caudate nucleus, and the ventral anterior nucleus in the thalamus. Conversely, for the lower-level episodic executive tasks, activations were located in the posterior region of the PFC, the body of the caudate nucleus, and the medial dorsal nucleus in the thalamus. When lacunar infarcts and WMH occur in these frontal-subcortical circuits, impairment in executive function is likely to follow.

Co-occurrence of vascular and neurodegenerative pathologies (such as AD [amyloidopathy and tauopathy] and Lewy body disease [α-synucleinopathy]) occurs frequently, especially with increasing age. Macro- and microinfarcts are each found in approximately 30% of elderly persons, often combined with AD conditions.[7–9] Converging evidence indicates that ischemic infarcts and neurodegenerative lesions

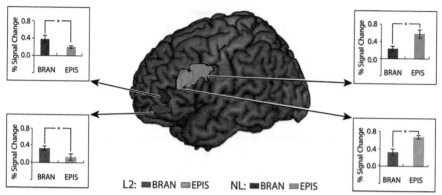

L2: ■BRAN ▨EPIS   NL: ■BRAN ▨EPIS

Fig. 1. Posterior-to-anterior pattern of activations depending on the levels of cognitive hierarchies across L2 and NL in the PFC. Brain activations elicited by the episodic and branching conditions across L2 and NL were rendered on a canonical brain provided with MRIcron software (http://www.mccauslandcenter.sc.edu/mricro/mricron/). Activations from the contextual condition in the left hemisphere and the branching condition in the right hemisphere are not displayed here (see **Table 1** for their coordinates). Bar graphs represent the mean percentage signal change within the sphere-shaped regions (radius 2 mm) centered on the peak voxels for each condition. Error bars denote SEM. n19, *p<0.05. BRAN, Branching condition; EPIS, episodic condition; NL, nonlanguage. (*From* Jeon HA, Anwander A, Friederici AD. Functional network mirrored in the prefrontal cortex, caudate nucleus, and thalamus: high-resolution functional imaging and structural connectivity. J Neurosci 2014;34(28):9207; with permission.)

combine in an additive fashion to increase the risk of cognitive impairment and dementia.[10-14] (For review, see Chui and Ramirez-Gomez[15]).

> Cognitive
> impairment = aging + amyloidopathy + tauopathy + synucleinopathy + vascular factors + systemic factors − cognitive reserve − neuroplasticity

The application of "either/or" diagnostic criteria in epidemiologic studies fosters a dichotomous view of VCI and AD (**Table 1**). Thus, a multifactorial approach that addresses neurodegenerative, vascular, and systemic factors may be more realistic when addressing cognitive impairment in late life (**Table 2**).

Epidemiology

From a public health perspective, VCI is the second most common cause of cognitive impairment in late life after AD. One of 3 persons meets criteria for dementia after their first stroke.[16] Persons with stroke who are not initially demented are twice as likely as normal controls to subsequently have dementia over the next 10 years.[17] The incidence of vascular dementia increases exponentially after 65 years of age, ranging from 3 to 19 per 1000 persons per year at age 80 years,[18-20] approximately half the rate of AD. In the Canadian Health & Aging Study of persons older than age 65 years, the prevalence of CIND (cognitive impairment not dementia) was 17%, similar to the combined persons with dementia or stroke (8% each).[21] In this study, the relative contributions of VBI to CIND were believed to be considerable.

To minimize survival bias, cohorts at risk should be established in midlife and followed longitudinally. In the Honolulu Heart Program, history of high systolic blood

Table 1
Dichotomous approach: clinical criteria for vascular dementia

Diagnostic Criteria		Dementia	VBI	Evidence of Causal Relationship
HIS (0–17 points)[100] HIS ≥7 suggests MID HIS 5–6 suggests MIX HIS ≤4 suggests AD		No specific criteria.	CVD risk factors (HTN, ASCVD). Sudden onset. Stepwise progression. Focal neurologic signs and symptoms.	Not specifically required.
DSM-IV (APA, 1994)		Memory loss Sufficient to interfere. No clouding of consciousness.	Stepwise deteriorating course, and "patchy" distribution of deficits, focal neurologic signs, and symptoms.	Evidence from the history, physical examination, or laboratory tests of significant CVD that is judged to be etiologically related to the disturbance.
ICD-10 (WHO, 1993)		Unequal distribution of deficits in higher cognitive functions with some affected and others relatively spared.	Evidence of focal brain damage, with at least 1 of the following: unilaterally increased tendon reflexes, an extensor plantar response, pseudobulbar palsy.	From the history, examination, or test, evidence of significant CVD, which may reasonably be judged to be etiologically related to the dementia.
ADDTC[103]	Probable	Multifaceted cognitive impairment sufficient to interfere with customary affairs of life.	Infarct outside cerebellum by imaging.	2 infarcts, or 1 infarct with temporal relationship to onset of cognitive impairment.
	Possible		1 infarct outside cerebellum by imaging OR confluent white matter change.	Not required.
NINDS-AIREN[104]	Probable	Memory loss plus impairment in 2 other cognitive domains.	Focal neurologic signs. Imaging findings	Abrupt onset, stepwise progression, temporal relationship to onset of cognitive impairment.
	Possible		Either imaging findings, abrupt onset, stepwise, OR temporal relationship.	

Criteria	Level	Cognitive Criteria	Imaging	Temporal/Other Relationship
AHA/ASA (2011)[105]	Probable	Decline in cognitive function in ≥2 domains sufficient to interfere with ADL. At least 4 domains tested. Decline in ADLs are independent from motor/sensory sequelae of the vascular event.	Imaging evidence of CVD.	Clear temporal relationship between vascular event and cognitive deficit onset, or clear relationship between severity and pattern of cognitive impairment and diffuse, subcortical CVD. No history of gradually progressive cognitive deficits before/after CVA to suggest nonvascular neurodegenerative etiology. Evidence of another potential cause for cognitive dysfunction in addition to CVD.
	Possible	See above. Severe aphasia precludes cognitive assessment.	Imaging findings, but no clear relationship (temporal, severity, or cognitive pattern) with cognitive impairment. No imaging available.	
DSM-5 (APA, 2013)[107] Major or mild NCD	Probable	Decline in cognitive function in ≥1 cognitive domains sufficient to interfere with ADL. No clouding of consciousness.	Imaging findings CT or MRI. Temporal relationship. Prominent decline in attention and executive function. Presence of clinical evidence plus genetic disorder (eg, CADASIL).	Evidence from the history, physical examination, or laboratory tests of significant CVD that is judged to be etiologically related to the neurocognitive deficits.
	Possible		Evidence of VBI without clear temporal relationship to cognitive deficits.	

Abbreviations: ADDTC, State of California Alzheimer's Disease Diagnostic and Treatment Centers; ADL, activities of daily living; AHA/ASA, American Heart Association/American Stroke Association; ASCVD, asymptomatic cardiovascular disease; CT, computed tomography scan; HIS, Hachinski Ischemic Score; HTN, hypertension; MID, multi-infarct dementia; MIX, mixed dementia (vascular and AD); NCD, Neurocognitive disorder; NINDS-AIREN, National Institute of Neurologic Disorders and Stroke and Association Internationale pour la Recherché et l'Enseignement en Neurosciences.

Table 2
Multifactorial approach to cognitive impairment

Common Etiologic Factors	Physical Pheno type	Cognitive Phenotype	Biomarker			Treatment Considerations
			MRI	CSF	Other	
Neurodegenerative factors	Tau (neurofibrillary tangles)		MEM>EXEC Amnestic memory impairment. Atypical focal presentations	Hippocampal atrophy, atrophy of multimodal association areas	Increased p-tau	Reduced FDG PET in precuneus, and parietal-temporal-frontal lobes	Symptomatic cognitive and behavioral treatment (acetylcholinesterase inhibitors, memantine)
	Amyloid-β (plaques)				Decreased Amyloid-β	Positive amyloid PET scan	
	α-synuclein (Lewy bodies)	Extra pyramidal signs	Decreased attention and EXEC, slowing			Decreased dopamine transporter on PET scans	Symptomatic motor and behavioral treatment. Caution: neuroleptic sensitivity
	TDP-43		Semantic PPA, hippocampal sclerosis	Temporal pole atrophy, hippocampal atrophy			

Vascular factors	Atherosclerosis	Ankle-brachial index	EXEC≥MEM	Generalized atrophy, territorial infarcts, microinfarcts	Carotid intima media thickening	Treat VRF (HTN, DM, HL, AFib). Secondary prevention of stroke. Caution: increased risk of cerebral hypotension with confluent WMH
	Arteriolosclerosis	Retinal artery changes	EXEC≥MEM slowing	WMH, lacunar infarcts, deep MBs		
	CAA			WMH, microinfarcts, lobar hemorrhage, peripheral MBs	Increased MMP-9	Caution: increased risk of brain hemorrhage with anticoagulation therapy
	Microvascular disease			Future DCE-MRI?	Retinal angiography	Treat VRF (eg, diabetes)
Systemic factors	Metabolic Endocrine Inflammation Toxic		Decreased attention and EXEC		Medication side-effects, metabolic, inflammatory abnormalities	Address polypharmacy Correct metabolic and inflammatory factors

Abbreviations: DCE, dynamic contrast enhanced; DM, diabetes mellitus; EXEC, executive function; HL, hyperlipidemia; HTN, hypertension; MEM, memory; MMP-9, methyl-metalloproteinase-9; VRF, vascular risk factors.

pressure[22] and diabetes mellitus[23] were associated with greater risk of dementia in late life (especially among persons with the apolipoprotein E ε4 allele). In the Framingham study,[24] duration of diabetes was related to poorer cognitive performance. In the CAIDE study, higher midlife cholesterol levels were associated with increased risk of dementia.[25,26] These epidemiologic studies underscore the importance of managing hypertension, diabetes mellitus, and cholesterol beginning in midlife.

MRI scans in longitudinal, population-based studies find SBI and WMH in approximately one-third of persons older than 65 years.[27–29] These lesions increase with age, are associated with hypertension, and increase the risk of stroke and dementia.[30,31] In the Framingham Offspring study of middle-age adults, SBI and severe WMH were associated with increased risk of stroke and dementia independent of vascular risk factors.[32] These studies identify subclinical VBI on MRI as relevant targets for early detection and primary prevention. Cerebral microbleeds (MBs) are also present in one-third of persons older than 80 years based on population studies, and are associated with increased risk of stroke, cognitive decline, and mortality.[33]

Genetic Epidemiology

Several forms of CVD are associated with genetic mutations or polymorphisms. CADASIL is caused by mutations or deletions in the Notch 3 gene (chromosome 19p13).[34,35] A similar autosomal recessive syndrome (CARASIL) results from mutations in the HtrA serine peptidase 1 (HTRA1).[36] Dutch, Icelandic, and Finnish forms of familial CAA are associated with hemorrhage (Hereditary Cerebral Hemorrhage with Amyloidosis [HCHWA]).[37] More commonly, the apolipoprotein E ε4 allele (present in approximately 25% of the general population) increases vascular deposition of the amyloid-β protein as the sporadic form of CAA.[38]

CLINICAL SUBTYPES OF VASCULAR COGNITIVE IMPAIRMENT

VCI has been categorized in many ways including heritability (eg, CADASIL), location (eg, subcortical vascular dementia [SVD], strategic location), clinical presentation (poststroke dementia, Binswanger syndrome), or MRI findings (eg, SBI). This article reviews several common syndromes that are not mutually exclusive.

Poststroke Dementia

In hospital- and community-based series, history of first stroke doubles the risk of subsequent dementia.[16] In Olmsted County, Minnesota, prevalent dementia was 30% immediately after stroke and incident dementia was 7% 1 year after stroke and increased to 48% 25 years after stroke.[39] Compared with normal controls, history of stroke doubles the risk of dementia over 10 years.[17] Risk factors for dementia at the time of stroke include fewer years of education, older age, diabetes mellitus, atrial fibrillation, and recurrent stroke.[40] Stroke locations associated with higher likelihood of cognitive impairment include left hemisphere, anterior and posterior cerebral artery distribution, multiple infarcts, and other strategic infarcts.[16] Neuroimaging variables associated with poststroke dementia (PSD) include SBI, WMH, and global and medial temporal atrophy.[16] Concomitant AD is also a major risk factor for PSD. A recent study by Liu and colleagues[41] in 72 subjects with cognitive impairment after stroke/transient ischemic attack found that those with positive amyloid-β deposition detected by C-PiB PET (carbon-11-labeled Pittsburgh compound B PET) after the index event experienced a more severe and rapid cognitive decline on the Mini Mental State Examination (MMSE) and the memory domain of the Montreal Cognitive Assessment (MoCA) during a 3-year follow-up compared with those with negative amyloid PET scans.[41] About 15% to 30% of persons with PSD have a history of dementia before stroke,[42,43] and approximately one-third have significant medial temporal atrophy.[44]

Strategic Infarct Dementia

A dementia syndrome may follow a single infarct placed in a strategic location. The left angular gyrus, inferomesial temporal, and medial frontal lobe are considered strategic locations perfused by large arteries. Frontal-subcortical loops are strategic networks for executive function. These networks include prefrontal cortex, head of the caudate, anterior and dorsomedial thalamic nuclei, capsular genu, and anterior limb of the internal capsule.[45,46] The dementia syndrome associated with thalamic infarcts is characterized by marked apathy, impaired attention and mental control, and anterograde and retrograde amnesia.[47-49]

Subcortical Vascular Dementia

SVD is defined by VBI confined mainly to subcortical white and gray matter. Small vessel infarcts account for 25% of subjects hospitalized for strokes and make up nearly 60% of asymptomatic strokes in community-based studies.[29] In addition to PSD and strategic infarct dementia caused by small vessel disease, lacunar state and Binswanger syndrome both fall under the umbrella of SVD.

Lacunar state is an extreme phenotype of SVD, characterized by multiple lacunar infarcts in the basal ganglia, thalamus, and white matter. Clinical features can include the sudden onset hemiparesis, lack of volition, akinetic mutism, dysarthria, pseudobulbar palsy and affect, small-stepped gait, and urinary incontinence.[50] Before MRI, the frontal predilection for subcortical gray matter and white matter was documented by autopsy.[50,51]

The pathologic hallmark of Binswanger syndrome (subcortical arteriosclerotic encephalopathy) is prominent demyelination of the deep white matter, ascribed to stenosis of the deep penetrating medullary arteries.[52,53] The clinical triad is typically a slowly progressive dementia, gait apraxia, and urinary incontinence. Subcortical arteriosclerotic encephalopathy may be mistaken for normal pressure hydrocephalus (NPH), although the pathophysiology differs. In the case of Binswanger, ventriculomegaly occurs secondary to brain atrophy rather than impairment of cerebrospinal fluid (CSF) absorption. Elevation of methyl-metalloproteinase-9 in CSF also supports a diagnosis of Binswanger rather than normal pressure hydrocephalus.[54]

Criteria for the SVD subtype of VCI emphasize slowing of cognition, executive dysfunction (impairment in selective attention, abstract reasoning, and mental flexibility), depression, extrapyramidal signs, and gait disturbance.[55] In an autopsy-confirmed study, a "low executive" profile was 67% sensitive and 86% specific in distinguishing SVD from AD (positive likelihood ratio, 4.7).[56] Score on word recall (higher in SVD) and difference between phonemic versus semantic verbal fluency (smaller in SVD) differentiated SVD from AD with a positive likelihood ratio of 2.57 (Ramirez Gomez unpublished data, 2014). Although the sample size was small, the reference groups were defined by neuropathology, thereby avoiding the circularity that often occurs when comparison groups are defined clinically. The study suggests modest clinical utility of executive versus memory impairment profiles for distinguishing SVD and AD.

Cerebral Autosomal Dominant Arteriopathy Subcortical Infarcts and Leukoencephalopathy

CADASIL offers a prototypic example of pure SVD without concomitant AD. Extracellular domains of the NOTCH3 protein accumulate in the smooth muscle walls of small arterioles.[57,58] CADASIL is associated with migraine, depression, and seizures beginning in early adulthood followed by recurrent ischemic events and progressive cognitive decline.[59,60] Prominent slowing and impairment in executive function, with relative preservation of recall and receptive language, are noted on neuropsychological testing.[61] Severity of cognitive impairment correlates better with lacunar infarcts, rather than WMH or MBs.[62,63] Increase of mean diffusivity in the thalamus has also been correlated with severity of cognitive impairment.[64]

Duering and colleagues[65] compared cortical thickness before and after the occurrence of new lacunar infarcts in 9 patients with CADASIL. They used probability analyses using diffusion tensor imaging to test for a causal relationship between incident subcortical infarct and morphologic alterations in connected cortical regions (**Fig. 2**). The results support the hypothesis that secondary neurodegeneration of cortical gray matter follows axonal damage to anatomically related white matter tracts.

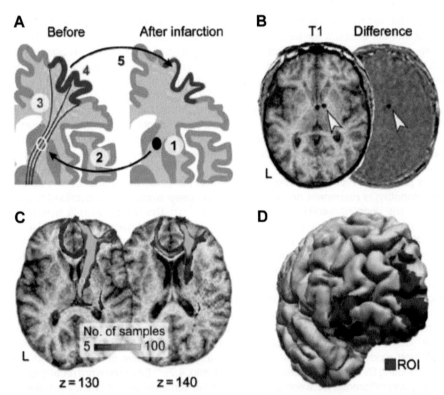

Fig. 2. (*A*) Location of the incident infarct (*black ovoid*) (*1*) is projected onto the healthy tissue (*white open ovoid*) on the last scan preceding the infarct (*2*) and used as a seed for probabilistic tractography (*3*) to identify the connected cortical region of interest (ROI). Cortical thickness within this ROI compared with cortex outside this region (reference region) is studied over time. (*B*) Difference image (right) between 2 time points highlights an incident lacunar infarct (*arrowhead*). T1 with incident infarct (left) is shown for comparison. (*C*) Probabilistic tractography in a single subject with an incident infarct in the right capsular genu (*open white ovoid*). Voxels harboring a minimum of 5 tractography samples are depicted. Tractography identifies the anterior thalamic radiation. (*D*) Connected cortical region from the same subject on a 3-dimensional pial surface model of the right hemisphere. (*From* Duering M, Righart R, Csanadi E, et al. Incident subcortical infarcts induce focal thinning in connected cortical regions. Neurology 2012;79(20):2026; with permission.)

Subclinical Vascular Brain Injury

Symptomatic stroke is the "tip of the iceberg" of VBI. In the Rotterdam study, the prevalence of SBIs was 5 times greater than that of symptomatic stroke.[29] SBI should be differentiated from CSF-filled perivascular spaces,[66] which are sometimes especially prominent in the putamen and infraputaminal regions and near the anterior commissure (**Fig. 3**).[67] Recently, the standards for reporting vascular changes on neuroimaging (STRIVE) criteria described enlarged perivascular space as smaller than 3 mm in diameter, linear or slitlike, and following the course of a blood vessel traveling through the gray or white matter.[68] Prominent perivascular spaces have been associated with other markers of SVD, stroke risk, CAA, AD, and cognitive dysfunction.[69–71] Can MRI help differentiate type of CVD: CAA versus atherosclerosis/lipohialinosis? Rarefaction of the periventricular and deep white matter can be seen as leukoaraiosis on computed tomography scan[72] and as WMH on fluid-attenuated inversion recovery or T2-weighted MRI.[73]

Semiquantitative white matter intensity scales are useful to communicate severity of WMH in clinical practice. In cross-sectional studies, WMH ratings are associated with mild impairment on the Modified MMSE.[74] In longitudinal MRI studies, incident SBI and worsening WMH correlate with cognitive decline, especially information processing speed,[75–77] supporting the relevance of SBI and WMH as presymptomatic targets for risk reduction. Recent studies in persons with subcortical VBI found that decreased fractional anisotropy of even normal-appearing white matter is associated with subtle cognitive decline.[78]

Cerebral MBs are small, round, or ovoid hypointensities, of less than 10 mm in diameter, evident on T2* gradient-recall echo and susceptibility-weighted MRI sequences.[33] The presence of MBs is considered a marker of small vessel conditions caused by either hypertensive vasculopathy or CAA. It is widely accepted that the location of MBs suggests underlying pathology.[79,80] Deep and lobar MBs have

Dilated giant infra-putaminal perivascular space

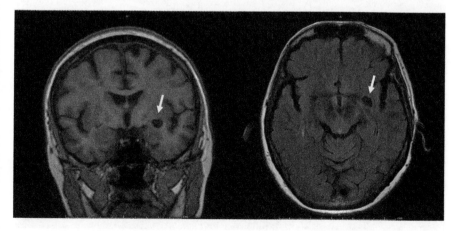

T-1 weighted   FLAIR

Fig. 3. An ovoid smoothly demarcated fluid-filled cyst (*white arrow*) shows the same CSF attenuation as observed on T1-weighted and Flair images, consistent with a giant dilated infraputaminal perivascular space.

been associated with hypertensive vasculopathy and strictly lobar MBs (mostly in the occipital and posterior temporo-parietal regions) with CAA (**Fig. 4**). The differentiation of atherosclerosis from CAA based on the distribution of MBs has been derived from clinical and imaging studies[81–85] rather than direct morphologic-pathologic correlations[81,86–90] (**Table 3**). This differentiation is based on the assumption that hemosiderin deposition, the pathologic basis of MRI MBs, indicates atherosclerosis or CAA depending on location.[91] However, more recent studies found that hemosiderin may also indicate decreased iron clearance[92] and microinfarcts,[93] suggesting more complex underlying neuropathologic mechanisms for MRI MB findings than previously

Lobar Cerebral Microbleeds

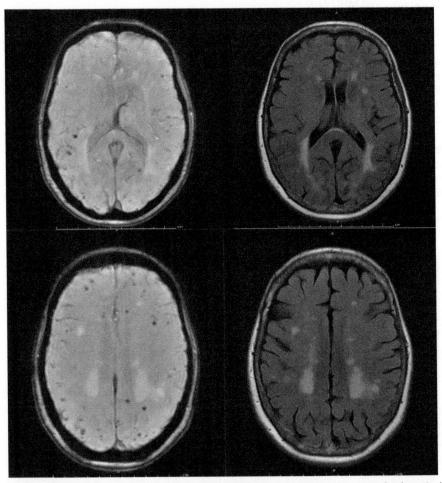

Fig. 4. Multiple small round hypointense lesions are seen on MRI in the cortical-subcortical junction on T2* gradient-recall echo sequences (upper and bottom left) consistent with multiple cerebral MBs and WMHs (upper and bottom right) in a 72-year-old white woman with mild cognitive impairment, amnestic subtype. ApoE ε4/ε4 homozygote. CSF: low amyloid-β (275 pg/mL), high p-tau (80 pg/mL).

Table 3
Can MRI help differentiate type of cerebrovascular disease: cerebral amyloid angiopathy versus atherosclerosis/lipohialinosis?

Pathology	MRI	CAA	AS/LH
White matter demyelination	WMH	+	+
Lacunar infarct	BI		++
Intracerebral hemorrhage	ICH	Lobar	Deep (basal ganglia, thalamus, pons, cerebellum)
MB	MB	+ Cortical (lobar)	++ Basal ganglia (deep)
Microinfarct	MI (7T MRI)	Cortical (barrel)	Basal ganglia and cortical (star-shaped)

Abbreviations: AS, atherosclerosis; BI, brain infarct; LH, lipohialinosis.

appreciated. It is still unclear if these microscopic lesions have the same biological significance and underlying mechanisms as radiologically defined MBs. Supporting this, a recent neuropathologic study did not find "a direct topographic relationship between location of cerebral MBs and CAA."[92] Clinically, MBs may be an independent contributor to cognitive impairment. Cognitive deficits associated with MBs may vary depending on the location of MBs, mostly affecting executive function, speed of processing, and other nonmemory cognitive domains.[94,95] Recently, in a Japanese cohort of subjects with vascular risk factors (n = 729), the presence of $\geq$2 MBs or mixed lobar and deep MBs, was associated with increased risk of all-cause dementia, independent of other risk factors (age, sex, education and *APOE* ε4 status).[96]

EVALUATION AND DIAGNOSIS
Clinical Evaluation

The clinical evaluation for VCI follows the established approach to the evaluation of cognitive impairment: a thorough history (from both the patient and a reliable informant); physical examination, including screening mental state examination, with emphasis on complete neurologic (focal neurologic signs, gait disturbance) and cardiovascular components (funduscopic examination of retinal vessels, carotid bruit, cardiac arrhythmia); laboratory testing (left ventricular hypertrophy, renal insufficiency); and neuroimaging (brain computed tomography scan or MRI). Currently, structural MRI provides the most sensitive and specific measure of VBI.[97] Emphasis is placed on identification by history of vascular risk factors (hypertension, hyperlipidemia, diabetes, heart disease) for risk reduction and on the pattern of cognitive and affective disturbance and functional decline for symptomatic treatment, management, and support.

Neuropsychological Testing

There is no single characteristic behavioral profile for VCI. Memory impairment in VCI is variable, tends to be of the dysexecutive rather than amnestic type, and responds better to cueing or recognition formats. WMH and SBI are often associated with decreased processing speed and executive function. In contrast to AD, in which semantic fluency usually is more affected than phonemic fluency, in VCI they generally are equally affected.[98] Microinfarcts have been associated with lower perceptual speed and semantic and episodic memory deficits independent of macroscopic infarcts or AD conditions.[8] Inclusion of Trail Making Test B, verbal fluency, clock drawing, digit symbol substitution, episodic memory (including free and cued recall), language, and visual-spatial domains has been recommended by a 2005 North American workshop.[99] **Table 4** emphasizes that the MoCA, Modified MMSE, and Mini-Cog (but not the MMSE) include assessment of executive function.

Clinical Diagnosis

A diagnosis of VCI is typically made using one of several diagnostic criteria (see **Table 1**). In comparing diagnostic criteria, it is useful to consider: (1) evidence of cognitive impairment/dementia, (2) evidence of VBI, and (3) likelihood that VBI is causing VCI. The Hachinski Ischemic Score[100] assigns 1 or 2 points to a list of risk factors, signs, and symptoms associated with stroke. The Diagnostic and Statistical Manual of Mental Disorders (DSM)-IV[101] and ICD-10[102] (World Health Organization 1993) leave assessment of causal relationship between VBI and VCI to the judgment of the clinician. For a diagnosis of probable vascular dementia, the State of California Alzheimer's Disease Diagnostic and Treatment Centers criteria[103] allow either a temporal relationship between VBI and VCI or evidence of 2 or more infarcts on a neuroimaging study. A temporal relationship between a vascular insult and cognitive decline is required for a diagnosis of probable vascular dementia by National Institute of Neurologic Disorders and Stroke and Association Internationale pour la Recherché et l'Enseignement en Neurosciences criteria,[104] thereby increasing the stringency of these criteria.

More recent clinical criteria were published for the diagnosis of VCI by the American Heart Association/American Stroke Association in 2011.[105] These rely on evidence of VBI present by structural neuroimaging and establish causality based on temporal relationship and correlation between type of VBI and cognitive deficits. In addition, the International Society for Vascular Behavioral and Cognitive Disorders (VASCOG) has recently proposed a new set of criteria.[106] Updated DSM-5 criteria have been released[107] and propose a change in terminology from vascular dementia or VCI to major or mild neurocognitive impairment due to CVD.

Mixed Alzheimer Disease/Vascular Cognitive Impairment

For the clinical diagnosis of mixed AD/VCI, the presence of AD can be recognized by neuropsychological profile, structural imaging, CSF biomarkers, glucose PET, and amyloid PET imaging. The diagnosis of VBI, however, still hinges predominantly on the structural MRI findings. With the notable exception of microinfarcts (which elude in vivo detection), infarcts, hemorrhages, and WMHs on structural MRI currently represent the best markers for VBI. Severe amnesia and atrophy of the hippocampus are characteristic of early AD; whereas the cognitive profile for VCI is highly variable and depends on size and location of VBI. In general, the cognitive profile of mixed AD/SVD is dominated by AD (for review, see Chui and Ramirez-Gomez15).

The advent of amyloid PET scans has provided a noninvasive means of differentiating pure from mixed SVD. The Seoul criteria for pure SVD[108] are based on a comparison of amyloid PET-positive versus PET-negative subgroups among 77 patients with cognitive impairment, lacunar infarcts, and WMH on MRI. The ideal model for identifying pure SVD (amyloid PET negative) was age ≤75 years, ≥5 lacunes, and medial temporal atrophy ≤3. This yielded an accuracy of 67.5% (49% sensitivity and 100% specificity) in differentiating pure versus mixed SVD. Amyloid PET could help differentiate pure VCI from mixed AD/VCI in general (**Fig. 5**).

Table 4
Brief cognitive assessment tools (5–10 minutes)

Instrument	Attention	Memory	Executive	Language	Visual Spatial	Speed
Mini-Cog	Registration	3-word recall	Clock drawing	—	Clock drawing	—
MMSE	Registration Reversal	3-word recall Orientation	—	Naming[2] Repeat 3-step command Read, write	Copy pentagons[1]	—
Modified MMSE	Registration Reversal	3-word recall Cued recall First and second recall Orientation	Animal fluency Similarities	Naming[7] Repeat 3-step command Read, write Animal fluency	Copy pentagons[10]	Animal fluency in 30 s
MoCA	Registration Reversal Selective attention	5-word recall Cued recall Orientation	Short Trails B Letter fluency Clock drawing Similarities	Naming[3] Repeat Letter fluency	Copy cube Clock drawing	Letter fluency in 60 s

Hippocampal amnestic pattern is characterized by poor response to cueing and rapid forgetting (between first and second recall).

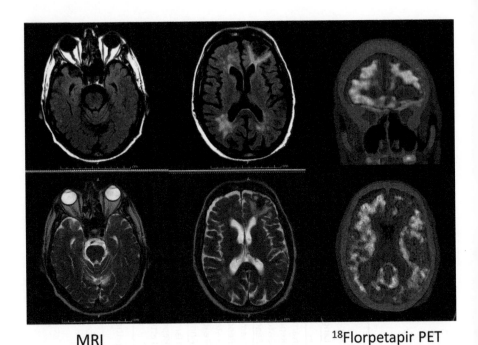

MRI ^{18}Florpetapir PET

Fig. 5. Mixed PSD plus AD. An 83-year-old man with history of hypertension and dyslipidemia, presented with progressive memory loss. Initial MRI showed moderate severe WMH. He subsequently had focal neurologic signs, and repeat MRI showed a left frontal cystic infarct. Memory continues to worsen gradually. Florbetapir amyloid PET scan is positive, suggesting mixed PSD plus AD.

Cerebrospinal Fluid Biomarkers

To date, no validated CSF biomarkers have been established to support the diagnosis of VCI, although a variety of substances have been proposed as measure of blood-brain barrier dysfunction in CVD, including the albumin index and methyl-metalloproteinase-9 levels.[54]

Cerebrovascular Disease Reactivity

Further studies to determine markers that reflect the health and reactivity of intracerebral blood vessels and blood-brain barrier integrity are needed. Arterial stiffness measured by carotid femoral pulse velocity was a stronger predictor of decline in executive function (Hajjar and colleagues, 2016).[109] Cerebrovascular reactivity has been assessed in research settings using transcranial Doppler, arterial spin labeling MRI, or blood oxygen level–dependent functional MRI in response to changes in CO_2 level and blood pressure.[110,111] Integrity of the blood-brain barrier can be assessed by dynamic contrast enhancement MRI, using gadolinium contrast and dynamic uptake modeling.[112]

Neuropathologic Contributions to Diagnosis and Understanding

Neuropathologic studies determine the type and severity of CVD and severity and distribution of AD pathologic conditions. In contrast to AD, there is no gold standard for the neuropathologic diagnosis of VCI. Typically, the reference standard is based on evidence of infarcts in neocortex, without considering the causal relationship between VBI and VCI. With these caveats, the clinical criteria for vascular dementia show high specificity and moderate sensitivity.[113] Several longitudinal cohort studies with high autopsy rates (Religious Orders Study, Honolulu Asia Aging Study, Baltimore Longitudinal Study of Aging) underscore (1) the high prevalence of mixed vascular and neurodegenerative pathologies in late life and (2) the additive risk of cerebral infarcts and AD conditions for cognitive impairment.[11–13] They also disclose the importance of microinfarcts[8] and hippocampal sclerosis[114] for cognitive impairment and memory loss, reminding us that these lesions often go undetected or unsuspected until autopsy.

Autopsy studies show the frequent co-occurrence of neurodegenerative and vascular conditions, which increases with age. We anticipate that evaluation and treatment will shift away from a dichotomous approach (eg, SVD vs AD) to a multifactorial approach (eg, to what extent neurodegenerative, vascular, and systemic factors are present in a given individual [see **Table 2**]). The presence of an amnestic pattern of memory impairment, hippocampal atrophy, and CSF/PET biomarkers would provide one means of ascertaining the presence of neurodegenerative factors. Evidence of infarcts, hemorrhages, and WMH would be used as a measure of vascular factors. Medical history, medications, and laboratory studies would assist in identifying the presence of systemic toxic, metabolic, endocrine, and inflammatory factors.

TREATMENT OF VASCULAR FACTORS
Primary Prevention: Identification and Reduction of Risk Factors for Atherosclerosis

The type of underlying CVD (eg, arteriosclerosis or CAA) should be considered. There are currently no proven treatments to prevent CAA, although preventative clinical trials could establish whether antiamyloid interventions (eg, a β-secretase inhibitor) retard the accumulation of amyloid-β in blood vessels and the brain parenchyma. In contrast, the beneficial effects of treating atherosclerotic risk factors (eg, hypertension, diabetes mellitus, and dyslipidemia) for stroke risk reduction are well established.[115] It has been estimated that an 8% reduction of vascular risk factors over 10 years would significantly reduce the incidence of dementia.[116] Over the last 3 decades, the incidence of vascular dementia, and to a lesser extent AD, has declined in successive cohort waves of the Framingham Heart Study, concomitant with more widespread pharmacologic treatment of hypertension and hyperlipidemia.[117]

Hypertension
Hypertension primary or secondary prevention trials that include cognitive outcome measures are still limited (**Table 5**), often begin late in life, and last for relatively short durations. Recently, the quality of cognitive and imaging outcome measures has greatly improved. In a meta-analysis of several placebo-controlled trials (SHEP, Sys-Eur, HYVET, and PROGRESS), treatment of hypertension was associated with reduction in the combined risk ratio (hazard ratio, 0.87; 95% confidence interval, 0.76–1.00; $P = .045$).[118] The Syst-Eur trial[119,120] suggested that treatment of 1000 patients for 5 years could prevent 20 cases of dementia (95% confidence interval, 7–33). In PROGRESS, a secondary prevention trial among persons with previous stroke or transient ischemic attack,[121] treatment with perindopril plus or minus indapamide showed a 19% relative risk reduction in cognitive decline and WMH progression over 4 years compared with placebo.[122] The Systolic Blood Pressure Intervention Trial—Memory and Cognition in Decreased Hypertension (SPRINT-MIND)[123] is designed to determine whether tighter blood pressure control over 5 years reduces the risk of incident dementia, rate of cognitive decline, and deceleration of brain volume loss in a subset of participants with SVD.

Table 5
Primary and secondary prevention: clinical trials that include a cognition outcome measure

Study	RX	Type of Intervention	Follow-up (y)	Main Results for Dementia	Significance
Primary Prevention					
SHEP (1991), N = 4736	Anti-HTN	Diuretic (chlorthalidone) and/or β-blocker (atenolol) or reserpine	4.5	16% reduction in dementia	NS
Syst-Eur (1998), N = 2418	Anti-HTN	Ca-channel blocker (dihydropyridine) with or without β-blocker (enalapril maleate) and/or diuretic (hydrochlorothiazide)	2.0	50% (0%–76%) reduction in dementia	$P = .05$
SCOPE (2003), N = 4937	Anti-HTN	ARB (candesartan cilexetil) and/or diuretics	3.7	7% increased risk in active arm (but only 3.2/1.6 mm Hg reduction in blood pressure in treatment vs control arm)	$P > .20$
HYVET (2008), N = 3336	Anti-HTN	Diuretic (indapamide) with or without ACEI (perindopril)	2.2	14% (−9% to 23%) reduction in dementia Trial stopped early because of significant reduction in stroke and mortality)	$P = .2$
PROSPER (2010), N = 5804	Statin	Pravastatin 40 mg vs placebo in elderly persons at high risk for cardiovascular events and stroke.	3.5	Significant reduction in composite death outcome (hazard ratio, 0.85, 95% CI 0.74–0.97, $P = .014$), but no difference in cognitive outcome	NS
ACCORD-MIND (2013), N = 2977	Antiglycemic	Tight vs loose glycemic control and cognitive decline	3.33	Rosiglitazone exposure but not insulin use was associated with greater decline in DSST performance in participants randomized to the intensive but not the standard glycemia group.	—

Trial	Intervention	Question/Description		Status	Result
ASPREE (2008), Target N = 18,000	Aspirin	Does aspirin use reduce incidence of cardiovascular events and vascular dementia?	5	Pending	—
MAPT (2014), N = 1680	DHA Cognitive Rx Exercise Rx	DHA, DHA + multidomain intervention (cognitive training, physical training, nutritional advice) for persons with subjective memory complaint.	3	Pending	—
SPRINT-MIND (2016), N = 9361	Anti-HTN	Does lower systolic blood pressure goal (120 mm Hg) result in a 20% reduction in cardiovascular disease events?	4-6	Pending	—
AIBL-Active (2012), N = 156	Exercise	Effect of exercise on progression of WMH for persons with memory complaint ± MCI	2	Pending	—
Secondary Prevention					
PROGRESS (2003), N = 6104	Anti-HTN	ACEI (perindopril) with or without diuretic (indapamide)	4.0	12% (−8% to 28%) reduction in dementia	$P = .2$
PRoFESS (2008), N = 20,332	Anti-HTN	ARB (telmisartan)	2.4	No reduction of the risk of dementia	$P = .48$

Abbreviations: ACEI, angiotensin-converting enzyme inhibitors; ARB, angiotensin receptor blockers; DSST, Digit Symbol Substitution Test; HTN, hypertension; MCL, mild cognitive impairment; NS, not significant.

Retrospective, observational studies have suggested the possibility that specific classes of antihypertensive medications may have differential effects on cognitive outcome. For example, In the National Alzheimer's Coordinating Center database, medications affecting the renin-angiotensin system (eg, angiotensin-converting enzyme inhibitors and angiotensin receptor blockers) were associated with fewer AD conditions[124] and less longitudinal cognitive decline.[125] A small pilot study suggested beneficial cognitive effects of an angiotensin receptor blocker versus angiotensin-converting enzyme inhibitor for hypertensive patients with mild executive impairment,[126] but this needs to be tested in a larger clinical trial.

Type 2 diabetes, statins, aspirin

The Memory in Diabetes (MIND) substudy of the ACCORD examined whether interventions for type 2 diabetes reduce cognitive decline and structural brain changes.[127] Rosiglitazone exposure but not insulin use was associated with greater decline in Digit Symbol Substitution Test performance over 40 months in participants randomly assigned to the intensive but not the standard glycemia group.[128] Imaging analyses have shown that longer duration of type 2 diabetes mellitus is associated with greater loss of gray matter, especially in the frontal lobes, and that rate of brain volume loss was less in the group with tighter glycemic control (**Fig. 6**).[129] In the PROSPER study,

MIND-ACCORD STUDY

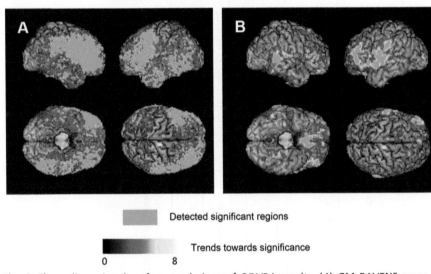

Detected significant regions

Trends towards significance

0   8

Fig. 6. Three-dimensional surface renderings of ODVBA results. (*A*) GM RAVENS maps in relationship with short versus long diabetes duration at baseline. Subjects with long diabetes duration (n = 100) had lower RAVENS values (ie, lower regional GM volume, in the highlighted areas) compared with subjects with short diabetes duration (n = 100). (*B*) GM dRAVENS maps in relationship with standard versus intensive glycemic treatment arm. Subjects in the intensive treatment arm (n = 221) had lower longitudinal decrease in GM tissue volume in the highlighted areas compared with subjects in the standard treatment arm (n = 267). The green color indicates the detected significant regions with FDR-corrected $q<0.05$. The hot color indicates the trends toward significance characterized by the $-\log$ (P) values shown in the color bar. (*From* Erus G, Battapady H, Zhang T, et al. Spatial patterns of structural brain changes in type 2 diabetic patients and their longitudinal progression with intensive control of blood glucose. Diabetes Care 2015;38(1):102; with permission.)

no difference in cognitive decline was found among subjects treated with pravastatin compared with placebo after a mean follow-up period of 42 months.[130] A recent meta-analysis of randomized clinical trials, case-control studies, and cohort studies, concluded that there is low to moderate quality evidence that statins have a neutral effect on cognition.[131] The ASPREE trial[132] is a clinical trial evaluating (every 6 months) the prevention of cardiovascular disease and vascular dementia with low-dose aspirin in the elderly (subjects ≥65 years); the study is expected to be completed in 2017.

Nutritional supplements and exercise

In the Women's Antioxidant Cardiovascular Study, antioxidant supplementation did not slow cognitive change among women with preexisting cardiovascular disease or risk factors.[133] Observational cohort studies have suggested potential benefits of omega-3-fatty acids[134] or exercise[135,136] in the prevention of cognitive decline among cognitively intact individuals. The Multi-domain Approach to Prevention Treatment (MAPT) study randomly assigned persons with subjective memory complaints to receive placebo versus docosahexaenoic acid (DHA) versus DHA plus cognitive training, physical training, and nutritional advice.[137] The effectiveness of exercise for prevention of WMH is underway as part of the Australian Imaging Biomarkers and Life-style Flagship Study of Aging (AIBL).[138]

Secondary Prevention After Stroke

For secondary prevention, a recent study evaluating outcomes of a large community-based stroke registry from London found that "appropriate vascular risk manage-ment," defined as clinically indicated use of antihypertensives, antithrombotic agents, and lipid-lowering drugs, was associated with reduced long-term risk of cognitive impairment assessed by the MMSE in patients with ischemic strokes without history of atrial fibrillation.[139] Independent effects were seen with antihypertensives, the com-bination of aspirin and dipyridamole, and statins. No effects on cognition were seen in patients with history of atrial fibrillation or hemorrhagic stroke.

Symptomatic Treatment of Vascular Cognitive Impairment

Positive effects of cholinesterase inhibitors and memantine have been reported in ran-domized, double-blind, placebo-controlled trials of vascular dementia. A meta-analysis showed favorable effects of cholinesterase inhibitors on cognitive outcomes, but not for global impressions of change.[140] Despite more rigorous implementation of diagnostic criteria, it remains difficult to parse out the contribution of mixed AD path-ologic conditions. Unlike AD, loss of cholinergic neurons in the basal forebrain is not characteristic of vascular dementia. Disruption of cholinergic pathways by severe WMH in Binswanger syndrome[141] and CADASIL,[142,143] however, has been seen. In CADASIL, treatment with donepezil was associated with improvement in a secondary measure of executive function.[144] Cholinesterase inhibitors were generally well toler-ated although associated with an increase in gastrointestinal side-effects; they should be avoided in patients with heart block. Cholinesterase inhibitors and memantine have been approved for the treatment of vascular dementia in some countries but not in the United States. At this time, guidelines for VCI should follow guidelines for the preven-tion and treatment of stroke.

SUMMARY

CVD is the second leading cause of cognitive impairment in late life. The manifesta-tions of VCI are widely heterogeneous in severity, pathophysiology, and neurobeha-vioral phenotype depending on site, size, and sum of VBI. MRI might show preclinical evidence of VBI (eg, SBI and WMH), which is associated with impairment in executive function. One-third of patients experience PSD and, if not initially affected, are at twice the risk of subsequent cognitive impairment over the ensuing 10 years. CADASIL represents the prototype for pure small vessel type of vascular cognitive impairment and has greatly advanced our understanding of underlying pathophysiology and brain-behavior correlations. Neuropathology studies show that AD and VBI often occur together and exert additive adverse effects on cognition.

Many risk factors for sporadic VBI (eg, hypertension, diabetes mellitus, dyslipidemia) are modifiable, although double-blind, placebo-controlled trials are often inconclusive because they are started too late, are too short in duration, or lack sufficiently sensitive cognitive outcome measures. Cholinesterase inhibitors and memantine show mild benefits for cognitive but not global endpoints in trials. They are not currently approved by the US Food and Drug Administration for the symptomatic treatment of VCI but are approved in some other countries. By and large, the means for early detection and prevention of VCI are known. The major challenge remains one of diligent clinical practice and public health implementation. It has been projected that a 10% reduction in 7 risk factors (including 5 vascular risk factors) for 10 years could result in an 8% reduction in incident dementia cases.

REFERENCES

1. Tomlinson BE, Blessed G, Roth M. Observations on the brains of demented old people. J Neurol Sci 1970;11(3):205–42.

2. Vermeer SE, Hollander M, van Dijk EJ, et al. Silent brain infarcts and white matter lesions increase stroke risk in the general population: the Rotterdam Scan Study. Stroke 2003;34(5):1126–9.

3. Grinberg LT, Thal DR. Vascular pathology in the aged human brain. Acta Neuropathol 2010;119(3):277–90.

4. Iadecola C. The pathobiology of vascular dementia. Neuron 2013;80(4):844–66.

5. Alexander GE, DeLong MR, Strick PL. Parallel organization of functionally segregated circuits linking basal ganglia and cortex. Annu Rev Neurosci 1986;9: 357–81.

6. Jeon HA, Anwander A, Friederici AD. Functional network mirrored in the prefrontal cortex, caudate nucleus, and thalamus: high-resolution functional imaging and structural connectivity. J Neurosci 2014;34(28):9202–12.

7. Schneider JA, Arvanitakis Z, Bang W, et al. Mixed brain pathologies account for most dementia cases in community-dwelling older persons. Neurology 2007; 69(24):2197–204.

8. Arvanitakis Z, Leurgans SE, Barnes LL, et al. Microinfarct pathology, dementia, and cognitive systems. Stroke 2011;42(3):722–7.

9. Soontornniyomkij V, Lynch MD, Mermash S, et al. Cerebral microinfarcts associated with severe cerebral beta-amyloid angiopathy. Brain Pathol 2010;20(2): 459–67.

10. Snowdon DA, Greiner LH, Mortimer JA, et al. Brain infarction and the clinical expression of Alzheimer disease. The Nun Study. JAMA 1997;277(10):813–7.

11. Schneider JA, Wilson RS, Bienias JL, et al. Cerebral infarctions and the likelihood of dementia from Alzheimer disease pathology. Neurology 2004;62(7): 1148–55.

12. White L. Brain lesions at autopsy in older Japanese-American men as related to cognitive impairment and dementia in the final years of life: a summary report from the Honolulu-Asia aging study. J Alzheimers Dis 2009;18(3):713–25.

13. Troncoso JC, Zonderman AB, Resnick SM, et al. Effect of infarcts on dementia in the Baltimore longitudinal study of aging. Ann Neurol 2008;64(2):168–76.
14. Toledo JB, Arnold SE, Raible K, et al. Contribution of cerebrovascular disease in autopsy confirmed neurodegenerative disease cases in the National Alzheimer's Coordinating centre. Brain 2013;136(Pt 9):2697–706.
15. Chui HC, Ramirez-Gomez L. Clinical and imaging features of mixed Alzheimer and vascular pathologies. Alzheimers Res Ther 2015;7(1):21.
16. Leys D, Henon H, Mackowiak-Cordoliani MA, et al. Poststroke dementia. Lancet Neurol 2005;4(11):752–9.
17. Ivan CS, Seshadri S, Beiser A, et al. Dementia after stroke: the Framingham Study. Stroke 2004;35(6):1264–8.
18. Rocca WA, Kokmen E. Frequency and distribution of vascular dementia. Alzheimer Dis Assoc Disord 1999;13(Suppl 3):S9–14.
19. Knopman DS, Rocca WA, Cha RH, et al. Incidence of vascular dementia in Rochester, Minn, 1985-1989. Arch Neurol 2002;59(10):1605–10.
20. Ravaglia G, Forti P, Maioli F, et al. Incidence and etiology of dementia in a large elderly Italian population. Neurology 2005;64(9):1525–30.
21. Jin YP, Di Legge S, Ostbye T, et al. The reciprocal risks of stroke and cognitive impairment in an elderly population. Alzheimers Dement 2006;2(3):171–8.
22. Peila R, White LR, Petrovich H, et al. Joint effect of the APOE gene and midlife systolic blood pressure on late-life cognitive impairment: the Honolulu-Asia aging study. Stroke 2001;32(12):2882–9.
23. Peila R, Rodriguez BL, Launer LJ. Type 2 diabetes, APOE gene, and the risk for dementia and related pathologies: The Honolulu-Asia Aging Study. Diabetes 2002;51(4):1256–62.
24. Elias MF, Elias PK, Sullivan LM, et al. Obesity, diabetes and cognitive deficit: The Framingham Heart Study. Neurobiol Aging 2005;26(Suppl 1):11–6.
25. Solomon A, Kivipelto M, Wolozin B, et al. Midlife serum cholesterol and increased risk of Alzheimer's and vascular dementia three decades later. Dement Geriatr Cogn Disord 2009;28(1):75–80.
26. Solomon A, Kareholt I, Ngandu T, et al. Serum total cholesterol, statins and cognition in non-demented elderly. Neurobiol Aging 2009;30(6):1006–9.
27. Longstreth WT Jr, Bernick C, Manolio TA, et al. Lacunar infarcts defined by magnetic resonance imaging of 3660 elderly people: the Cardiovascular Health Study. Arch Neurol 1998;55(9):1217–25.
28. Longstreth WT Jr, Manolio TA, Arnold A, et al. Clinical correlates of white matter findings on cranial magnetic resonance imaging of 3301 elderly people. The Cardiovascular Health Study. Stroke 1996;27(8):1274–82.
29. Vermeer SE, Koudstaal PJ, Oudkerk M, et al. Prevalence and risk factors of silent brain infarcts in the population-based Rotterdam Scan Study. Stroke 2002;33(1):21–5.
30. Vermeer SE, Den Heijer T, Koudstaal PJ, et al. Incidence and risk factors of silent brain infarcts in the population-based Rotterdam Scan Study. Stroke 2003;34(2):392–6.
31. Vermeer SE, Prins ND, den Heijer T, et al. Silent brain infarcts and the risk of dementia and cognitive decline. N Engl J Med 2003;348(13):1215–22.
32. Debette S, Beiser A, DeCarli C, et al. Association of MRI markers of vascular brain injury with incident stroke, mild cognitive impairment, dementia, and mortality: the Framingham Offspring Study. Stroke 2010;41(4):600–6.
33. Yates PA, Villemagne VL, Ellis KA, et al. Cerebral microbleeds: a review of clinical, genetic, and neuroimaging associations. Front Neurol 2014;4:205.

34. Tournier-Lasserve E, Joutel A, Melki J, et al. Cerebral autosomal dominant arteriopathy with subcortical infarcts and leukoencephalopathy maps to chromosome 19q12. Nat Genet 1993;3(3):256–9.

35. Joutel A, Corpechot C, Ducros A, et al. Notch3 mutations in CADASIL, a hereditary adult-onset condition causing stroke and dementia. Nature 1996; 383(6602):707–10.

36. Hara K, Shiga A, Fukutake T, et al. Association of HTRA1 mutations and familial ischemic cerebral small-vessel disease. N Engl J Med 2009;360(17):1729–39.

37. Revesz T, Holton JL, Lashley T, et al. Genetics and molecular pathogenesis of sporadic and hereditary cerebral amyloid angiopathies. Acta Neuropathol 2009;118(1):115–30.

38. Greenberg SM, Rebeck GW, Vonsattel JP, et al. Apolipoprotein E epsilon 4 and cerebral hemorrhage associated with amyloid angiopathy. Ann Neurol 1995; 38(2):254–9.

39. Kokmen E, Whisnant JP, O'Fallon WM, et al. Dementia after ischemic stroke: a population-based study in Rochester, Minnesota (1960-1984). Neurology 1996;46(1):154–9.

40. Srikanth VK, Quinn SJ, Donnan GA, et al. Long-term cognitive transitions, rates of cognitive change, and predictors of incident dementia in a population-based first-ever stroke cohort. Stroke 2006;37(10):2479–83.

41. Liu W, Wong A, Au L, et al. Influence of Amyloid-beta on Cognitive Decline After Stroke/Transient Ischemic Attack: Three-Year Longitudinal Study. Stroke 2015; 46(11):3074–80.

42. Pohjasvaara T, Mantyla R, Aronen HJ, et al. Clinical and radiological determinants of prestroke cognitive decline in a stroke cohort. J Neurol Neurosurg Psychiatry 1999;67(6):742–8.

43. Cordoliani-Mackowiak MA, Henon H, Pruvo JP, et al. Poststroke dementia: influence of hippocampal atrophy. Arch Neurol 2003;60(4):585–90.

44. Bastos-Leite AJ, van der Flier WM, van Straaten EC, et al. The contribution of medial temporal lobe atrophy and vascular pathology to cognitive impairment in vascular dementia. Stroke 2007;38(12):3182–5.

45. Cummings JL. Frontal-subcortical circuits and human behavior. Arch Neurol 1993;50(8):873–80.

46. Tatemichi TK, Desmond DW, Prohovnik I. Strategic infarcts in vascular dementia. A clinical and brain imaging experience. Arzneimittelforschung 1995;45(3A): 371–85.

47. Katz DI, Alexander MP, Mandell AM. Dementia following strokes in the mesencephalon and diencephalon. Arch Neurol 1987;44(11):1127–33.

48. Stuss DT, Guberman A, Nelson R, et al. The neuropsychology of paramedian thalamic infarction. Brain Cogn 1988;8(3):348–78.

49. Bogousslavsky J, Regli F, Uske A. Thalamic infarcts: clinical syndromes, etiology, and prognosis. Neurology 1988;38(6):837–48.

50. Ishii N, Nishihara Y, Imamura T. Why do frontal lobe symptoms predominate in vascular dementia with lacunes? Neurology 1986;36(3):340–5.

51. Dozono K, Ishii N, Nishihara Y, et al. An autopsy study of the incidence of lacunes in relation to age, hypertension, and arteriosclerosis. Stroke 1991;22(8): 993–6.

52. Roman GC. Senile dementia of the Binswanger type. A vascular form of dementia in the elderly. JAMA 1987;258(13):1782–8.

53. Bennett DA, Wilson RS, Gilley DW, et al. Clinical diagnosis of Binswanger's disease. J Neurol Neurosurg Psychiatry 1990;53(11):961–5.

54. Rosenberg GA, Bjerke M, Wallin A. Multimodal markers of inflammation in the subcortical ischemic vascular disease type of vascular cognitive impairment. Stroke 2014;45(5):1531–8.

55. Erkinjuntti T, Inzitari D, Pantoni L, et al. Research criteria for subcortical vascular dementia in clinical trials. J Neural Transm Suppl 2000;59:23–30.

56. Reed BR, Mungas DM, Kramer JH, et al. Profiles of neuropsychological impairment in autopsy-defined Alzheimer's disease and cerebrovascular disease. Brain 2007;130(Pt 3):731–9.

57. Okeda R, Arima K, Kawai M. Arterial changes in cerebral autosomal dominant arteriopathy with subcortical infarcts and leukoencephalopathy (CADASIL) in relation to pathogenesis of diffuse myelin loss of cerebral white matter: examination of cerebral medullary arteries by reconstruction of serial sections of an autopsy case. Stroke 2002;33(11):2565–9.

58. Miao Q, Paloneva T, Tuisku S, et al. Arterioles of the lenticular nucleus in CADASIL. Stroke 2006;37(9):2242–7.

59. Dichgans M, Mayer M, Uttner I, et al. The phenotypic spectrum of CADASIL: clinical findings in 102 cases. Ann Neurol 1998;44(5):731–9.

60. Desmond DW, Moroney JT, Lynch T, et al. The natural history of CADASIL: a pooled analysis of previously published cases. Stroke 1999;30(6):1230–3.

61. Peters N, Opherk C, Danek A, et al. The pattern of cognitive performance in CADASIL: a monogenic condition leading to subcortical ischemic vascular dementia. Am J Psychiatry 2005;162(11):2078–85.

62. Liem MK, van der Grond J, Haan J, et al. Lacunar infarcts are the main correlate with cognitive dysfunction in CADASIL. Stroke 2007;38(3):923–8.

63. Viswanathan A, Gschwendtner A, Guichard JP, et al. Lacunar lesions are independently associated with disability and cognitive impairment in CADASIL. Neurology 2007;69(2):172–9.

64. O'Sullivan M, Singhal S, Charlton R, et al. Diffusion tensor imaging of thalamus correlates with cognition in CADASIL without dementia. Neurology 2004;62(5):702–7.

65. Duering M, Righart R, Csanadi E, et al. Incident subcortical infarcts induce focal thinning in connected cortical regions. Neurology 2012;79(20):2025–8.

66. van Swieten JC, van den Hout JH, van Ketel BA, et al. Periventricular lesions in the white matter on magnetic resonance imaging in the elderly. A morphometric correlation with arteriolosclerosis and dilated perivascular spaces. Brain 1991;114(Pt 2):761–74.

67. Pullicino PM, Miller LL, Alexandrov AV, et al. Infraputaminal 'lacunes'. Clinical and pathological correlations. Stroke 1995;26(9):1598–602.

68. Wardlaw JM, Smith EE, Biessels GJ, et al. Neuroimaging standards for research into small vessel disease and its contribution to ageing and neurodegeneration. Lancet Neurol 2013;12(8):822–38.

69. Arba F, Quinn TJ, Hankey GJ, et al. Enlarged perivascular spaces and cognitive impairment after stroke and transient ischemic attack. Int J Stroke 2016. [Epub ahead of print].

70. Maclullich AM, Wardlaw JM, Ferguson KJ, et al. Enlarged perivascular spaces are associated with cognitive function in healthy elderly men. J Neurol Neurosurg Psychiatry 2004;75(11):1519–23.

71. Ramirez J, Berezuk C, McNeely AA, et al. Imaging the perivascular space as a potential biomarker of neurovascular and neurodegenerative diseases. Cell Mol Neurobiol 2016;36(2):289–99.

72. Hachinski VC, Potter P, Merskey H. Leuko-araiosis. Arch Neurol 1987;44(1): 21–3.
73. Fazekas F, Schmidt R, Scheltens P. Pathophysiologic mechanisms in the development of age-related white matter changes of the brain. Dement Geriatr Cogn Disord 1998;9(Suppl 1):2–5.
74. van Straaten EC, Fazekas F, Rostrup E, et al. Impact of white matter hyperintensities scoring method on correlations with clinical data: the LADIS study. Stroke 2006;37(3):836–40.
75. Longstreth WT Jr, Arnold AM, Beauchamp NJ Jr, et al. Incidence, manifestations, and predictors of worsening white matter on serial cranial magnetic resonance imaging in the elderly: the Cardiovascular Health Study. Stroke 2005; 36(1):56–61.
76. van Dijk EJ, Prins ND, Vrooman HA, et al. Progression of cerebral small vessel disease in relation to risk factors and cognitive consequences: Rotterdam Scan study. Stroke 2008;39(10):2712–9.
77. Carey CL, Kramer JH, Josephson SA, et al. Subcortical lacunes are associated with executive dysfunction in cognitively normal elderly. Stroke 2008;39(2):397–402.
78. Tuladhar AM, van Norden AG, de Laat KF, et al. White matter integrity in small vessel disease is related to cognition. Neuroimage Clin 2015;7:518–24.
79. McAleese KE, Alafuzoff I, Charidimou A, et al. Post-mortem assessment in vascular dementia: advances and aspirations. BMC Med 2016;14(1):129.
80. Greenberg SM, Vernooij MW, Cordonnier C, et al. Cerebral microbleeds: a guide to detection and interpretation. Lancet Neurol 2009;8(2):165–74.
81. Greenberg SM, Nandigam RN, Delgado P, et al. Microbleeds versus macrobleeds: evidence for distinct entities. Stroke 2009;40(7):2382–6.
82. Poels MM, Vernooij MW, Ikram MA, et al. Prevalence and risk factors of cerebral microbleeds: an update of the Rotterdam scan study. Stroke 2010;41(10 Suppl): S103–6.
83. Vernooij MW, van der Lugt A, Ikram MA, et al. Prevalence and risk factors of cerebral microbleeds: the Rotterdam Scan Study. Neurology 2008;70(14): 1208–14.
84. O'Donnell HC, Rosand J, Knudsen KA, et al. Apolipoprotein E genotype and the risk of recurrent lobar intracerebral hemorrhage. N Engl J Med 2000;342(4): 240–5.
85. Dierksen GA, Skehan ME, Khan MA, et al. Spatial relation between microbleeds and amyloid deposits in amyloid angiopathy. Ann Neurol 2010;68(4):545–8.
86. Fazekas F, Kleinert R, Roob G, et al. Histopathologic analysis of foci of signal loss on gradient-echo T2*-weighted MR images in patients with spontaneous intracerebral hemorrhage: evidence of microangiopathy-related microbleeds. AJNR Am J Neuroradiol 1999;20(4):637–42.
87. Schrag M, McAuley G, Pomakian J, et al. Correlation of hypointensities in susceptibility-weighted images to tissue histology in dementia patients with cerebral amyloid angiopathy: a postmortem MRI study. Acta Neuropathol 2010; 119(3):291–302.
88. Tatsumi S, Shinohara M, Yamamoto T. Direct comparison of histology of microbleeds with postmortem MR images: a case report. Cerebrovasc Dis 2008; 26(2):142–6.
89. De Reuck J, Auger F, Cordonnier C, et al. Comparison of 7.0-T T(2)*-magnetic resonance imaging of cerebral bleeds in post-mortem brain sections of Alzheimer patients with their neuropathological correlates. Cerebrovasc Dis 2011;31(5):511–7.

90. De Reuck J, Auger F, Durieux N, et al. Topography of Cortical Microbleeds in Alzheimer's Disease with and without Cerebral Amyloid Angiopathy: A Post-Mortem 7.0-Tesla MRI Study. Aging Dis 2015;6(6):437–43.
91. Charidimou A, Werring DJ. Letter by Charidimou and Werring regarding article, "Cerebral microbleeds in the elderly". Stroke 2011;42(4):e368.
92. Kovari E, Charidimou A, Herrmann FR, et al. No neuropathological evidence for a direct topographical relation between microbleeds and cerebral amyloid angiopathy. Acta Neuropathol Commun 2015;3:49.
93. Tanskanen M, Makela M, Myllykangas L, et al. Intracerebral hemorrhage in the oldest old: a population-based study (vantaa 85+). Front Neurol 2012;3:103.
94. Martinez-Ramirez S, Greenberg SM, Viswanathan A. Cerebral microbleeds: overview and implications in cognitive impairment. Alzheimers Res Ther 2014; 6(3):33.
95. Charidimou A, Werring DJ. Cerebral microbleeds and cognition in cerebrovascular disease: an update. J Neurol Sci 2012;322(1–2):50–5.
96. Miwa K, Tanaka M, Okazaki S, et al. Multiple or mixed cerebral microbleeds and dementia in patients with vascular risk factors. Neurology 2014;83(7):646–53.
97. Jagust WJ, Zheng L, Harvey DJ, et al. Neuropathological basis of magnetic resonance images in aging and dementia. Ann Neurol 2008;63(1):72–80.
98. Tierney MC, Black SE, Szalai JP, et al. Recognition memory and verbal fluency differentiate probable Alzheimer disease from subcortical ischemic vascular dementia. Arch Neurol 2001;58(10):1654–9.
99. Hachinski V, Iadecola C, Petersen RC, et al. National Institute of Neurological Disorders and Stroke-Canadian Stroke Network vascular cognitive impairment harmonization standards. Stroke 2006;37(9):2220–41.
100. Hachinski VC, Lassen NA, Marshall J. Multi-infarct dementia. A cause of mental deterioration in the elderly. Lancet 1974;2(7874):207–10.
101. American Psychiatric Association, American Psychiatric Association. Task Force on DSM-IV. Diagnostic and statistical manual of mental disorders: DSM-IV. 4th edition. Washington, DC: American Psychiatric Association; 1994.
102. World Health Organization. The ICD-10 classification of mental and behavioural disorders diagnostic criteria for research. Geneva (Switzerland): World Health Organization; 1993. xiii, 248 p. 24 cm.
103. Chui HC, Victoroff JI, Margolin D, et al. Criteria for the diagnosis of ischemic vascular dementia proposed by the State of California Alzheimer's Disease Diagnostic and Treatment centers. Neurology 1992;42(3 Pt 1):473–80.
104. Roman GC, Tatemichi TK, Erkinjuntti T, et al. Vascular dementia: diagnostic criteria for research studies. Report of the NINDS-AIREN International workshop. Neurology 1993;43(2):250–60.
105. Gorelick PB, Scuteri A, Black SE, et al. Vascular contributions to cognitive impairment and dementia: a statement for healthcare professionals from the american heart association/american stroke association. Stroke 2011;42(9):2672–713.
106. Sachdev P, Kalaria R, O'Brien J, et al. Diagnostic criteria for vascular cognitive disorders: A VASCOG Statement. Alzheimer Dis Assoc Disord 2014;28(3):206–18.
107. American Psychiatric Association. Diagnostic and statistical manual of mental disorders. 5th edition. Arlington (VA): American Psychiatric Publishing; 2013.
108. Kim GH, Lee JH, Seo SW, et al. Seoul criteria for PiB(-) subcortical vascular dementia based on clinical and MRI variables. Neurology 2014;82(17):1529–35.
109. Hajjar I, Goldstein FC, Martin GS, et al. Roles of arterial stiffness and blood pressure in hypertension-associated cognitive decline in healthy adults. Hypertension 2016;67(1):171–5.

110. Hajjar I, Marmerelis V, Shin DC, et al. Assessment of cerebrovascular reactivity during resting state breathing and its correlation with cognitive function in hypertension. Cerebrovasc Dis 2014;38(1):10–6.
111. Yan L, Liu CY, Smith RX, et al. Assessing intracranial vascular compliance using dynamic arterial spin labeling. Neuroimage 2016;124(Pt A):433–41.
112. Montagne A, Barnes SR, Sweeney MD, et al. Blood-brain barrier breakdown in the aging human hippocampus. Neuron 2015;85(2):296–302.
113. Gold G, Bouras C, Canuto A, et al. Clinicopathological validation study of four sets of clinical criteria for vascular dementia. Am J Psychiatry 2002;159(1):82–7.
114. Zarow C, Sitzer TE, Chui HC. Understanding hippocampal sclerosis in the elderly: epidemiology, characterization, and diagnostic issues. Curr Neurol Neurosci Rep 2008;8(5):363–70.
115. Goldstein LB, American Heart Association, American Stroke Association. A primer on stroke prevention and treatment: an overview based on AHA/ASA guidelines. Chichester (United Kingdom); Hoboken (NJ): Wiley-Blackwell; 2009.
116. Barnes DE, Yaffe K. The projected effect of risk factor reduction on Alzheimer's disease prevalence. Lancet Neurol 2011;10(9):819–28.
117. Satizabal CL, Beiser AS, Chouraki V, et al. Incidence of Dementia over Three Decades in the Framingham Heart Study. N Engl J Med 2016;374(6):523–32.
118. Peters R, Beckett N, Forette F, et al. Incident dementia and blood pressure lowering in the Hypertension in the Very Elderly Trial cognitive function assessment (HYVET-COG): a double-blind, placebo controlled trial. Lancet Neurol 2008;7(8):683–9.
119. Forette F, Seux ML, Staessen JA, et al. Prevention of dementia in randomised double-blind placebo-controlled Systolic Hypertension in Europe (Syst-Eur) trial. Lancet 1998;352(9137):1347–51.
120. Forette F, Seux ML, Staessen JA, et al. The prevention of dementia with antihypertensive treatment: new evidence from the Systolic Hypertension in Europe (Syst-Eur) study. Arch Intern Med 2002;162(18):2046–52.
121. Tzourio C, Anderson C, Chapman N, et al. Effects of blood pressure lowering with perindopril and indapamide therapy on dementia and cognitive decline in patients with cerebrovascular disease. Arch Intern Med 2003;163(9):1069–75.
122. Dufouil C, Chalmers J, Coskun O, et al. Effects of blood pressure lowering on cerebral white matter hyperintensities in patients with stroke: the PROGRESS (Perindopril Protection Against Recurrent Stroke Study) Magnetic Resonance Imaging Substudy. Circulation 2005;112(11):1644–50.
123. Ramsey TM, Snyder JK, Lovato LC, et al. Recruitment strategies and challenges in a large intervention trial: Systolic blood pressure intervention trial. Clin Trials 2016;13(3):319–30.
124. Hajjar I, Brown L, Mack WJ, et al. Impact of angiotensin receptor blockers on Alzheimer disease neuropathology in a large brain autopsy series. Arch Neurol 2012;69(12):1632–8.
125. Wharton W, Goldstein FC, Zhao L, et al. Modulation of Renin-Angiotensin system may slow conversion from mild cognitive impairment to Alzheimer's disease. J Am Geriatr Soc 2015;63(9):1749–56.
126. Hajjar I, Hart M, Chen YL, et al. Antihypertensive therapy and cerebral hemodynamics in executive mild cognitive impairment: results of a pilot randomized clinical trial. J Am Geriatr Soc 2013;61(2):194–201.
127. Cukierman-Yaffe T, Gerstein HC, Williamson JD, et al. Relationship between baseline glycemic control and cognitive function in individuals with type 2 diabetes and other cardiovascular risk factors: the action to control cardiovascular

risk in diabetes-memory in diabetes (ACCORD-MIND) trial. Diabetes Care 2009; 32(2):221–6.

128. Seaquist ER, Miller ME, Fonseca V, et al. Effect of thiazolidinediones and insulin on cognitive outcomes in ACCORD-MIND. J Diabetes Complications 2013; 27(5):485–91.

129. Erus G, Battapady H, Zhang T, et al. Spatial patterns of structural brain changes in type 2 diabetic patients and their longitudinal progression with intensive control of blood glucose. Diabetes Care 2015;38(1):97–104.

130. Trompet S, van Vliet P, de Craen AJ, et al. Pravastatin and cognitive function in the elderly. Results of the PROSPER study. J Neurol 2010;257(1):85–90.

131. Richardson K, Schoen M, French B, et al. Statins and cognitive function: a systematic review. Ann Intern Med 2013;159(10):688–97.

132. Nelson MR, Reid CM, Ames DA, et al. Feasibility of conducting a primary prevention trial of low-dose aspirin for major adverse cardiovascular events in older people in Australia: results from the ASPirin in Reducing Events in the Elderly (ASPREE) pilot study. Med J Aust 2008;189(2):105–9.

133. Kang JH, Cook NR, Manson JE, et al. Vitamin E, vitamin C, beta carotene, and cognitive function among women with or at risk of cardiovascular disease: The Women's Antioxidant and Cardiovascular Study. Circulation 2009;119(21):2772–80.

134. Beydoun MA, Kaufman JS, Satia JA, et al. Plasma n-3 fatty acids and the risk of cognitive decline in older adults: the Atherosclerosis Risk in Communities Study. Am J Clin Nutr 2007;85(4):1103–11.

135. Sturman MT, Morris MC. Mendes de Leon CF, Bienias JL, Wilson RS, Evans DA. Physical activity, cognitive activity, and cognitive decline in a biracial community population. Arch Neurol 2005;62(11):1750–4.

136. Ravaglia G, Forti P, Lucicesare A, et al. Physical activity and dementia risk in the elderly: findings from a prospective Italian study. Neurology 2008;70(19 Pt 2): 1786–94.

137. Vellas B, Carrie I, Gillette-Guyonnet S, et al. Mapt Study: A Multidomain Approach for Preventing Alzheimer's disease: design and baseline data. J Prev Alzheimers Dis 2014;1(1):13–22.

138. Cyarto EV, Lautenschlager NT, Desmond PM, et al. Protocol for a randomized controlled trial evaluating the effect of physical activity on delaying the progression of white matter changes on MRI in older adults with memory complaints and mild cognitive impairment: the AIBL Active trial. BMC Psychiatry 2012;12:167.

139. Douiri A, McKevitt C, Emmett ES, et al. Long-term effects of secondary prevention on cognitive function in stroke patients. Circulation 2013;128(12):1341–8.

140. Kavirajan H, Schneider LS. Efficacy and adverse effects of cholinesterase inhibitors and memantine in vascular dementia: a meta-analysis of randomised controlled trials. Lancet Neurol 2007;6(9):782–92.

141. Tomimoto H, Ohtani R, Shibata M, et al. Loss of cholinergic pathways in vascular dementia of the Binswanger type. Dement Geriatr Cogn Disord 2005;19(5–6): 282–8.

142. Mesulam M, Siddique T, Cohen B. Cholinergic denervation in a pure multi-infarct state: observations on CADASIL. Neurology 2003;60(7):1183–5.

143. Keverne JS, Low WC, Ziabreva I, et al. Cholinergic neuronal deficits in CADASIL. Stroke 2007;38(1):188–91.

144. Dichgans M, Markus HS, Salloway S, et al. Donepezil in patients with subcortical vascular cognitive impairment: a randomised double-blind trial in CADASIL. Lancet Neurol 2008;7(4):310–8.

Lewy Body Disorders

Douglas Galasko, MD

KEYWORDS

- Lewy body • α-synuclein • Dementia • Diagnosis • Management

KEY POINTS

- Cognitive disorders associated with Lewy Bodies are arbitrarily divided into Parkinson's Disease-Dementia and Dementia with Lewy bodies depending on the order in which symptoms arise.
- Clinical evaluation should include movement, cognition, behavior, sleep and autonomic function.
- Biomarkers including brain imaging and polysomnography may be helpful diagnostic tools.
- Medications can help to manage many of the diverse symptoms.

INTRODUCTION

Dementia syndromes associated with Lewy body pathology are subdivided into dementia with Lewy bodies (DLB) and Parkinson disease with dementia (PDD), arbitrarily based on the timing of cognitive decline in relation to motor symptoms. DLB is an underdiagnosed cause of dementia in the elderly. In addition to symptoms of Alzheimer disease (AD) and Parkinson disease (PD), DLB has distinctive neurobehavioral and cognitive features.[1,2] A major clinical diagnostic question is how to distinguish DLB and AD. PDD starts with the movement disorder characteristic of PD, followed by cognitive decline after years or even decades. PDD, therefore, is not a diagnostic puzzle. The distribution of pathology in DLB and PDD helps to explain the diversity of symptoms.[3,4] The key pathologic feature in these disorders is aggregation of the protein α-synuclein, forming structures called Lewy bodies (LB) in neuronal cell bodies and neurites in neuronal processes. Much evidence implicates the spread of α-synuclein between neurons in the progression of disease.

Disclosures: Dr D. Galasko has received research funding from the National Institute on Aging, the California Institute for Regenerative Medicine, the Alzheimer's Drug Discovery Foundation, and from the Michael J. Fox Foundation. He has received honoraria for serving as an advisor to vTv Therapeutics. He is a paid editor for the journal *Alzheimer's Research and Therapy*. He has served on data safety boards for Eli Lilly and Company and Prothena Inc.

Department of Neurosciences, University of California, San Diego, 9500 Gilman Drive, La Jolla, CA 92093-0948, USA
E-mail address: dgalasko@ucsd.edu

THE WHAT AND WHERE OF DEMENTIA WITH LEWY BODIES PATHOLOGY

In addition to the classic involvement of the substantia nigra in PD, α-synuclein pathology has a predilection for the olfactory nerve, branches and nuclei of the vagus nerve, and the locus ceruleus and other brainstem nuclei.[5] Dysfunction of these structures results in loss of sense of smell, constipation and autonomic dysfunction, altered alertness, and rapid eye movement (REM) sleep behavior disorder (RBD), which are common to both PD and DLB and may precede motor or cognitive symptoms by years.[6] In DLB and PDD, α-synuclein pathology includes cortical regions of the brain.

In DLB, there are 3 variations of α-synuclein pathology: brainstem predominant, limbic (also called transitional), and neocortical. Brainstem lesions affect the substantia nigra, nuclei of the vagus and glossopharyngeal nerves, reticular nuclei, and locus ceruleus. Limbic or transitional pathology occurs in the amygdala, transentorhinal cortex, and cingulate. Neocortical pathology is found in areas such as the temporal, frontal, and parietal cortex. Limbic and neocortical α-synuclein lesions are associated with clinical features characteristic of DLB and also distinguish PDD from PD.[4] AD pathology often coexists in DLB and PDD. Concomitant AD pathology contributes to cognitive impairment and may mask or attenuate the neurobehavioral features of DLB. Unlike AD pathology, LB and Lewy neurites in the neocortex are not obviously associated with neuron loss or atrophy.

Is the association of AD and α-synuclein lesions a coincidence? In sporadic DLB and PDD, AD pathology may also be present simply because of age. However, about 20% to 30% of patients with autosomal dominant early onset familial AD have widespread α-synuclein pathology,[7] and a similar proportion of people with Down syndrome (DS), who develop accelerated AD pathology, also have α-synuclein lesions. This finding suggests more than a chance relationship because the onset of dementia in familial AD and DS is younger than the typical age of onset of PD. How amyloid pathology may accelerate α-synuclein aggregation in a subset of people is unknown.

EPIDEMIOLOGY AND RISK FACTORS

Autopsy studies from research centers suggest that DLB pathology occurs in about 20% to 25% of cases of dementia in the elderly. However, more thorough studies using antibodies against α-synuclein reveal amygdala pathology in as many as 40% to 50% of cases. The clinical significance of amygdala-only α-synuclein pathology is unclear, as no unique or characteristic features identify these patients during life. In brains originating from community-based studies, the frequency of DLB pathology is lower, about 10%.[8] The prevalence of DLB has rarely been assessed in population-based clinical studies. It is estimated to account for about 4% of cases of dementia in community-based studies and about 7% in clinic series.[9] Clinical and pathologic studies indicate that age is a risk factor for DLB: the typical age at onset ranges from about 70 years to 85 years. DLB is more common in men than women, as is RBD, one of the characteristic symptoms associated with brainstem LB. DLB has been studied mainly among Caucasian and Japanese populations, and its worldwide occurrence is unknown. Although there are no environmental factors that have been definitively shown to modify the risk of DLB or PDD, one study has suggested that caffeine intake may be a protective factor.[10]

Cognitive impairment is common in PD, and dementia may eventually affect as many as 80% of patients.[11,12] Age and PD duration are the leading risk factors for PDD. The underpinnings of PDD include degeneration of nuclei and pathways involving cholinergic, dopaminergic and noradrenergic pathways,[13] α-synuclein pathology in the medial temporal lobe, and coexisting AD pathology in more than 50% of cases.[14]

Many genetic alterations contribute to PD. The most common of these are leucine rich receptor kinase 2 (*LRRK2*) mutations (particularly G2019S, which is found world-wide, with an increased frequency in people of Ashkenazi Jewish or North African descent) and glucocerebrosidase A (*GBA*) mutations. Mutations in the gene for α-syn-uclein (*SNCA*) are rare. People with PD due to *GBA* and *SNCA* mutations have a high likelihood of developing cognitive decline and a clinical picture of DLB. Genome-wide association studies for late-life DLB or PDD have identified 5 genes linked to PD that are also associated with the risk for DLB and/or PDD, namely, *GBA, LRRK2*, microtu-bule-associated protein tau (*MAPT*), scavenger receptor class B member 2 (*SCARB2*) and *SNCA*.[15] Also, apolipoprotein E (*APOE*) e4, the strongest genetic risk factor for late-onset AD, is linked to DLB and PDD.[16] Shared PD and AD genetic risk is consis-tent with the admixture of α-synuclein and AD pathology in DLB. Although genetic fac-tors may shed light on mechanisms of disease, there is no role for clinical genetic testing in DLB or PDD at present.

DIAGNOSTIC CRITERIA AND A CLINICAL APPROACH TO PARKINSON DISEASE WITH DEMENTIA AND DEMENTIA WITH LEWY BODIES

Diagnostic criteria for PDD[17] focus on the assessment of cognitive decline and its impact on functional abilities. At the stage of PD when dementia typically occurs, neuropsychiatric, sleep, movement, and autonomic symptoms may be present. The difficult part of the diagnosis is determining whether functional impairment results from cognitive changes and is not solely due to advanced motor features of PD. By contrast, the major clinical problem in DLB is distinguishing it from AD. Diagnostic clin-ical criteria for DLB were developed in 1996[1] and updated in 2005.[2] The 1-year rule was proposed to split DLB and PDD: PDD is diagnosed if motor symptoms precede cognitive decline by more than a year; DLB is used if cognitive decline precedes or ac-companies the first motor symptoms. These distinctions are arbitrary, and it may sometimes be difficult to judge which symptom started first. Separating DLB and PDD has been questioned because the clinical features and brain pathology overlap. However, for research purposes and to enhance diagnostic awareness, DLB remains a useful concept. **Table 1** lists the clinical features and **Table 2** the biomarkers that may be used to evaluate patients with PDD and DLB. The discussion that follows fo-cuses on DLB, but the approach to PDD is similar.

CORE CLINICAL FEATURES

The essential feature of DLB is the *D* (dementia), referring to cognitive decline sufficient to interfere with independence in complex daily activities. This cognitive decline typi-cally has a gradual onset. Progression is similar to that of AD, although sometimes DLB may progress more rapidly. The pattern of cognitive impairment in DLB may differ from AD, with selective deficits on tests of attention, visuospatial, and executive func-tion.[18] Symptoms related to visuospatial difficulty include sitting down on the edges of chairs, tripping on stairs, or misjudging distances while driving. General cognitive symptoms in DLB include forgetfulness; impaired judgment, organization, and plan-ning; and getting lost. Memory impairment may not be prominent early in DLB, although patients with significant concomitant AD pathology show deficits on tests of memory and learning. Brief screening tests, such as the Mini-Mental State Examination (MMSE), may be insensitive to the early cognitive changes of DLB or PDD. Formal neu-ropsychologic testing can more clearly identify deficits characteristic of DLB.

The clinical features of fluctuation, hallucinations, and parkinsonism are called core features of DLB.[1] The original diagnostic criteria for DLB specified that dementia plus 2

Table 1
Clinical and diagnostic features of dementia with Lewy bodies and Parkinson disease with dementia

	DLB	PDD
Major clinical features		
Chronology of symptoms	Dementia precedes or occurs together with onset of motor features of parkinsonism.	Motor symptoms precede dementia by 12 mo or longer, often by many years.
Dementia	It may have prominent deficits on tests of attention, executive function, and visuospatial ability. Memory impairment is often less prominent at onset but occurs with progression and if there is concomitant AD.	It is similar to DLB.
Fluctuating cognition	There is marked variation in alertness and attention.	It may be present.
Hallucinations	It is recurrent, most often visual, well formed (eg, people, animals), and detailed.	It is often present.
Motor parkinsonism	It is variable, may be mild; tremor is often absent.	It is more likely to be moderate to severe when dementia develops.
RBD	RBD is more common in men. It may precede DLB or PDD.	
Associated clinical features	Features include daytime sleepiness, transient episodes of unresponsiveness, neuroleptic sensitivity, orthostatic hypotension, urine incontinence, constipation, falls, and anosmia.	

Clinical features grouped as associated have been called supportive or suggestive in consensus criteria for DLB and also occur commonly in PDD but are not essential for diagnosis.
Adapted from Refs.[2,15,57]

or more core features (fluctuation, hallucinations, parkinsonism) defined probable DLB. One core feature indicated possible DLB, whereby there is a lower likelihood that α-synuclein pathology contributes to dementia. These criteria are currently under revision and will elevate RBD to a core feature and include the use of biomarkers to support a diagnosis of probable DLB.

Fluctuation refers to changes in alertness, attention, and cognition and includes periods of decreased attention, staring spells, or confusion, lasting from seconds to hours. Although it is sometimes striking, fluctuation may be difficult to identify in DLB. Research tools to assess fluctuation include a detailed informant-based diary or the use of psychometric tests that measure variability in choice reaction time. A brief questionnaire about fluctuation[19] and a set of 4 questions about daytime drowsiness, sleeping 2 hours or more per day, staring into space, or episodes of disorganized speech[20] are more practical. In patients with varying alertness, delirium may need to be considered; the workup should include factors such as infection, dehydration,

Table 2
Neuroimaging and other biomarkers in the diagnosis of Lewy body dementia

Biomarker	DLB	PDD
Dopamine transporter imaging using SPECT or PET	Low dopamine transporter uptake in basal ganglia	Not needed for diagnosis unless PD has not been previously diagnosed
MIBG cardiac scintigraphy	Decreased uptake	
Polysomnography	Confirms RBD Can identify other sleep problems, for example, obstructive sleep apnea, periodic movements of sleep	
MRI structural imaging	Relative preservation of medial temporal lobe structures, unless AD is also present	
EEG	Prominent posterior slow-wave activity on EEG with periodic fluctuations in the prealpha/theta range	—
CSF Aβ42, tau, P-tau 181	Concomitant AD pathology indicated by decreased CSF Aβ42 and increased tau or P-tau 181	
CSF α-synuclein	Decreased levels of α-synuclein in CSF in DLB or PDD not diagnostically helpful because of extensive overlap with controls and with AD	

Abbreviations: CSF, cerebrospinal fluid; EEG, electroencephalogram; MIBG, metaiodobenzylguanidine; SPECT, single-photon emission computed tomography.

uncontrolled medical disorders, and the effects of central nervous system–active medications.

Hallucinations, most commonly visual, are characteristic of DLB. Patients typically report recurrent, complex visual hallucinations, for example, seeing people, animals, or insects, and may describe them in great detail.[1] Patients may misinterpret shadows or patterns as people or objects, referred to as illusions. Patients with DLB with visual hallucinations have more severe visuospatial dysfunction than those without.[21] Patients may find the hallucinations frightening and can develop delusions related to them. In PD, hallucinations occur in about 30% of patients, persist even after doses of dopaminergic medications are decreased, and may be a predictor of dementia. The anatomic basis of hallucinations is not clear, although weakening of interactions between neural networks for attention and conscious perception may be important.[22] The burden of LB in the inferior temporal lobe plus cholinergic deficits in the temporal lobe and other cortical areas may play a role. Visual hallucinations occurring only in a setting of delirium are not evidence for a diagnosis of DLB. In the presence of severe vision loss, recurrent and vivid visual hallucinations suggest Charles Bonnet syndrome rather than DLB.

In DLB, parkinsonian motor signs may be milder than those typically found in idiopathic PD.[23,24] Rest tremor may be less common in DLB than in PD/PDD; axial signs, such as stooped posture, slowing of gait, and postural instability, may be more prominent. Tremor in DLB may worsen with walking or show overflow (involvement of a wider distribution of muscles) when standing.[25] Assessment of parkinsonism in patients with advanced dementia may be difficult because cognitive impairment and apraxia limit their ability to follow instructions to perform motor tasks. Assessment of gait and postural instability are an important part of the examination regardless of diagnostic specificity. Patients with DLB do not always show a good or prolonged response to L-dopa, but a trial of treatment is warranted.[26] This point may be explained by widespread pathology in DLB that directly affects the striatum and also by deficits in nondopamine neurotransmitter pathways. Other causes of slowing of gait and impaired balance in elderly people include vascular pathology affecting subcortical structures (eg, extensive white matter hyperintensities on MRI or lacunar infarcts) as well as arthritis, pain, deconditioning, and fear of falling. Parkinsonian findings may also be secondary to dopamine receptor blocking actions of potent neuroleptic drugs.

RBD occurs frequently in patients with α-synuclein pathology, including DLB, PD, and multisystem atrophy.[27] It may precede these diagnoses by years, consistent with the idea that α-synuclein pathology spreads or advances from the reticular activating system and nuclei such as the locus ceruleus to the substantia nigra and later to limbic and cortical regions. RBD is much more common in men than women. Its symptoms are due to the lack of motor inhibition during REM sleep. During periods of REM sleep, patients make vocalizations and movements, such as shouting, grunting, thrashing, punching, or kicking, and seem to act out their dreams. They may describe frightening dreams if awakened, such as being chased. Symptoms of RBD can be disturbing to the patients' bed partner and can result in injuries if patients fall out of bed. The history alone may strongly indicate RBD. A formal sleep study may be needed to confirm RBD if there is serious sleep disruption. Other disturbances during sleep and arousal are common in DLB and PDD, including daytime drowsiness, obstructive sleep apnea, and periodic limb movements in sleep, and may warrant polysomnography.

SUGGESTIVE FEATURES FOR DEMENTIA WITH LEWY BODIES

Several clinical features in patients with DLB are either less specific or not common enough to be considered as core features. These features have been termed *suggestive* in consensus criteria for DLB and include neuroleptic sensitivity, autonomic symptoms, repeated falls, delusions, and depression. Neuroleptic sensitivity was first reported in elderly patients with DLB treated with typical antipsychotic medications but later in some patients treated with atypical agents.[1,2] Sensitivity included marked cognitive and motor deterioration that could require hospitalization and was sometimes fatal. Therefore, use of neuroleptics in DLB is discouraged and a neuroleptic challenge should not be considered as a diagnostic test. Dysfunction of the autonomic nervous system is common in DLB, PD, and PDD and due to α-synuclein pathology in central autonomic pathways, such as branches of the vagal nerve or in neurons in paraspinal autonomic ganglia. The most prominent symptoms are orthostatic hypotension and syncope, whereas others may include erectile dysfunction, excess salivation, constipation, altered sweating, and seborrhea. Transient loss of consciousness or awareness may be due to presyncope or to fluctuation. Urine incontinence is common in dementia and aging from a variety of causes and is not a specific indicator of autonomic problems in DLB. Patients with DLB and PDD may have repeated falls because of parkinsonism, impaired postural reflexes, autonomic impairment and impaired visuospatial judgment, and also general factors, such as aging, deconditioning due to lack of activity, and dementia. Delusions are fairly common in DLB, as in other dementias. In some patients they may relate to the visual hallucinations and may be systematized. Depression is common in DLB. Apathy without a depressed mood may be prominent, although not specific. With the progression of dementia, anxiety and agitation often develop and may require treatment.

EARLY STAGES OF PARKINSON DISEASE WITH DEMENTIA AND DEMENTIA WITH LEWY BODIES

Disease-modifying treatment of PDD and DLB is more likely to succeed when started as early as possible; therefore, early diagnosis is a priority. For PD, a stage of mild cognitive impairment (MCI) was recently defined[28] and prodromal DLB is being studied.[29] Loss of sense of smell and constipation are overrepresented in patients with DLB and PD, and may occur years before cognitive or motor symptoms. However, these symptoms are nonspecific. RBD is a strong predictor of PD or DLB.[30] The cognitive profile of MCI that progresses to PDD or DLB varies: in some patients, mild deficits on visuospatial and executive tests occur, but others show an amnestic picture. Fluctuations and hallucinations rarely precede the general picture of DLB.

BIOMARKERS

Neuroimaging markers can help in the diagnostic workup of DLB. For PDD, they have research utility, because dementia is a clinical diagnosis in the setting of an established diagnosis of PD. Although there is no way to image or biochemically detect aggregates of α-synuclein in the brain, imaging may provide indirect evidence of α-synuclein pathology. Dopamine nerve terminal density in the basal ganglia, reflecting projections from the substantia nigra, can be imaged using single-photon emission computed tomography (eg, DaTscan) or PET. Decreased binding has sensitivity of about 80% for DLB and high specificity to distinguish DLB from AD.[31,32] Peripheral sympathetic cardiac denervation, imaged using metaiodobenzylguanidine scintigraphy, is highly sensitive and specific for DLB.[33,34] Occipital lobe hypometabolism occurs on fluorodeoxyglucose (FDG) PET imaging in about 70% to 80% of patients with DLB but not in AD.[35] The pathologic basis of this finding is not clear. The cingulate island sign, an area of preserved normal uptake in the midcingulate or posterior cingulate, is another FDG PET feature that is characteristic of DLB.[36]

MRI shows relative preservation of the hippocampus and medial temporal lobe in DLB compared with AD and cannot clearly distinguish DLB from other causes of dementia.[37] Longitudinal MRI studies show similar rates of atrophy in patients with AD and those with DLB with concomitant AD.[38] In PD-MCI and PDD, changes on MRI include cortical atrophy, often with preservation of medial temporal lobe structures, and changes in white matter tracts.[39] PET imaging methods that detect fibrillar amyloid beta protein allow AD plaque pathology to be diagnosed during life. In one of the larger studies to date that examined people with a spectrum of α-synuclein disorders, those with DLB had a higher amyloid burden than those with PDD, PD-MCI, PD, or age-comparable controls. In DLB but not the other groups, the extent of amyloid burden correlated with scores on tests of semantic memory but not other cognitive domains.[40] This finding suggests that fibrillar amyloid pathology may be more relevant to DLB than to PDD. PET imaging probes of abnormal fibrillar forms of tau were recently developed. In a preliminary study in PD/DLB/PDD, some patients showed increased tau uptake in areas, such as the inferior temporal gyrus, precuneus, and neocortex, which correlated with impaired cognition. This finding reaffirms that tau pathology may contribute to cognitive deficits across the PD/PDD/DLB spectrum.[41]

Analysis of electroencephalogram shows differences between DLB and AD, particularly in posterior regions (reviewed in Ref.[42]), but measures and methods have not been validated for routine use. Cerebrospinal fluid (CSF) biomarkers can provide evidence of AD-related pathophysiology (low CSF Aβ42 and high tau). Patients with DLB are more likely to have low CSF Aβ42, sometimes with increased total tau or phospho-tau (P-tau) 181.[43] In a recent multicenter study, about two-thirds of patients with DLB had decreased CSF Aβ42 and almost one-third had increased tau or P-tau levels. Abnormally low Aβ42 or increased tau or P-tau was associated with more rapid cognitive decline over 24 months.[44] In patients with PD, decreased CSF Aβ42 is related to a higher risk of progressive cognitive decline,[45] consistent with amyloid PET studies indicating that coincidental AD amyloid pathology is associated with faster clinical progression. CSF levels of α-synuclein may be slightly decreased in DLB or PD relative to AD and controls, but these are not diagnostically useful.[45] Recently, it was found that oligomeric α-synuclein is increased in CSF in DLB and PDD[46]; this promising initial finding requires validation.

MANAGEMENT AND TREATMENT OF PARKINSON DISEASE WITH DEMENTIA AND DEMENTIA WITH LEWY BODIES

Overall management begins with a detailed evaluation of cognitive, behavioral, sleep, movement, and autonomic symptoms. Education of the family and caregivers about PDD or DLB, and about general concerns for patients with dementia, such as managing finances and medications, home safety, caregiving needs, and the importance of cognitive and social stimulation and maintaining physical strength and walking skills, are important. Organizations such as the Lewy Body Disorders Association (www. lbda.org) and the Alzheimer's Association (www.alz.org) are excellent resources for information about DLB, PDD, and caregiving.

Medications should be selected according to target symptoms. The decision to use a medication depends on the severity of the symptoms; for example, mild, nonthreatening, visual hallucinations may not require treatment. **Table 3** shows target symptoms and lists some suggested medications. Of note, high-level evidence to support treatment of the diverse symptoms associated with DLB or PDD does not exist because there have been few clinical trials in this area.[47] Some options can be extrapolated from clinical trials on patients with AD or PD. In general, symptomatic medications should be started at low doses and titrated in light of target symptoms and side effects. It is best to introduce one new medication at a time to be able to clearly interpret benefits and side effects. The diverse symptoms associated with DLB and PDD often require use of multiple medications, some of which may interact. For example, an acetylcholinesterase inhibitor (AChEI) for cognition, a selective serotonin reuptake inhibitor (SSRI) for depression or apathy, an appropriate dose of L-dopa for parkinsonism, and an atypical antipsychotic to control hallucinations may all be needed. To limit the potential for drug-drug interactions, medications that do not clearly help after a reasonable trial should be stopped.

For parkinsonism in DLB, a trial of L-dopa is recommended. Because L-dopa may worsen neurobehavioral symptoms, a low dose should be started and increased slowly. The clinical response to L-dopa may be less dramatic in DLB than in idiopathic PD,[26] although some patients show improvement in gait, movement speed, and even alertness. Dopamine agonists are problematic in DLB because of their high risk of provoking behavioral symptoms or other side effects. In PDD, similar careful titration of L-dopa and other medications is needed to obtain the best balance between benefits and side effects.

For cognitive impairment, a trial of an AChEI, such as donepezil, rivastigmine, or galantamine, is worthwhile. Neuropathologic studies report a severe cholinergic deficit in limbic and cortical regions in DLB, suggesting that these patients may be particularly

Table 3
Medications to treat symptoms of Lewy body dementia (Parkinson disease with dementia and dementia with Lewy bodies)

Symptoms	Medications	Comments
Cognitive impairment		
Forgetfulness, poor attention, fluctuation	AChEIs: Donepezil Rivastigmine Galantamine	Tolerability of AChEIs possibly limited by gastrointestinal side effects
		Minimize concomitant medications with anticholinergic effects
	Memantine	Well tolerated, but small effect
Apathy, decreased initiative, psychomotor slowing	Antidepressants, for example, SSRI or SNRI drugs Stimulants, for example, modafinil	Sometimes improves on L-dopa and/or AChEIs
		Possible side effects, such as orthostasis, with older antidepressants, for example, tricyclic antidepressants
Motor impairment		
Bradykinesia, slowing of gait, increased tone, tremor	L-dopa/carbidopa	Hallucinations, anxiety, agitation, sleepiness
	Dopamine agonists, for example, ropinirole	Higher risk of hallucinations in DLB and PDD
Neuropsychiatric symptoms		
Hallucinations, delusions	AChEIs	Small effects on these symptoms
	Clozapine	Needs regular monitoring of blood count
	Risperidone, olanzapine, aripiprazole	Black box warning, risk of neuroleptic sensitivity
	Quetiapine	Black box warning
		Short acting, wide dose range
	Pimavanserine	Effective in 6-wk RCT; lacks postmarketing safety data
Agitation, insomnia	Atypical antipsychotics Trazodone, gabapentin, topiramate, valproic acid	Black box risks
		No evidence from RCTs, but widely used, for example, in AD
Depression	Fluoxetine, paroxetine, sertraline, citalopram	Tolerance of SSRIs potentially better than TCAs in PD
Anxiety	Paroxetine, sertraline, buspirone	Minimal study in RCTs in PD
		Benzodiazepines not recommended because of potential for confusion and falls
RBD	Melatonin Clonazepam	—
Daytime hypersomnolence	Stimulants, for example, modafinil	—
Autonomic impairment		
Orthostasis	Fludrocortisone Midodrine	Fluid retention, edema

Abbreviations: AChEIs, acetylcholinesterase inhibitors; RCT, randomized clinical trial; SNRI, serotonin-norepinephrine reuptake inhibitor; SSRI, selective serotonin reuptake inhibitor; TCA, tricyclic antidepressant.

responsive to AChEI treatment. Randomized clinical trials of AChEIs have been conducted in DLB[48,49] and PDD.[50] The first trial in DLB assessed rivastigmine and found no major effect on the MMSE but significant improvement on computerized tests of attention and a trend for benefit on behavioral symptoms. A later trial of donepezil found benefits relative to placebo on the MMSE that were maintained with open-label follow-up for 52 weeks.[49] A trial of rivastigmine in PDD showed favorable treatment-placebo differences in measures of cognition (including computerized timed tests of attention), global ratings, and activities of daily living. Rivastigmine did not affect parkinsonism, although 10% of patients showed worsening of tremor.[47] Gastrointestinal side effects were the most common reason to discontinue AChEIs in all of these trials. Although evidence is limited,[47] it is reasonable to try an AChEI for cognition or fluctuation in DLB or PDD. Memantine is approved for the treatment of AD. In DLB and PDD, randomized clinical trials found that memantine was safe and well tolerated and had small effects on global ratings and tests of attention but not on other cognitive or behavioral symptoms.[51,52]

Apathy and decreased initiative may contribute to cognitive and functional impairment and are not necessarily part of depression. Although L-dopa may incidentally help these symptoms, other medications may be worth considering if apathy and inertia are disabling. SSRI or serotonin-norepinephrine reuptake inhibitor antidepressants may be tried, with experience drawn from their extensive use in depression in PD.[53] Sometimes apathy is accompanied by daytime hypersomnia. Additional treatment possibilities in this situation may include stimulants, such as methylphenidate or modafinil. Anxiety and depression may co-occur in PDD and DLB. Although evidence from formal clinical trials is limited, analyses suggest that SSRIs are better tolerated and may be more efficacious than tricyclic antidepressants in PD.[54]

For behavioral symptoms, such as hallucinations, psychosis, and agitation, non-medication approaches, for example, distraction, should be tried. For delusions and agitation, the impact of general health factors (eg, pain, infections) and environmental and interpersonal triggers should be explored. If high doses of L-dopa are being used, reduction may lead to improvement. Visual hallucinations may require drug treatment only if they are disturbing to patients. Sometimes AChEI treatment may help with hallucinations.[48] Typical neuroleptics should be avoided because of risks of worsening parkinsonism or causing severe reactions with cognitive and motor decline (neuroleptic sensitivity). Atypical antipsychotic agents, such as olanzapine or risperidone, should be used cautiously because they have weak D-2 receptor blocking activity. Atypical antipsychotic agents, such as quetiapine or clozapine, have support from clinical trials in PD with psychotic symptoms (reviewed in Refs.[47,53]), although the blood monitoring required for clozapine makes it impractical. Many classes of medications have been tried for delusions and agitation in patients with dementia but lack evidence from randomized clinical trials. Medications, such as trazodone, and anticonvulsants, such as valproate, gabapentin, or topiramate, may be considered. Sedatives, such as alprazolam, should be avoided because of risks of confusion and falls. Meta-analyses of elderly patients treated with neuroleptic medications have shown increases in morbidity and mortality,[55] and these medications carry a black box warning from the Food and Drug Administration (FDA). Nevertheless, the judicious use of atypical antipsychotic agents, such as quetiapine (which has an advantage of being short acting), can be considered, at least as a short-term intervention, with careful clinical monitoring for potential side effects, such as drowsiness. Pimavanserin, a serotonin inverse agonist, recently received FDA approval for treatment of hallucinations and delusions associated with PD psychosis[56] based on 6 weeks of treatment in a randomized clinical trial. Postmarketing data will be important to determine its longer-term benefits and safety.

Sleep disorders in patients with DLB/PDD should be carefully characterized to determine the best treatment. If the clinical description is inadequate or uncertain, polysomnography is helpful. For obstructive sleep apnea, standard approaches, such as nasal continuous positive airway pressure or bi–positive airway pressure, may improve symptoms. To control RBD symptoms, melatonin or clonazepam are worthwhile.[27] For insomnia, similar medications to those used for agitation may be considered as well as low doses of benzodiazepines, such as zolpidem. Newer sleep-promoting agents, such as eszopiclone, zaleplon, and extended-release zolpidem, have a theoretic advantage of lower risk of tolerance but have not been formally studied in patients with DLB.

FUTURE DIRECTIONS

Revised diagnostic criteria and use of biomarkers may help to develop earlier and more accurate diagnosis of DLB and stronger predictors of PDD. Further studies will clarify whether there are biological and meaningful clinical differences between DLB and PDD. Genetic studies may improve our understanding of mechanisms of disease and suggest new treatment targets. Biomarkers that allow monitoring of α-synuclein pathology would greatly help with disease staging and development of disease-modifying treatment. Because the pathology of many patients with DLB includes deposition of amyloid beta protein, it is likely that antiamyloid treatments will be useful in DLB and in some patients with PDD.

REFERENCES

1. McKeith IG, Galasko D, Kosaka K, et al. Consensus guidelines for the clinical and pathological diagnosis of dementia with Lewy bodies (DLB). Neurology 1996;67: 1113–24.
2. McKeith IG, Dickson DW, Lowe J, et al. Diagnosis and management of dementia with Lewy bodies. Neurology 2005;65:1863–72.
3. Aarsland D, Ballard CG, Halliday G. Are Parkinson's disease with dementia and dementia with Lewy bodies the same entity? J Geriatr Psychiatry Neurol 2004;17: 137–45.
4. Toledo JB, Gopal P, Raible K, et al. Pathological α-synuclein distribution in subjects with coincident Alzheimer's and Lewy body pathology. Acta Neuropathol 2016;131:393–409.
5. Braak H, Del Tredici K, Rub U, et al. Staging of brain pathology related to sporadic Parkinson's disease. Neurobiol Aging 2003;24:197–211.
6. Walker Z, Possin KL, Boeve BF, et al. Lewy body dementias. Lancet 2015;386: 1683–97.
7. Ringman JM, Monsell S, Ng DW, et al. Neuropathology of autosomal dominant Alzheimer disease in the National Alzheimer Coordinating Center database. J Neuropathol Exp Neurol 2016;75:284–90.
8. Bennett DA, Schneider JA, Arvanitakis Z, et al. Neuropathology of older persons without cognitive impairment from two community-based studies. Neurology 2006;66:1837–44.
9. Vann Jones SA, O' Brien JT. The prevalence and incidence of dementia with Lewy bodies: a systematic review of population and clinical studies. Psychol Med 2014;44:673–83.

10. Boot BP, Orr CF, Ahlskog JE, et al. Risk factors for dementia with Lewy bodies: a case-control study. Neurology 2013;81:833–40.

11. Hely MA, Reid WG, Adena MA, et al. The Sydney multicenter study of Parkinson's disease: the inevitability of dementia at 20 years. Mov Disord 2008;23:837–44.

12. Aarsland D, Andersen K, Larsen JP, et al. Prevalence and characteristics of dementia in Parkinson disease: an 8-year prospective study. Arch Neurol 2003;60:387–92.

13. Gratwicke J, Jahanshahi M, Foltynie T. Parkinson's disease dementia: a neural networks perspective. Brain 2015;138:1454–76.

14. Irwin DJ, Lee VM, Trojanowski JQ. Parkinson's disease dementia: convergence of alpha-synuclein, tau and amyloid-beta pathologies. Nat Rev Neurosci 2013;14:626–36.

15. Bras J, Guerreiro R, Darwent L, et al. Genetic analysis implicates APOE, SNCA and suggests lysosomal dysfunction in the etiology of dementia with Lewy bodies. Hum Mol Genet 2014;23:6139–46.

16. Tsuang D, Leverenz JB, Lopez OL, et al. APOE epsilon4 increases risk for dementia in pure synucleinopathies. JAMA Neurol 2013;70:223–8.

17. Emre M. Dementia associated with Parkinson's disease. Lancet Neurol 2003;2:229–37.

18. Collerton D, Burn D, McKeith I, et al. Systemic review and meta-analysis show that dementia with Lewy bodies is a visual-perceptual and attentional-executive dementia. Dementia 2003;16:229–37.

19. Walker MP, Ayre GA, Cummings JL, et al. The clinician assessment of fluctuation and the one day fluctuation assessment scale. Two methods to assess fluctuating confusion in dementia. Br J Psychiatry 2000;177:252–6.

20. Ferman TJ, Smith GE, Boeve BF, et al. DLB fluctuations: specific features that reliably differentiate DLB from AD and normal aging. Neurology 2004;62:1804–9.

21. Bronnick K, Emrat M, Tekin S, et al. Cognitive correlates of visual hallucinations in dementia associated with Parkinson's disease. Mov Disord 2011;26:824–9.

22. Weil RS, Schrag AE, Warren JD, et al. Visual dysfunction in Parkinson's disease. Brain 2016;139:2827–43.

23. Burn DJ, Rowan EN, Allan LM, et al. Motor subtype and cognitive decline in Parkinson's disease, Parkinson's disease with dementia, and dementia with Lewy bodies. J Neurol Neurosurg Psychiatry 2006;77:585–9.

24. Petrova M, Mehrabian-Spasova S, Aarsland D, et al. Clinical and neuropsychological differences between mild Parkinson's disease dementia and dementia with Lewy bodies. Dement Geriatr Cogn Dis Extra 2015;5:212–20.

25. Onofrj M, Varanese S, Bonanni L, et al. Cohort study of prevalence and phenomenology of tremor in dementia with Lewy bodies. J Neurol 2013;260:1731–42.

26. Molloy S, McKeith IG, O'Brien JT, et al. The role of levodopa in the management of dementia with Lewy bodies. J Neurol Neurosurg Psychiatry 2005;76:1200–3.

27. Boeve BF, Silber MH, Ferman TJ. REM sleep behavior disorder in Parkinson's disease and dementia with Lewy bodies. J Geriatr Psychiatry Neurol 2004;17:146–57.

28. Litvan I, Goldman JG, Troster AI, et al. Diagnostic criteria for mild cognitive impairment in Parkinson's disease: movement disorder society task force guidelines. Mov Disord 2012;27:349–56.

29. Donaghy PG, O'Brien JT, Thomas AJ. Prodromal dementia with Lewy bodies. Psychol Med 2015;45:259–68.

30. Boeve BF, Silber MH, Ferman TJ, et al. REM sleep behavior disorder and degenerative dementia. An association likely reflecting Lewy body disease. Neurology 1998;51:363–70.

31. O'Brien JT, Colloby S, Fenwick J, et al. Dopamine transporter loss visualized with FP-CIT SPECT in the differential diagnosis of dementia with Lewy bodies. Arch Neurol 2004;61:919–25.
32. McKeith I, O'Brien J, Walker Z, et al. Sensitivity and specificity of dopamine transporter imaging with 123I-FP-CIT SPECT in dementia with Lewy bodies: a phase III, multicentre study. Lancet Neurol 2007;6:305–13.
33. Taki J, Yoshita M, Yamada M, et al. Significance of I-123-MIBG scintigraphy as a pathophysiological indicator in the assessment of Parkinson's disease and related disorders: it can be a specific marker for Lewy body disease. Ann Nucl Med 2004;18:453–61.
34. Tiraboschi P, Corso A, Guerra UP, et al. I-2β-carbomethoxy-3β-(4-iodophenyl)-N-(3-fluoropropyl) nortropane single photon emission computed tomography and (123) I-metaiodobenzylguanidine myocardial scintigraphy in differentiating dementia with Lewy bodies from other dementias: a comparative study. Ann Neurol 2016;80:368–78.
35. Minoshima S, Foster NL, Sima AAF, et al. Alzheimer's disease versus dementia with Lewy bodies: cerebral metabolic distinction with autopsy confirmation. Ann Neurol 2001;50:358–65.
36. Graff-Radford J, Murray ME, Lowe VJ, et al. Dementia with Lewy bodies: basis of cingulate island sign. Neurology 2014;83:801–9.
37. Koikkalainen J, Rhodius-Meester H, Tolonen A, et al. Differential diagnosis of neurodegenerative diseases using structural MRI data. Neuroimage Clin 2016; 11:435–49.
38. Nedelska Z, Ferman TJ, Boeve BF, et al. Pattern of brain atrophy rates in autopsy-confirmed dementia with Lewy bodies. Neurobiol Aging 2015;36:452–61.
39. Duncan GW, Firbank MJ, O'Brien JT, et al. Magnetic resonance imaging: a biomarker for cognitive impairment in Parkinson's disease? Mov Disord 2013; 28:425–38.
40. Gomperts SN, Locascio JJ, Marque M, et al. Brain amyloid and cognition in Lewy body diseases. Mov Disord 2012;27:965–73.
41. Gomperts SN, Locascio JJ, Makaretz SJ. Tau positron emission tomographic imaging in the Lewy body diseases. JAMA Neurol 2016;73(11):1334–41.
42. Cromarty RA, Elder GJ, Graziadio S, et al. Neurophysiological biomarkers for Lewy body dementias. Clin Neurophysiol 2016;127:349–59.
43. Vanderstichele H, De Vreese K, Blennow K, et al. Analytical performance and clinical utility of the INNOTESTVR PHOSPHO-TAU (181P) assay for discrimination between Alzheimer's disease and dementia with Lewy bodies. Clin Chem Lab Med 2006;44:1472–80.
44. Abdelnour C, van Steenoven I, Londos E, et al. Alzheimer's disease cerebrospinal fluid biomarkers predict cognitive decline in Lewy body dementia. Mov Disord 2016;31:1203–8.
45. Delgado-Alvarado M, Gago B, Navalpotro-Gomez I, et al. Biomarkers for dementia and mild cognitive impairment in Parkinson's disease. Mov Disord 2016;31: 861–81.
46. Hansson O, Hall S, Ohrfelt A, et al. Levels of cerebrospinal fluid α-synuclein oligomers are increased in Parkinson's disease with dementia and dementia with Lewy bodies compared to Alzheimer's disease. Alzheimers Res Ther 2014;6:25.
47. Stinton C, McKeith I, Taylor JP, et al. Pharmacological management of Lewy body dementias: a systematic review and meta-analysis. Am J Psychiatry 2015;172: 731–42.

48. McKeith I, Del-Ser T, Spano PF, et al. Efficacy of rivastigmine in dementia with Lewy bodies: a randomized, double-blind, placebo-controlled international study. Lancet 2000;356:2031–6.

49. Mori E, Ikeda M, Nagai R, et al. Long-term donepezil use for dementia with Lewy bodies: results from an open-label extension of phase III trial. Alzheimers Res Ther 2015;7:5.

50. Emre M, Aarsland D, Albanese A, et al. Rivastigmine for dementia associated with Parkinson's disease. N Engl J Med 2004;351:2509–18.

51. Matsunaga S, Kishi T, Iwata N. Memantine for Lewy body disorders: systematic review and meta-analysis. Am J Geriatr Psychiatry 2015;23:373–83.

52. Stubendorff K, Larsson V, Ballard C, et al. Treatment effect of memantine on survival in dementia with Lewy bodies and Parkinson's disease with dementia: a prospective study. BMJ Open 2014;4:e005158.

53. Miyasaki JM, Shannon K, Voon V, et al. Practice parameter: evaluation and treatment of depression, psychosis and dementia in Parkinson's disease (an evidenced-based review). Neurology 2006;66:996–1002.

54. Bomasang-Layno E, Fadlon I, Murray AN, et al. Antidepressive treatments for Parkinson's disease: a systematic review and meta-analysis. Parkinsonism Relat Disord 2015;21:833–42.

55. Schneider LS, Dagerman K, Insel PS. Efficacy and adverse effects of atypical antipsychotics for dementia: meta-analysis of randomized, placebo-controlled trials. Am J Geriatr Psychiatry 2006;14:191–210.

56. Cummings J, Isaacson S, Mills R, et al. Pimavanserin for patients with Parkinson's disease psychosis: a randomised, placebo-controlled phase 3 trial. Lancet 2014; 383(9916):533–40.

57. Revisions proposed at the 4th International DLB Symposium. Lauderdale (FL), December 1-4, 2015.

Frontotemporal Dementia

Nicholas T. Olney, MD[a],*, Salvatore Spina, MD, PhD[a],
Bruce L. Miller, MD[a],[b]

KEYWORDS

- Frontotemporal dementia (FTD) • Primary progressive aphasia • Nonfluent PPA
- Semantic PPA • Motor neuron disease • Progressive supranuclear palsy (PSP)
- Corticobasal syndrome (CBS)

KEY POINTS

- The core frontotemporal dementia (FTD) spectrum disorders include behavioral variant FTD, nonfluent/agrammatic variant primary progressive aphasia, and semantic variant PPA.
- Related FTD disorders include frontotemporal dementia with motor neuron disease, progressive supranuclear palsy, and corticobasal syndrome.
- The most common neuropathologic substrates of frontotemporal lobar degeneration (FTLD) are FTLD-tau, FTLD-TDP, and FTLD-FET.
- The 3 genes most commonly associated with FTD are *C9ORF72*, *MAPT*, and *GRN*.
- There are currently no US Food and Drug Administration -approved treatments for FTD.

INTRODUCTION

Frontotemporal dementia (FTD) has undergone numerous changes in nomenclature and categorization schemes since it was first described by Pick in 1892. Presently, FTD encompasses clinical disorders that include changes in behavior, language, executive control, and motor symptoms. Here, the term is used to characterize the core FTD spectrum disorders: behavioral variant FTD (bvFTD), nonfluent/agrammatic variant primary progressive aphasia (nfvPPA), and semantic variant PPA (svPPA). Related FTD disorders discussed include frontotemporal dementia with motor neuron disease (FTD-MND), progressive supranuclear palsy syndrome (PSP-S), and corticobasal syndrome (CBS). The term frontotemporal lobar degeneration (FTLD) is used for pathologic conditions that cause degeneration of frontal and temporal lobes. FTD is a heterogeneous disorder with distinct clinical phenotypes associated with multiple neuropathologic substrates.

Disclosure: See last page of article.
[a] Department of Neurology, UCSF Memory and Aging Center, San Francisco, CA, USA; [b] UCSF School of Medicine, San Francisco, CA, USA
* Corresponding author. 675 Nelson Rising Lane, Suite 190, San Francisco, CA 94158.
E-mail address: Nicholas.Olney@ucsf.edu

Neurol Clin 35 (2017) 339–374
http://dx.doi.org/10.1016/j.ncl.2017.01.008
0733-8619/17/© 2017 Elsevier Inc. All rights reserved.

neurologic.theclinics.com

A BRIEF HISTORY OF FRONTOTEMPORAL DEMENTIA

In 1892, Pick,[1] a Czech neurologist, provided the first known description of a patient with FTD. He depicted a patient with progressive deterioration of language associated with left temporal lobe atrophy, a process that would presently be classified as svPPA.[2] Histologic analysis of Pick's clinical cases, performed by Alois Alzheimer in 1911, showed silver staining argyrophilic cytoplasmic inclusions within neurons.[3] In 1923, Gans described "Pick's atrophy" to characterize unique cases with atrophy in the frontal and temporal lobes.[4] By 1926, Pick's students Onari and Spatz expanded on Alzheimer's pathologic description by delineating Pick's bodies from Pick's cells identifying "Pick's disease" as a neuropathologic entity.[4,5]

There was then a dearth of research into dementia until the 1970s. During this period, most clinical, anatomic, and pathologic patterns gleaned by these early pioneers was largely overlooked.[6] Until the late 1950s to early 1960s, a vascular cause was the accepted cause of "senility," purportedly emanating from decreased cerebral blood flow and miniature infarctions and deemed "arteriosclerotic dementia."[7,8] Only a few groups continued Pick's work during this time, using accurate clinical descriptions correlated with neuroanatomical and pathologic analysis. The perseverance of these researchers would not be appreciated until decades afterward. Marginal progress in FTD research was made until Delay, Brion and Escourolle, a French group of researchers, published their seminal paper emphasizing the clinical and neuropathologic differences between (AD) and Pick's disease. Pick's disease was described to feature frontotemporal atrophy with sparing of the posterior lobes with histology revealing ballooned cells and cortical-subcortical gliosis.[4] The clinical syndrome of Pick's disease showed increased behavioral alterations, lack of insight, and relative freedom from apraxia and agnosia.[4] In contrast, AD featured more diffuse cerebral atrophy and on histology showed neurofibrillary tangles and senile plaques. Clinically, Alzheimer patients had symptoms of agnosia, apraxia, and problems with spatial orientation. In 1974, Constantinidis and colleagues[9] divided Pick's disease into 3 subtypes. Only one of the 3 subtypes had classic Pick bodies, suggesting that Pick bodies were not required for a diagnosis of Pick's disease.

By the 1970s, there was a major shift in reasoning: arteriosclerotic dementia was no longer considered the underlying abnormality for senility, and the concept of dementia became associated with Alzheimer neuropathology.[8,10] In 1976, Katzman[11] wrote about an Alzheimer epidemic, suggesting that in the United States 880,000 to 1,200,000 people over the age of 65 may have AD. During this period, the phrase, "don't pick Pick's disease" was often repeated to young researchers looking for careers in neurology, based on the misconception that Pick's disease was both very rare and indistinguishable from AD during life.[6] Although most dementia research in the United States was focused on AD, 2 groups in Europe started following large cohorts of persons with non-Alzheimer dementias. In Lund, Sweden, Ingvar, Gustafson, and Brun found clinical correlation of frontal lobe atrophy with hypoperfusion in the frontal lobes, and only 20% of cases had classic Pick bodies on autopsy.[12,13] In Manchester, England, Neary, Snowden, and Mann described a large cohort of patients with dementia of the frontal type and found clinical correlations with neuroimaging (single-photon emission computed tomography, SPECT), neuropsychiatric testing, and neuropathology.[5] Around the same time, Mesulam[14] described patients with nonfluent and fluent aphasia without Alzheimer abnormality.[5] Mesulam eventually coined the term primary progressive aphasia (PPA).[15] In 1989, Snowden and colleagues[16] suggested the term "semantic dementia" to describe the patient with predominant left temporal atrophy and aphasia that Pick originally described, whereas predominant right temporal lobe atrophy was not associated with behavioral disturbances and less language involvement until later.[17] Collaboration between the 2 groups in Manchester, England and Lund, Sweden led to the first research criteria for FTD.[18] The clinical diagnostic criteria were revised in the late 1990s, when the FTD spectrum was divided into a behavioral variant, a nonfluent aphasia variant, and a semantic dementia variant.[19] With modernized neuroimaging techniques and neuropsychological evaluations, these groups proved that FTD was distinct from AD during life and that FTD-specific subtypes could better characterize patients.

Further advances in neuroimaging, genetics, and neuropathology have been incorporated in the most recent revision of the clinical research criteria.[2,20] This article focuses on providing the most up-to-date information on the FTD clinical spectrum and its neuropathologic and genetic substrates.

EPIDEMIOLOGY

The incidence of FTD is estimated to be 1.61 to 4.1 cases per 100,000 people annually.[21,22] One study showed the prevalence of FTD, PSP, and CBS was 10.8 per 100,000 with peak prevalence at the age range of 65 to 69 years.[21] There is an estimated 20,000 to 30,000 people in the United States with FTD at one time.[22] FTD is the second most common dementia in persons under the age of 65 and is thought to be less frequent that AD.[22,23] The average age of onset is between 45 and 65, but there have been documented cases younger than age 30 and in the elderly.[24] In a systematic review of 26 studies on FTD prevalence, men and women were found to be equally affected, and the diagnosis of bvFTD was 4 times more prevalent than the PPA diagnoses.[25] BvFTD accounts for roughly 60% of FTD cases, and the other 40% are language variants of FTD.[26] FTD is likely underdiagnosed among nonneurologists because of the lack of recognition and the overlap with a multitude of psychiatric disorders.[22,27]

BEHAVIORAL VARIANT FRONTOTEMPORAL DEMENTIA

bvFTD presents with early changes in behavior, personality, emotion, and executive control.[20] These changes can include new behavioral symptoms such as disinhibition, new compulsions, dietary changes, or symptoms like apathy and lack of empathy. Many of these initial symptoms are easily mistaken for a psychiatric illness, making bvFTD patients at high risk for misdiagnosis.[28] In order to meet clinical criteria for a diagnosis of bvFTD, there needs to be a constellation of at least 3 symptoms fitting into the 6 categories, which include disinhibition, apathy, lack of empathy, compulsions, hyperorality, and executive dysfunction[20] (**Box 1**). These categories are discussed later in further detail.

The behavioral symptoms of bvFTD correlate with dysfunction in the paralimbic areas, including medial frontal, orbital frontal, anterior cingulate, and frontoinsular cortices.[29,30] Right hemisphere atrophy is associated more with behavior changes.[29] Von Economo neurons (VENs), present primarily in large-brained, socially complex animals,[31] are found in the pregenual anterior cingulate cortex, frontoinsular and orbital frontal cortex.[31,32] Seeley and colleagues[33–35] has shown that VENs are selectively vulnerable in bvFTD but not AD. These VEN-containing areas within the salience network are selectively vulnerable and do not represent the epicenter of bvFTD abnormality, before there is spread to other areas within the network. Neurodegeneration is thought to spread within the network with toxic protein aggregates moving from cell to cell in a prionlike manner.[36,37]

Box 1
Diagnostic criteria for behavioral variant frontotemporal dementia

I. Neurodegenerative disease

The following symptom must be present to meet criteria for bvFTD

A. Shows progressive deterioration of behavior and/or cognition by observation or history (as provided by a knowledgeable informant).

II. POSSIBLE bvFTD

Three of the following behavioral/cognitive symptoms (A–F) must be present to meet criteria. Ascertainment requires that symptoms be persistent or recurrent, rather than single or rare events.

A. Early behavioral disinhibition (one of the following symptoms [A.1–A.3] must be present):
  A.1. Socially inappropriate behavior
  A.2. Loss of manners or decorum
  A.3. Impulsive, rash or careless actions

B. Early apathy or inertia (one of the following symptoms [B.1–B.2] must be present):
  B.1. Apathy
  B.2. Inertia

C. Early loss of sympathy or empathy (one of the following symptoms [C.1–C.2] must be present):
  C.1. Diminished response to other people's needs and feelings
  C.2. Diminished social interest, interrelatedness or personal warmth

D. Early perseverative, stereotyped, or compulsive/ritualistic behavior (one of the following symptoms [D.1–D.3] must be present):
  D.1. Simple repetitive movements
  D.2. Complex, compulsive, or ritualistic behaviors
  D.3. Stereotypy of speech

E. Hyperorality and dietary changes (one of the following symptoms [E.1–E.3] must be present):
  E.1. Altered food preferences
  E.2. Binge eating, increased consumption of alcohol or cigarettes
  E.3. Oral exploration or consumption of inedible objects

F. Neuropsychological profile: executive/generation deficits with relative sparing of memory and visuospatial functions (all of the following symptoms [F.1–F.3] must be present):
  F.1. Deficits in executive tasks
  F.2. Relative sparing of episodic memory
  F.3. Relative sparing of visuospatial skills

III. PROBABLE bvFTD

All of the following symptoms (A–C) must be present to meet criteria.

A. Meets criteria for possible bvFTD

B. Exhibits significant functional decline (by caregiver report or as evidenced by Clinical Dementia Rating Scale or Functional Activities Questionnaire scores)

C. Imaging results consistent with bvFTD (one of the following [C.1–C.2] must be present):
  C.1. Frontal and/or anterior temporal atrophy on MRI or CT
  C.2. Frontal and/or anterior temporal hypoperfusion or hypometabolism on PET or SPECT

IV. bvFTD WITH DEFINITE FTLD PATHOLOGY

Criterion A and either criterion B or C must be present to meet criteria.

A. Meets criteria for possible or probable bvFTD

B. Histopathological evidence of FTLD on biopsy or at postmortem

C. Presence of a known pathogenic mutation

V. Exclusionary criteria for bvFTD

Criteria A and B must be answered negatively for any bvFTD diagnosis. Criterion C can be positive for possible bvFTD but must be negative for probable bvFTD.

A. Pattern of deficits is better accounted for by other nondegenerative nervous system or medical disorders

B. Behavioral disturbance is better accounted for by a psychiatric diagnosis

C. Biomarkers strongly indicative of Alzheimer disease or other neurodegenerative process

From Rascovsky K, Hodges JR, Knopman D, et al. Sensitivity of revised diagnostic criteria for the behavioural variant of frontotemporal dementia. Brain 2011;134(Pt 9):2460; with permission.

It is imperative to take an excellent and thorough clinical history with the goal of identifying the brain region where the disease begins. New symptoms developing through time can localize the spread of neuropathologic changes with disease progression. There are heterogeneous clinical phenotypes with bvFTD based on the regional spread in the individual patient. Executive control is lost once the neuropathology involves the dorsal lateral prefrontal cortex that interacts with bilateral parietal lobes.[34,38]

Disinhibition includes socially inappropriate behavior such as invading interpersonal space, inappropriate touching, or overfamiliarity with strangers. There can be impulsive or careless actions like new onset gambling, stealing, poor decision-making without regards to the consequences (eg, buying matching motorcycles for themselves and their 7-year-old son). Disinhibition is linked to right orbital frontal cortex degeneration.[39,40] New criminal behaviors are seen in 37% to 54% of bvFTD patients.[41,42] Loss of social decorum such as telling off-color jokes, using crude language, and rudeness with lack of embarrassment is common in bvFTD. There can be dramatic change in self-awareness, with lack of insight into one's disease.[43]

Apathy can present in many ways.[44] Affective apathy presents as indifference or not caring. Motor apathy manifests as decreased drive to move and less movement overall,[45] whereas cognitive apathy is a loss of desire to engage in goal-oriented activities.[44] Symptoms of apathy may also include social withdrawal in work activities, family functions, or hobbies. Patients often need prompting to stay engaged in conversation, do chores, or even to move. Apathy is easily misinterpreted as depression. Atrophy in the medial prefrontal lobes and anterior cingulate have been correlated with apathy in bvFTD.[29,46,47]

Lack of empathy or sympathy is common. In one scenario, a bvFTD patient has an improper response to a family member being diagnosed with a serious medical condition. Other responses that fit this category include insensitivity and lack of interest toward others or making cruel comments toward others. Another symptom included within this category is a patient's indifference toward their own diagnosis of bvFTD and the impact it may have on others, which has been called "frontal anosodiaphoria."[48] Lack of empathy has been more strongly correlated with atrophy in the right temporal lobe in right svPPA patients and the subcallosal gyrus in bvFTD patients.[49]

Perseverative, stereotyped, or compulsive behaviors often ritualistic in quality can occur in bvFTD.[50–53] Simple repetitive motor behaviors include tapping, clapping, rubbing, picking, and lip smacking. More complex behaviors included in this category are collecting cigarette butts, counting rituals, walking fixed routes, or repetitive trips to the bathroom. Speech can also become stereotyped with specific repetitive patterns. Stereotyped and compulsive behaviors have been associated with several brain areas. Aberrant motor behavior has been affiliated with atrophy in the right dorsal anterior cingulate and left premotor cortex.[29] Atrophy in the striatum has been associated with stereotypes (tapping, rocking, protruding one's tongue).[51] Complex compulsions have been associated with asymmetric temporal lobe atrophy.[53] Obsessive compulsive behaviors in bvFTD have been correlated with loss of gray matter in bilateral globus pallidus, left putamen, and lateral temporal pole (left middle and inferior temporal gyri).[52]

Hyperorality and major changes in dietary habits can also manifest in bvFTD. Changes in food preference, particularly an inclination toward sweets or carbohydrates, are common and lead to weight gain.[54] Patients may overeat, stuffing food in their mouth, and in such cases, satiety will be an insufficient cue to stop. One study showed that bvFTD patients continued to eat sweet sandwiches despite claiming to be full.[55] As patients become more disinhibited, they may grab food off other people's plates. Later in the course of bvFTD, hyperorality can occur, with oral exploration or eating inedible objects. Changes in eating behavior have been associated with atrophy in the orbital frontal cortex, right insular cortex, and the striatum.[55,56] Some suggest involvement of the hypothalamus.[57]

Neuropsychological testing of patients with bvFTD should test multiple domains and be anatomically oriented to target specific brain structures.[6] Notation of abnormal behaviors and impaired emotional processing should be described by the examiner if present. Formal neuropsychological testing can be normal in early stages of the disease.[58] As abnormality involves the dorsal lateral prefrontal cortex, executive function will emerge on neuropsychological testing and can help differentiate bvFTD patients from those with AD.[38]

There is subset of patients that exhibit a clinical presentation called "FTD-phenocopy," or slowly progressive bvFTD, that meets clinical criteria for possible bvFTD. In some instances, these patients do not suffer from a neurodegenerative condition.[59] However, in one study, 2 of 4 patients identified as slowly progressive bvFTD, carried the pathogenic repeat in the chromosome 9 open reading frame 72 (C9ORF72) gene.[60] Recently, at University of California, San Francisco (UCSF), a new subgroup was identified with slow progression associated with minimal cortical atrophy but with subcortical atrophy, of whom 88% carry the C9ORF72 repeat.[61] This finding suggests that patients with slowly progressive bvFTD, or the "FTD-phenocopy" presentation, should be tested for the C9ORF72 repeat as a possible cause for neurodegeneration.

Frontal and/or anterior temporal lobe atrophy on structural (MRI or CT) neuroimaging or hypometabolism on PET or SPECT can further support a diagnosis of bvFTD (**Fig. 1**).[20] Neurologists are encouraged to interpret their patients' MRI images, as radiologists may underestimate atrophy patterns that are suggestive of bvFTD.[62]

PRIMARY PROGRESSIVE APHASIAS

The PPAs are neurodegenerative syndromes, where language is the primary impairment in the first 2 years of symptom onset, that Mesulam[14,63] initially described as a "slowly progressive aphasia" and later renamed primary progressive aphasia. For approximately 2 decades, PPAs were divided into semantic dementia and progressive nonfluent aphasia, although several PPA cases did not fit into this binary

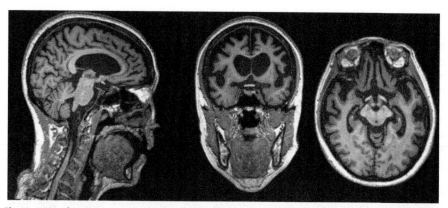

Fig. 1. MRI of a patient with bvFTD showing severe frontal and temporal lobe atrophy. The patient is a 60-year-old woman who developed symptoms of withdrawal, not taking care of her farm animals, 8 years before. Her symptoms progressed to impaired hygiene, lack of empathy, and disobeying the rules of the road. In the last 2 years, she developed repetitive behaviors, hyperorality, incontinence, and a nonfluent aphasia.

categorization.[2] A third type of variant that was fluent with syntactically simple sentences but frequent word finding pauses was described by Gorno-Tempini and colleagues[2,64] and called logopenic primary progressive aphasia (lvPPA). The most recent clinical research criteria for PPAs include svPPA, nfvPPA, and logopenic variant PPA.[2] The logopenic variant of PPA has been correlated predominantly with AD abnormality so will not be discussed in detail in this article.[65,66] The other 2 types of PPA, svPPA and nfvPPA, are considered part of the FTD spectrum and are predominantly associated with FTD neuropathology.

SEMANTIC VARIANT PRIMARY PROGRESSIVE APHASIA

The study of temporal lobe variants of FTD has furthered the understanding of language and behavior. If the left temporal lobe is involved, as in left svPPA, symptoms are predominantly language based with a slow loss of semantic knowledge. When the right temporal lobe is primarily involved (right svPPA), behavioral symptoms predominate. As time progresses, both temporal lobes become involved, and symptoms begin to overlap.[67] By 5 to 7 years, patients get more frontal lobe structures involved and develop symptoms of bvFTD with disinhibition, change in food preference, and weight gain.[67] Patients with svPPA tend to have slow progression and can live a decade or more after symptom onset.[68] Of the core clinical phenotypes in FTD, svPPA is the least likely to have a genetic cause underlying the cause.[69,70]

The initial features of classic left temporal svPPA are anomia and single-word comprehension deficits.[2] The earliest symptom is often poor comprehension of single low-frequency words, such as "giraffe," with initial preservation of higher frequency words like "dog." Neuropsychological testing must include semantic screening for low-frequency words, with a test like the Boston Naming Test (BNT), as the 2 words (pen, watch) in the Mini–Mental State Examination (MMSE) are not sensitive enough to detect early svPPA.[6,38] As symptoms progress, patients also lose semantic knowledge about objects,[2] so if a patient does not know the word "giraffe," they will not improve with phonemic cues or semantic hints like "animal with a long neck." When svPPA patients are asked to read irregularly spelled words (yacht, gnat), they will sound them out, attempting phonetic "regularization," having lost the knowledge or their unconventional sound (ie, y-act, ga-nat), a phenomenon known as surface dyslexia.[2] In svPPA, repetition is spared; speech apraxia is not present, and syntax and grammar remain impressively intact. If the mesial temporal lobes are involved, memory can be affected, but executive function and visuospatial skills typically are preserved.[71] Clinical research criteria for language predominant (left) svPPA must include the core features of impaired confrontational naming and impaired single-word comprehension. There also must be 3 of the following 4 criteria: impaired object knowledge, surface dyslexia, spared repetition, and spared speech production[2] (**Box 2**).

Right temporal svPPA patients present with prominent behavioral changes that include emotional distance, irritability, social isolation, bizarre alterations in dress, compulsions, disruption of sleep, appetite, and libido.[17,67,72] Patients with right temporal svPPA often lack social pragmatics. They can be viscous, with telling

---

Box 2
Diagnostic criteria for the semantic variant primary progressive aphasia

I. Clinical diagnosis of semantic variant PPA

Both of the following core features must be present:

A. Impaired confrontation naming

B. Impaired single-word comprehension

At least 3 of the following other diagnostic features must be present:

A. Impaired object knowledge, particularly for low-frequency or low-familiarity items

B. Surface dyslexia or dysgraphia

C. Spared repetition

D. Spared speech production (grammar and motor speech)

II. IMAGING-SUPPORTED SEMANTIC VARIANT PPA DIAGNOSIS

Both of the following criteria must be present:

A. Clinical diagnosis of semantic variant PPA

B. Imaging must show one or more of the following results:
   1. Predominant anterior temporal lobe atrophy
   2. Predominant anterior temporal hypoperfusion or hypometabolism on SPECT or PET

III. SEMANTIC VARIANT PPA WITH DEFINITE PATHOLOGY

Clinical diagnosis (criterion A below) and either criterion B or C must be present:

A. Clinical diagnosis of semantic variant PPA

B. Histopathologic evidence of a specific neurodegenerative pathology (eg, FTLD-tau, FTLD-TDP, AD, other)

C. Presence of a known pathogenic mutation

From Gorno-Tempini ML, Hillis AE, Weintraub S, et al. Classification of primary progressive aphasia and its variants. Neurology 2011;76(11):1009; with permission.

long-winded stories, interrupting loved ones, and not picking up on normal social cues that they may be acting inappropriately. It is thought that this inability to pick up social cues has to do with an inability to read the emotions on faces. Worsening degrees of right amygdala atrophy has been correlated with impairment in processing facial emotions.[73]

Patients with either left or right temporal svPPA can have new compulsions. Left svPPA patients have been shown to have compulsions directed toward visual or nonverbal stimuli where objects are devoid of verbal information like coins or pictures. Right svPPA have compulsions around games with words and symbols.[67]

An interesting phenomenon is the development of new artistic abilities that has been observed in svPPA. Left svPPA patients have developed new visual abilities in painting, drawing, music, and gardening.[74–76] Right svPPA patients can have emergent abilities in writing despite their progressive neurodegenerative condition.[6] One patient with bilateral, right worse than left, svPPA was studied in depth at UCSF. As the right temporal lobe became more involved, he showed decline in emotional perception displayed through his new skill of painting.[77] The topics of the painting would show couples and landscapes, but as his disease progressed, the facial expressions became less genuine. Painted couples would stand next to each other, not holding hands, with bizarre smiles showing teeth.[77] One could theorize that this case illustrates the difficulty the patient had understanding emotions in others as the right temporal lobe involvement progressed (**Fig. 2**).

Neuroimaging can further support a diagnosis of svPPA, with anterior temporal pole atrophy on structural imaging or hypoperfusion on functional imaging[2] (**Figs. 3** and **4**). Traditionally, early symptoms originate from anterior and inferior temporal lobes involving the amygdala, with later symptoms deriving from pathologic spread into the contralateral temporal lobe and then into the ventromedial frontal cortex and insula.[47,67,78]

NONFLUENT/AGRAMMATIC PRIMARY PROGRESSIVE APHASIA

Patients with nfvPPA first present with effortful speech and often endorse word-finding problems. Over time, the speech becomes labored, slow, slurred, and choppy with disrupted prosody. The patient begins making inconsistent speech sound errors without awareness of this deficit. There can be inconsistent insertions, deletions, distortions, and substitutions in speech sounds. If a patient is asked to repeat a

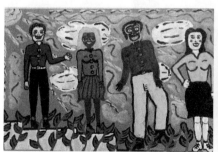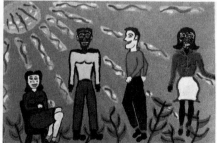

Fig. 2. Paintings made by a 53-year-old man with FTLD that had both language and behavioral symptoms. He developed compulsions for painting as one of his early symptoms, and it is postulated that as his right temporal lobe become more involved that the faces in his work became less detailed and began to have a more generic smile with teeth. (*Courtesy of* the UCSF Memory and Aging Center, San Francisco, CA; with permission.)

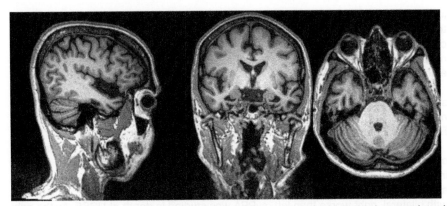

Fig. 3. Left svPPA MRI. MRI showing left temporal lobe atrophy in sagittal, coronal, and axial cuts. The patient is a 61-year-old man, whose first symptom was 6 years before with the inability to name apples in a fruit bowl. His problems with semantics and naming progressed, and 3 years before he had difficulty recognizing faces of neighbors. More recent symptoms include the urge to lick people and things (hyperorality).

complexly structured word like "catastrophe" 5 times in a row, he or she will demonstrate a motor speech apraxia by repeating this word differently each time.[79] Improper use of grammar is frequently present in nfvPPA, but can be subtle, or even absent in the early stages of the illness. Patients can often have an aphemia, but can still communicate correctly with written language. Eventually agrammatism will involve both verbal and written language. Effortful speech often occurs before clear apraxia of speech or agrammatism.[2] The neuroanatomical correlate for the symptoms of nfvPPA are Broadman Area 44, 45 (Broca area) in the left inferior frontal gyrus and the anterior insula.[64] As time progresses, patients will have decreased verbal output

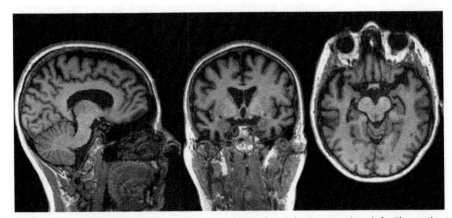

Fig. 4. Right svPPA MRI. MRI shows bitemporal atrophy right greater than left. The patient is a 64-year-old woman, whose first symptom was 10 years before, telling repetitive stories that slowly became less appropriate and embarrassed her friends and family. Six years before, she developed an obsession of taking specific walking routes to collect cigarette butts. More recently, she has shown lack of empathy toward her family and dog.

and eventually become nonverbal. Mutism in nfvPPA is correlated to a larger lesion expanding beyond the typical inferior frontal and insular regions involved early in nfvPPA.[80]

On neuropsychological testing, patients with nfvPPA eventually show deficits on the BNT and will still show retained semantic knowledge for these pictures.[64] Usually, at least during the early stages, word-finding difficulty is common, but frank anomia is rare. Comprehension typically remains intact, except for longer complex sentences. Executive function can show subtle dysfunction, but memory and visuospatial skills remain relatively spared early in the disease course.[64]

For a patient to meet clinical criteria for nfvPPA, they must have effortful speech with motor speech apraxia or agrammatism as well as supporting features of nfvPPA (**Box 3**).[2] Neuroimaging support for nfvPPA consists of atrophy on MRI or hypometabolism on PET or SPECT scan in the left inferior frontal gyrus, near the perisylvian area and involving Broca area[64] (**Fig. 5**).

Box 3
Diagnostic criteria for nonfluent/agrammatic variant primary progressive aphasia

I. Clinical diagnosis of nonfluent/agrammatic variant PPA:

At least one of the following core features must be present:

A. Agrammatism in language production

B. Effortful, halting speech with inconsistent speech sound errors and distortions (apraxia of speech)

At least 2 of 3 of the following other features must be present:

A. Impaired comprehension of syntactically complex sentences

B. Spared single-word comprehension

C. Spared object knowledge

II. IMAGING-SUPPORTED NONFLUENT/AGRAMMATIC VARIANT DIAGNOSIS

Both of the following criteria must be present:

A. Clinical diagnosis of nonfluent/agrammatic variant PPA

B. Imaging must show one or more of the following results:
1. Predominant left posterior frontoinsular atrophy on MRI or
2. Predominant left posterior frontoinsular hypoperfusion or hypometabolism on SPECT or PET

III. NONFLUENT/AGRAMMATIC VARIANT PPA WITH DEFINITE PATHOLOGY

Clinical diagnosis (criterion A below) and either criterion B or C must be present:

A. Clinical diagnosis of nonfluent/agrammatic variant PPA

B. Histopathologic evidence of a specific neurodegenerative pathology (eg, FTLD-tau, FTLD-TDP, AD, other)

C. Presence of a known pathogenic mutation

From Gorno-Tempini ML, Hillis AE, Weintraub S, et al. Classification of primary progressive aphasia and its variants. Neurology 2011;76(11):1009; with permission.

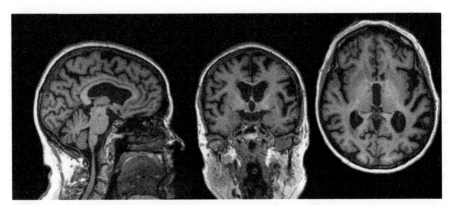

Fig. 5. nfvPPA MRI. MRI showing predominant left posterior frontoinsular atrophy. The patient is an 84-year-old woman, whose first symptom was word-finding difficulties 7 years before. Over time, she developed impaired grammar and a speech apraxia as her speech output diminished.

RELATED FRONTOTEMPORAL DEMENTIA SYNDROMES

The core FTD disorders are bvFTD, svPPA (right and left temporal variants), and nfvPPA, but there are other disorders within the FTD spectrum that include FTD-MND, PSP-S, and CBS.

Frontotemporal Dementia with Motor Neuron Disease

The relationship of dementia, motor neuron disease (MND), and parkinsonism was first noted in the Guamanian Chamorros, after World War II, in the amyotrophic lateral sclerosis (ALS)-parkinsonism dementia complex of Guam.[81,82] Up to 15% of FTD patients and up to 30% of patients with MND experience overlap between the 2 syndromes.[83] The coexistence of the 2 disorders may be underrecognized, as patients tend to present to either a neuromuscular disease clinic or a dementia clinic.[83] To meet criteria for MND, an FTD patient needs upper and lower motor neuron signs on physical examination or electromyogram (EMG).[84] The El Escorial criteria are one of the most widely accepted criteria for the diagnosis of ALS but the Awaji criteria are also used, which de-emphasizes the use of EMG to make an earlier diagnosis.[84–86] If an FTD patient presents with fasciculations, muscle weakness, trouble swallowing, spastic tone, hyperreflexia, or pathologic laughing or crying, this should raise concern for MND and prompt a neuromuscular workup. If patients with ALS present with symptoms concerning for bvFTD, this should prompt a cognitive workup. There is a shorter survival in patients with both FTD and MND because patients with FTD symptoms are less compliant with standard ALS treatments.[87]

The overlap story between FTD and MND became much richer in 2005, when Mackenzie[88] used ubiquitin immunohistochemistry to show that MND, FTD-MND, and FTD were related pathologically and fit on a spectrum. Then in 2006, TAR DNA-binding protein 43 (TDP-43) was shown to be the major disease protein in the neuropathology of tau-negative FTD and MND.[89–91] In 2009, human genetic studies and postmortem analysis linked mutations in the Fused in sarcoma (FUS) gene to a familial form of MND.[92–94] This finding prompted researchers to look for FUS abnormality in FTD patients. FUS inclusions were found in patients with FTD that did not have a mutation in the *FUS* gene.[95–98] A genetic linkage between FTD-MND and chromosome 9q21-q22 had been known since 2000,[99] but a hexanucleotide repeat, GGGGCC, in the noncoding region of C9ORF72 was not discovered until 2011.[100,101]

Corticobasal Degeneration

Corticobasal degeneration (CBD) was first described by Rebeiz and colleagues[102] in 1968, in 3 patients with progressive asymmetric symptoms of movement and posturing that were found to have "corticodentatonigral degeneration with neuronal achromasia" on autopsy. Despite numerous revisions in diagnostic criteria, predicting CBD neuropathology has proven to be a diagnostic challenge for clinicians with the correct CBD abnormality predicted before death in only 56% of cases.[103] Currently, the term CBS is used to describe the "canonical" clinical entity associated with CBD, understanding that many cases of CBS are not associated with CBD neuropathology and vice versa. Many cases of CBD abnormality have early clinical presentations different than CBS.[104] The clinical syndrome of CBS has been associated with AD, PSP, CBD, Pick's disease, TDP type A, Lewy body, and rarely, prion abnormality.[103–107] The term CBD is today only used to refer to the 4R tau-specific neuropathologic entity.

To meet the most recent clinical criteria for probable CBS, a patient must have an asymmetric presentation with 2 of the following motor symptoms: limb rigidity or akinesia, limb dystonia, or limb myoclonus, as well as 2 of the following higher cortical symptoms: orobuccal or limb apraxia, cortical sensory deficit, or alien limb phenomena.[103] Although asymmetry occurs with CBD, data have shown that CBD is not more likely to be asymmetric than any other neurodegenerative condition.[106,108] CBD tends to affect a dorsal frontal network involved with drive, movement, language, and behavior. In a paper by Lee and colleagues,[106] CBD was predicted by clinical syndromes bvFTD, nfvPPA, and an executive motor disorder. Typically, patients first present with a behavioral, language, or executive dysfunction, leading to suspicion of bvFTD or nfvPPA. Eventually, they exhibit motor dysfunction, often parkinsonism with axial rigidity.[109,110] The absence of early motor symptoms should not exclude CBD.[106] There is significant overlap with PSP clinically, and in some cases series, more than 50% of patients diagnosed with CBS in life had PSP abnormality.[111] Patients with an H1H1 haplotype of the MAPT gene are associated with an increased risk for CBD and PSP abnormality.[112] In general, if the disease begins in the parietal region or there is a parietally predominant syndrome, the diagnosis is more likely to be AD than CBD.

There are no specific biomarkers that allow the prediction of CBD abnormality. In patients who meet CBS criteria, current PET scan technology and cerebrospinal fluid (CSF) biomarkers can identify patients with Alzheimer abnormality, and those considered amyloid negative can be considered more likely to have 4R CBD neuropathology.[113] Neuroimaging with MRI is associated with more posterior atrophy in CBS associated with Alzheimer abnormality, and there is more frontal atrophy associated with CBD tau abnormality.[106,114] Dorsal atrophy can help predict underlying CBD 4R tau abnormality, especially in cases presenting as bvFTD.[115,116]

Progressive Supranuclear Palsy

PSP-S, previously known as Steele-Richardson-Olszewski syndrome, was first described in 1964.[117] The initial description of 9 patients displayed vertical greater than horizontal supranuclear gaze palsy, axial rigidity, dysarthria, frequent falls, pseudobulbar affect, lack of tremor, and mild dementia with vague changes in personality and psychiatric symptoms.[117] Neuropathologically, nerve cells loss and neurofibrillary tangles in the basal ganglia, brainstem, and cerebellum were reported decades before the identification of PSP as a 4R tau abnormality.[118] PSP-S can be a difficult diagnosis to make in the early stages because it can overlap with many syndromes, but by the final examination, clinicians have had accuracy as high as more than 80% in predicting the correct PSP abnormality.[119,120] At UCSF, nearly all cases (>92%) with a clinical diagnosis of PSP-S showed PSP abnormality. Most of the other PSP-S cases had CBD.

The 1996 consensus clinical research criteria for possible PSP define the following core features: onset after age 40, gradual progression, either vertical supranuclear gaze palsy or slow vertical saccades, and postural instability with falls in the first year.[121] Patients must also have no exclusion criteria. Probable PSP is inclusive of both a vertical supranuclear gaze palsy and a postural instability with falls.[121] Severe impairment of postural reflexes and bradykinesia make PSP falls extremely dangerous because patients are often unable to protect themselves from objects during the fall. The falls in PSP can be multifactorial from either the impaired eye movements, postural instability, impulsivity, or all 3 symptoms.

Patients can present with predominant executive dysfunction, personality changes, reduced mental speed, and attention deficits giving a more frontal behavior syndrome that is not emphasized in the current PSP criteria.[122] Patients presenting with frontal behavior symptoms and without falls or supranuclear gaze palsy in their first year of presentation are likely to be among the 20% of PSP patients that are clinically mis-diagnosed.[122,123] Clinical presentations of bvFTD or nfvPPA can progress to PSP, or alternatively, an initial presentation of PSP can progress into bvFTD or nfvPPA.[110,122,124] Williams and Lee[123] has proposed a system to further differentiate PSP. They classifies Richardson syndrome as the classic PSP-S described above. PSP-Parkinsonism (PSP-P) is the most common non–Steele-Richardson PSP sub-type, which is similar to Richardson syndrome but has tremor and mild responsive-ness to Levodopa. PSP-pure akinesia with gait freezing is a PSP-S subtype that can have a slower disease course despite severe atrophy in the globus pallidus, sub-stantia nigra, and subthalamic nucleus. There is also PSP-corticobasal syndrome (PSP-CBS) as well as PSP-progressive nonfluent aphasia.[123]

There are no definitive biomarkers for PSP. Recently, levels of neurofilament light chain in serum have been correlated with PSP disease severity, but this marker is not specific for PSP and has been associated with other neurodegenerative disor-ders.[125-128] Midbrain atrophy and the hummingbird sign on neuroimaging have been associated with PSP. The utility of the hummingbird sign in predicting midbrain atrophy has been debated, but there is evidence showing it can help differentiate PSP from idiopathic Parkinson disease and multisystem atrophy.[129] Boxer and col-leagues[115] showed that with neuroimaging, one can differentiate CBD from PSP with 93% accuracy using only the differences between atrophy of the midbrain and left frontal eye fields.

Neuropathology of Frontotemporal Lobar Degeneration

"Frontotemporal lobar degeneration" (FTLD) is defined as the neurodegenerative pro-cess causing selective neuronal loss and gliosis of the frontal and temporal lobes of the brain.[130] The term is also used, less strictly, to encompass the diverse group of neuropathologic substrates of disease associated with the clinical phenotypes of FTD, although some of these pathologic processes display a wider range of neurode-generation than the one limited to the frontal and temporal lobes of the brain. The cur-rent classification of "FTLD" subtypes is based on the immunohistochemical staining for specific intracellular protein accumulations associated with distinct molecular de-fects.[90,131] The basic groupings of FTLD-tau, FTLD-TDP, FTLD-FET, and FTLD-UPS are discussed as well as clinicopathologic correlations that are known for these neuropathologic entities (**Fig. 6**).

Frontotemporal Lobar Degeneration-Tau

The protein tau was first discovered in 1975 as an essential protein in microtubule assembly.[132] It was later found to assist in cellular transport and stabilization of the structure of the cell.[133] More recently, it has been established that tau is also involved in cellular signaling pathways.[134–136] The tau gene, *MAPT*, was found to be on chromosome 17q21 and over 50 mutations have been linked to FTLD-tau abnormality.[133,137–141] Alternative splicing of *MAPT* generates 6 different isoforms of tau. Alternative inclusion of exon 10 generates tau isoform with either 4 (4R tau) (3R tau) microtubule binding domain repeats.[133] Neurodegenerative diseases characterized by predominant accumulation of hyperphosphorylated tau inclusions are also called tauopathies. Neurofibrillary tangles in AD are composed of both hyperphosphorylated 4R tau and 3R tau inclusions. In FTLD-tau, Pick's disease is characterized by predominant deposition of 3R tau aggregates, whereas CBD, PSP, globular glial tauopathy (GGT), and argyrophilic grain disease (AGD) are 4R tauopathies. Distinct tauopathies have unique patterns of immunohistochemistry and Western blot profiles.[142]

Pick's Disease (3R Tau)

The neuropathology of Pick's disease displays ballooned neurons, known as Pick cells, as well as large spherical argyrophilic neuronal cytoplasmic inclusions, known as Pick bodies (**Fig. 7**). Pick bodies are predominantly composed of 3R tau, although

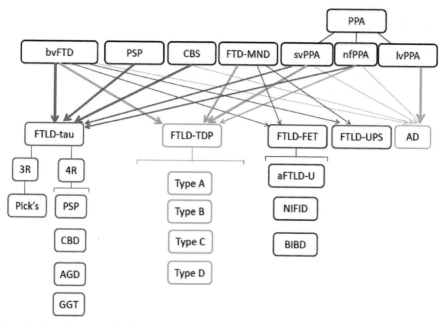

Fig. 6. Clinical and pathologic correlations in FTD spectrum disorders. This figure summarizes the overlap of FTD spectrum disorders (bvFTD, PSP, CBS, FTD-MND, svPPA, nfPPA) and their neuropathology (FTLD-tau, FTLD-TDP, FTLD-FET, FTLD-UPS) with a small portion of clinical syndromes being caused by AD abnormality. The clinical syndrome of lvPPA is highly correlated with AD abnormality.

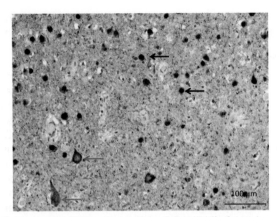

Fig. 7. 3R tau in Pick's disease. Photomicrograph of the middle frontal gyrus from a patient with Pick's disease. Tau immunohistochemistry demonstrates numerous Pick bodies (*black arrow*) and ballooned neurons or Pick's cells (*red arrows*). Tau stain CP13 (original magnification was 10×).

4R can be present.[143] Pick's disease is associated with severe atrophy of the ventral regions of the frontal and temporal lobes as well as anterior cingulate gyrus and insula. Pick's disease occurs predominantly sporadically, although it has been rarely reported in association with specific *MAPT* mutations: L315R, S320F, Q336H, and G389R.[142,144] Pick's presents more commonly as bvFTD, although nfvPPA and svPPA phenotypes are not infrequent.[145–147] In autopsy-confirmed cases within the UCSF cohort, 23% of patients with a clinical diagnosis of nfvPPA and 9% of svPPA had Pick 3R tau.

Progressive Supranuclear Palsy (4R Tau)

The neuropathology of PSP is characterized by the presence of tufted astrocytes, thorny astrocytes, and spherical "globose" neurofibrillary tangles in subcortical nuclei (**Fig. 8**).[105,148–150] Outside the brainstem, flame-shaped neurofibrillary tangles are seen, along with diffuse granular "pretangles."[151] Oligodendroglial cytoplasmic

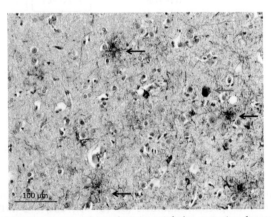

Fig. 8. 4R tau in PSP. Tau immunohistochemistry of the superior frontal sulcus showing tufted astrocytes (*black arrows*) and a globose tangle (*red arrow*). Tau stain CP13 (original magnification was 10×).

inclusions known as coiled bodies are seen in the cortex and more abundantly in the subcortical white matter.[151] The tau inclusions are predominantly composed of 4R tau and are present in the brainstem more than the cortex.[152] Cortical involvement can be variable, with the primary motor cortex and the frontal eye fields being more often involved, whereas worse cognitive performance is associated with wider cortical involvement.[153]

Corticobasal Degeneration (4R Tau)

Astrocytic plaques (**Fig. 9**) are the most characteristic neuropathologic hallmark of CBD.[154] Just like in tufted astrocytes of PSP, astrocytic plaques are made of hyper-phosphorylated 4R tau deposits in astrocytic processes.[152] In astrocytic plaques, these deposits localize in the most distal portion of the process as opposed to the localization of deposits (proximal to the cell body) in tufted astrocytes.[151] Neuronal inclusions in the form of granular cytoplasmic accumulation of tau or neurofibrillary tangles are seen in the cortex.[148] Ballooned neurons are a common feature of CBD, although they are also seen in Pick's disease.[148] A distinctive feature of CBD is the extensive involvement of the subcortical white matter with tau deposits in neurites and oligodendroglial coiled bodies.[151] CBD abnormality affects a wider range of cortical involvement than PSP abnormality, involving more dorsal regions, and tends to be found in the precentral and postcentral gyri.[148]

Globular Glial Tauopathy

GGT is a rare 4R tauopathy, whose pathologic classification has been recently revised. Proposed criteria describe 3 different pathologic subtypes that are variably associated with the clinical phenotypes of bvFTD and/or MND, with or without extrapyramidal signs.[155] Microscopically, the disease is characterized by the presence of large 4R tau inclusions with globular morphology in oligodendrocytes and astrocytes, particularly abundant within the white matter.[155]

Argyrophilic Grain Disease

AGD is a 4R tauopathy mainly characterized by the accumulation of small dotlike, commalike argyrophilic 4R tau positive inclusions ("grains"), predominantly seen in the temporal lobes and limbic structures. AGD can occur alone or contextually to other

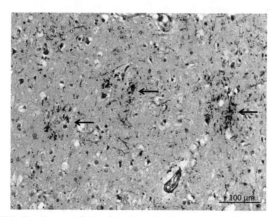

Fig. 9. 4R tau in CBD. Tau immunohistochemistry in the paracentral gyrus showing astrocytic plaques (*black arrows*). Tau stain CP13 (original magnification was 10×).

neurodegenerative diseases, more often AD abnormality.[156,157] The clinical presentation ranges from mild cognitive impairment to AD-like dementia and a slowly progressive bvFTD.[158–160] Tau deposits in AGD lack acetylation, a posttranslational modification step thought to be essential for the acquisition of pathogenic features by tau species in AD; hence, the hypothesis of a potential protective role of AGD in AD that may explain the more benign clinical phenotype (slow disease course) often associated with this underlying neuropathology.[158]

Frontotemporal lobar degeneration–TAR DNA-binding protein

In 2006, TDP-43 was shown to be the major disease protein in the neuropathology of both FTLD-U (tau negative, ubiquitin-positive FTLD) and ALS.[89–91] TDP-43 belongs to the heterogeneous nuclear ribonucleoproteins family and has been shown to be involved with microRNA processing, messenger RNA (mRNA) stabilization, transport, and translation.[161] The exact role of TDP-43 is unknown, but it has been associated with thousands of mRNA targets and thought to be vital for cell function.[162] Pathologic TDP-43 in neurodegenerative diseases is found as aggregates in the cytoplasm leading to phosphorylation, ubiquitination, and its degradation.[163] In 2011, a harmonized classification of FTLD-TDP abnormality was proposed to categorize TDP-43 neuropathology into 4 groups (A, B, C, D), which has since been widely accepted.[90]

TDP-43 type A neuropathology is characterized by an abundance of neuronal rounded or crescentlike cytoplasmic inclusions, and short dystrophic neurites and rare lentiform neuronal intranuclear inclusions (**Fig. 10**), which are more commonly found in cortical layer II.[90] TDP-43 type A neuropathology can present with the clinical phenotypes of bvFTD, nfvPPA, and CBS, whereas MND is less common.[90] Pathogenic mutations in *GRN* on chromosome 17 are associated with TDP-43 type A abnormality.[164]

TDP-43 type B neuropathology is characterized by much less frequent neuronal cytoplasmic inclusions and dystrophic neurites found in both superficial and deep cortical layers (**Fig. 11**).[90] TDP-43 type B abnormality is the most common subtype associated with the presence of neuronal cytoplasmic inclusions in lower motor neurons, with or without clinical signs of MND.[90] Clinical phenotypes of FTD, MND, and

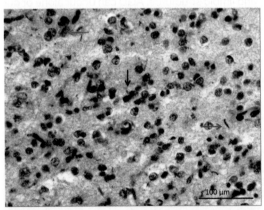

Fig. 10. TDP-43 type A. Orbitofrontal gyrus showing many short dystrophic neurites (*black arrow*), neuronal cytoplasmic inclusions (*green arrow*), and a lentiform neuronal intranuclear inclusions (*red arrow*). TDP immunohistochemistry. (*Courtesy of* Lea Grinberg, MD, PhD, UCSF.)

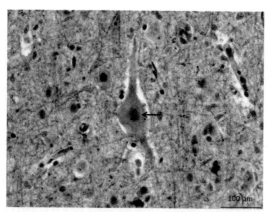

Fig. 11. TDP-43 type B. TDP immunohistochemistry of the precentral gyrus showing moderate neuronal cytoplasmic inclusions (*black arrow*). TDP immunohistochemistry. (*Courtesy of Lea Grinberg, MD, PhD, UCSF.*)

FTD-MND can have TDP-43 type B neuropathology.[90,165] Patients with C9ORF72 repeat expansions most often have TDP-43 type B, although TDP-43 type A is seen as well.[166]

TDP-43 type C neuropathology is characterized by long tortuous dystrophic neurites and few neuronal intracytoplasmic inclusions (**Fig. 12**),[90] whereas neuronal intranuclear inclusions are uncommon. TDP-43 type C is the most common neuropathology substrate of svPPA, and in the UCSF autopsy cohort, its abnormality confirmed in 90% of the cases.

TDP-43 type D is characterized by the presence of frequent lentiform neuronal intranuclear inclusions as well as short dystrophic neurites and rare neuronal cytoplasmic inclusions in all layers,[90] although these findings are more common in superficial layers. This subtype of FTLD-TDP is uniquely associated with mutations in the *VCP* gene and the clinical phenotype of inclusion body myopathy with Paget disease and FTD.[90,167]

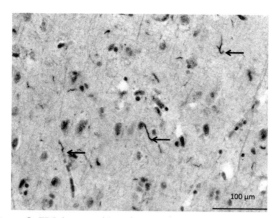

Fig. 12. TDP-43 type C. TDP immunohistochemistry of the insula showing long tortuous dystrophic neurites (*black arrows*), and few neuronal intranuclear inclusions. (*Courtesy of Lea Grinberg, MD, PhD, UCSF.*)

Frontotemporal Lobar Degeneration-FET

In 2009, human genetic studies found mutations in the FUS gene were linked to familial MND, and FUS cytoplasmic inclusions were found in postmortem analyses.[92–94] The role of FUS is not fully understood, but it has DNA/RNA binding properties and is thought to be similar to TDP-43.[94,168,169] Given the known overlap of MND and FTD, involvement of FUS in FTD was explored and FUS cytoplasmic inclusions were found in patients with FTD.[96,98,131] MND were correlated with mutations in the *FUS* gene, but FUS abnormality in FTD was shown to be sporadic and not affiliated with a mutation in FUS.[97] FUS is a member of the FUS, EWS, and TAF15 (FET) protein family, which also consists of other RNA/DNA binding proteins, Ewing sarcoma (EWS), and TATA-binding protein-associated factor 15 (TAF15).[169] In 2011, immunohistochemical analysis of FUS inclusions in FTLD showed that the whole FET family (FUS, EWS, and TAF15) were found in FTLD abnormality but not in MND FUS inclusions.[93] This finding suggests different mechanisms for FTLD and MND with FUS abnormality.[169] FET proteins were also found in neuronal intermediate filament inclusion disease (NIFID) and basophilic inclusion body disease (BIBD).[93,96,170] Previously, atypical FTLD-U (aFTLD-U), NIFID, and BIBD were considered FTLD-FUS subtypes, but because they are all positive for FET-positive inclusions, they can now grouped together under FTLD-FET.[169,171]

aFTLD-U neuropathology is characterized by neuronal cytoplasmic inclusions containing FET proteins and most distinctively by the presence of rare and unique neuronal intranuclear inclusions with a peculiar vermiform shape[171] (**Fig. 13**).

NIFID is a rare neurodegenerative disorder with distinct neuropathology due to immunoreactive neurofilament inclusions that were later found to bind all class IV intermediate filaments.[172] In 2009, NIFID was found to have intracellular FUS accumulation,[172] and in 2011, it was found to have widespread FET proteins accumulation.[93]

BIBD displays pathognomonic basophilic round inclusions, when stained with hematoxylin and eosin. Basophilic inclusions are more common in subcortical regions, such as the basal ganglia and brainstem tegmentum. There is severe frontotemporal atrophy in FTD cases and spinal cord involvement in MND cases.[173]

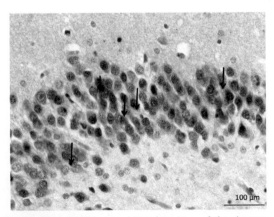

Fig. 13. aFTLD-U binding FUS. FUS immunohistochemistry of the dentate fascia (hippocampus) showing many FUS-positive neuronal cytoplasmic inclusions (*black arrows*). (*Courtesy of* Lea Grinberg, MD, PhD, UCSF.)

Frontotemporal Lobar Degeneration-Ubiquitin Proteasome System (UPS)

A rare form of FTD has been linked to chromosome 3 in a large Danish family[174] and was later associated with a mutation in the *CHMP2B* (charged multivesicular body protein 2B) gene.[175] *CHMP2B* mutations have been associated with familial FTD and ALS. The neuropathology is characterized by the presence of inclusions that are immunoreactive for ubiquitin and negative for tau, TDP-43, and FET proteins, although the exact nature of an eventual pathogenic protein remains unknown.[174]

Genetics

FTD frequently has a strong genetic component contributing to its pathogenesis. More than half of FTD cases are sporadic, but up to 40% of cases have a family history of dementia, psychiatric disease, or motor symptoms, with at least 10% of cases having an autosomal dominant pattern.[70,176] Of the clinical syndromes, FTD-MND is the most heritable, and svPPA is the least heritable.[70] The 3 most common genes associated with FTD are *C9ORF72*, *MAPT*, and *GRN*. Other less common genes associated with FTD include *VCP*, *CHMP2B*, *TARDBP*, *FUS*, *EXT2*, *TBK1*, and *SQSTM1*.

Microtubule-Associated Protein Tau

In the mid 1900s, FTD was observed by Malamud, Waggoner,[177] and Sjogren[178] to have a genetic contribution; some families had an autosomal dominant pattern of inheritance.[6] In 1994, Wilhelmsen and colleagues[179] linked a family that had an autosomal dominant pattern of FTD, which they called disinhibition-dementia-parkinsonism-amyotrophy-complex, to a region on chromosome 17. In 1998, as more FTD families were linked to chromosome 17, missense mutations in tau exons 9 to 13 and a splice site mutation in intron 10 were linked to increased 4R tau production as a possible mechanism for the tau abnormality.[138,180]

Clinical presentations of patients with *MAPT* mutations vary with bvFTD, nfPPA, PSP-S, and CBS are described.[181] Symptoms of MND are rarely associated with *MAPT* mutations.[166] The phenotype can vary between family members affected with the same mutation.[182] The neuroimaging of patients with MAPT mutations tends to show a more symmetric pattern of atrophy than other genetic causes of FTD.[181,183]

An H1H1 haplotype of the *MAPT* gene increases a patient's risk for PSP and CBD.[112,184] The rare sequence variant in *MAPT*, p.A152T, was found initially in patients with PSP, but in a larger study was shown to increase the risk of developing AD and FTD spectrum disorders, when compared with controls.[185] This finding of p.A152T in MAPT is the first time a tau polymorphism has been linked to both FTD and AD.

Progranulin (GRN)

In 2006, mutations in *GRN*, also on chromosome 17, were linked to FTLD.[186,187] Further research of GRN revealed that the haploinsufficiency was the mechanism for the neurodegeneration.[188,189] Patients with mutations in *GRN* have 50% less GRN mRNA progranulin levels in both CSF and plasma supporting the haploinsufficiency theory.[190,191] The exact role of progranulin is not fully understood, but it has been linked to neuronal growth, lysosomal function, plus inflammation and stress response.[188,189] The neuropathology associated with *GRN* is predominantly TDP-43 type A.[164,192]

Patients with *GRN* mutations most often present with bvFTD or nfvPPA, but CBS is also common and MND is rare.[192,193] On average, patients tend to be older at age of onset, mean age 60, and apathy is often a predominant symptom.[166] MRI can show asymmetry with atrophy in the frontotemporoparietal atrophy, suggesting a *GRN* mutation.[181] Only 70% to 90% of families with a *GRN* mutation have a family history of neurodegenerative disease, suggesting it has lower penetrance than other FTD genes.[194] Homozygote GRN carriers develop a syndrome suggestive of neuronal ceroid lipofuscinosis with early onset retinal degeneration, seizures, and cerebellar ataxia.[195]

Chromosome 9 Open Reading Frame 72

A genetic linkage between FTD-MND and chromosome 9q21-q22 had been known since 2000,[99] but a mutation was not discovered until 2011.[100,101] This mutation is a hexanucleotide repeat, GGGGCC, in a noncoding region of C9ORF72.[100,101] The pathologic C9ORF72 hexanucleotide repeat expansion is the most frequent genetic cause of familial FTD (11.7%) and familial ALS (23.5%).[100] The maximum size of hexanucleotide repeats in controls was 2 to 23. Expansion sizes from 700 to 1600 have been associated with pathogenesis causing FTD, MND, or FTD-MND.[100] The exact role of C9ORF72 is still being studied, but the repeat expansions of C9ORF72 are thought to cause loss of function in transcription as well as possible gain of function due to toxic RNA foci.[100] Dipeptides are produced by the abnormal expansions that also likely contribute to the neurodegeneration.[196]

The most common neuropathology associated with the pathologic C9ORF72 hexanucleotide repeat expansions (C9+) is TDP-43 type B.[166,197] There is current debate over the significance of inclusions with dipeptide repeat (DPR) proteins that are specifically found in all C9+ phenotypes.[196–199] The DPR proteins have not been correlated specifically with neurodegeneration, and cases of C9+ patients that died prematurely had DPR abnormality, no TDP-43 abnormality, and no symptoms of FTD or MND, suggesting DPR accumulates early.[198,200,201] C9+ patients show RNA aggregates, and these RNA foci have sparked theories about mechanism of neurotoxicity.[100,198]

The most common clinical phenotype with C9+ patients is bvFTD, although MND and FTD-MND are also common.[166,202] When compared with other gene FTD gene carriers, C9+ patients showed a higher likelihood of exhibiting psychotic symptoms and delusions.[166,203] In one study, C9+ patients were less likely to exhibit dietary changes but were more socially appropriate and warm.[166] C9+ patients can have a long disease course.[60,203]

MRI imaging of C9+ patients has shown typical FTD atrophy patterns when compared with controls, but when compared with other FTD genes, the atrophy pattern is atypical.[203,204] Patients with FTD-MND have shown more atrophy in dorsal frontal, parietal, the thalamus, and cerebellum.[203,204] Functional connectivity studies associated diminished salience network connectivity with atrophy of the left medial pulvinar thalamic nucleus in C9+ patients.[205]

Rare Genetic Causes of Frontotemporal Dementia

A rare autosomal dominant disorder with inclusion body myositis, Paget disease of the bone and FTD, has been linked to a mutation in VCP on chromosome 9.[206,207] Exome studies have linked VCP mutations to MND.[208] Mutations in VCP are linked to a unique form of neuropathology, TDP-43 type D.[206]

Mutations in FUS are rare and predominantly associated with familial ALS. Neuropathologically, they present as FTLD-FUS diseases with inclusions made of FUS protein in the absence of other FET proteins.[92,93]

There are numerous other genes that have been associated with FTLD that are uncommon which include mutations in TARDBP,[209–211] CHMP2B,[175] TBK1,[212,213] OPTN,[213,214] SQMSTM1,[214,215] UBQLN2,[216] and EXT-2.[217]

Treatments

There are currently no US Food and Drug Administration (FDA) -approved treatments for FTD, but off-label pharmacologic and behavioral modification techniques can be used to manage symptoms in FTD.

The FDA-approved treatments for AD have not shown benefit in FTD. There is evidence that acetylcholinesterase inhibitors actually make symptoms in FTD worse.[218,219] Memantine was tolerated in patients with FTD, but in a double-blind, placebo-controlled trial there was no benefit to behavior or cognition.[220,221]

It is accepted that FTD symptoms and behavior can improve with selective serotonin uptake inhibitors.[222–225] A small randomized, placebo-controlled double-blinded trial with Trazadone showed improvement in Neuropsychiatric Inventory (NPI) scores of FTD patients but no change in MMSE.[226]

Atypical antipsychotics should be used with caution in patients with FTLD given that they may have increased vulnerability to the extrapyramidal side effects and there is a black box warning for use in the elderly.[227] There is little evidence for benefit from mood stabilizers in FTLD, and evidence is limited.[228,229] Oxytocin has been proposed as a potential therapy targeting the emotional changes in FTD, and a small study showed mild improvement on the NPI after its use.[230,231]

There are also important nonpharmacological therapies to treat FTD symptoms. FTD symptoms can improve with caregiver education about behavioral, environmental, and physical techniques to minimize or redirect unwanted behaviors.[232] Benefits from physical exercise have been shown to delay cognitive decline and should be recommended to all FTD patients that can safely tolerate it.[233] Patients with nfvPPA, svPPA, and language deficits may benefit from speech therapy.[234]

Although there are no FDA-approved treatments for FTD, this is a hopeful time for FTD treatments to come to fruition. There are currently active clinical trials targeting specific FTD mechanisms and abnormality. There are trials targeted at tau abnormality with therapeutics aimed at preventing tau aggregation, tau microtubule stabilization, and removal of tau with tau-targeted antibodies.[235–237] There are trials currently targeting the haploinsufficiency in GRN gene expression by using different methods of increasing progranulin.[238–240] Antisense oligonucleotide therapies are being developed to target the toxin gain of function with *C9ORF72* genetic mutation.[240] Molecular-based treatments for FTD are closer than they have ever been.

DISCLOSURE

The authors have nothing to disclose.

Dr N.T. Olney has received grant support from the National Institutes of Health/National Institute of Aging T32AG023481-11S1 grant. Dr S. Spina receives research support from the National Institutes of Health/National Institute of Aging grant K08AG052648. Dr B.L. Miller has served as an Advisor/Director to The Tau Consortium, The John Douglas French Foundation, The Larry L. Hillblom Foundation, Medical Advisory Board, National Institute for Health Research, Cambridge Biomedical Research Center and its subunit, the Biomedical Research Unit in Dementia (UK); he has served as an External Advisor to University of Washington ADRC, Stanford University ADRC, and University of Pittsburgh ADRC; he has received grant/research support from National Institutes of Health/National Institute of Aging grants P50AG023501, P01AG019724, and P50AG1657303, Centers for Medicare & Medicaid Services (CMS) Dementia Care Ecosystem 1C1CMS3313460100, and a UCSF/Quest Diagnostics Dementia Pathway Collaboration Research Grant; he receives royalties from Cambridge University Press, Guilford Publications, Inc, and Neurocase.

REFERENCES

1. Pick A. Uber die Beziehungen der Senilen Hirnatrophie zur Aphasie. Prager Medizinische Wochenschrift 1892;17:165–7.
2. Gorno-Tempini ML, Hillis AE, Weintraub S, et al. Classification of primary progressive aphasia and its variants. Neurology 2011;76(11):1006–14.
3. Alzheimer A. Uber Eigenartige Krankheitsfalle des Spateren Alters. Z Gesamte Neruol Psychiatr 1911;4:356–85.
4. Thibodeau MP, Miller BL. 'Limits and current knowledge of Pick's disease: its differential diagnosis'. A translation of the 1957 Delay, Brion, Escourolle article. Neurocase 2013;19(5):417–22.
5. Rosen HJ, Lengenfelder J, Miller B. Frontotemporal dementia. Neurol Clin 2000; 18(4):979–92.
6. Miller BL. Frontotemporal dementia. New York: Oxford University Press; 2014.
7. Jellinger KA. The enigma of vascular cognitive disorder and vascular dementia. Acta Neuropathol 2007;113(4):349–88.
8. Roman G. Vascular dementia: a historical background. Int Psychogeriatr 2003; 15(Suppl 1):11–3.
9. Constantinidis J, Richard J, Tissot R. Pick's disease: histological and clinical correlations. Eur Neurol 1974;11:208–17.
10. Ryan NS, Rossor MN, Fox NC. Alzheimer's disease in the 100 years since Alzheimer's death. Brain 2015;138(Pt 12):3816–21.
11. Katzman R. Editorial: the prevalence and malignancy of Alzheimer disease. A major killer. Arch Neurol 1976;33(4):217–8.
12. Brun A. Frontal lobe degeneration of non-Alzheimer type revisited. Dementia 1993;4:126–31.
13. Ingvar DH, Gustafson L. Regional cerebral blood flow in organic dementia with early onset. Acta Neurol Scand 1970;46(Suppl 43):42+.
14. Mesulam MM. Slowly progressive aphasia without generalized dementia. Ann Neurol 1982;11(6):592–8.
15. Mesulam MM. Primary progressive aphasia. Ann Neurol 2001;49(4):425–32.
16. Snowden JS, Goulding PJ, Neary D. Semantic dementia: a form of circumscribed cerebral atrophy. Behav Neurol 1989;2:167–82.
17. Edwards-Lee T, Miller BL, Benson DF, et al. The temporal variant of frontotemporal dementia. Brain 1997;120(Pt 6):1027–40.
18. Clinical and neuropathological criteria for frontotemporal dementia. The Lund and Manchester Groups. J Neurol Neurosurg Psychiatr 1994;57(4):416–8.
19. Neary D, Snowden JS, Gustafson L, et al. Frontotemporal lobar degeneration: a consensus on clinical diagnostic criteria. Neurology 1998;51(6):1546–54.
20. Rascovsky K, Hodges JR, Knopman D, et al. Sensitivity of revised diagnostic criteria for the behavioural variant of frontotemporal dementia. Brain 2011; 134(Pt 9):2456–77.
21. Coyle-Gilchrist IT, Dick KM, Patterson K, et al. Prevalence, characteristics, and survival of frontotemporal lobar degeneration syndromes. Neurology 2016; 86(18):1736–43.
22. Knopman DS, Roberts RO. Estimating the number of persons with frontotemporal lobar degeneration in the US population. J Mol Neurosci 2011;45(3):330–5.
23. Hodges JR, Davies R, Xuereb J, et al. Survival in frontotemporal dementia. Neurology 2003;61(3):349–54.
24. Snowden JS, Neary D, Mann DM. Frontotemporal dementia. Br J Psychiatry 2002;180:140–3.

25. Hogan DB, Jette N, Fiest KM, et al. The prevalence and incidence of frontotemporal dementia: a systematic review. Can J Neurol Sci 2016;43(Suppl 1): S96–109.

26. Onyike CU, Diehl-Schmid J. The epidemiology of frontotemporal dementia. Int Rev Psychiatry 2013;25(2):130–7.

27. Lanata SC, Miller BL. The behavioural variant frontotemporal dementia (bvFTD) syndrome in psychiatry. J Neurol Neurosurg Psychiatr 2016;87(5):501–11.

28. Woolley JD, Khan BK, Murthy NK, et al. The diagnostic challenge of psychiatric symptoms in neurodegenerative disease: rates of and risk factors for prior psychiatric diagnosis in patients with early neurodegenerative disease. J Clin Psychiatry 2011;72(2):126–33.

29. Rosen HJ, Allison SC, Schauer GF, et al. Neuroanatomical correlates of behavioural disorders in dementia. Brain 2005;128(Pt 11):2612–25.

30. Seeley WW, Crawford R, Rascovsky K, et al. Frontal paralimbic network atrophy in very mild behavioral variant frontotemporal dementia. Arch Neurol 2008;65(2): 249–55.

31. Seeley WW, Carlin DA, Allman JM, et al. Early frontotemporal dementia targets neurons unique to apes and humans. Ann Neurol 2006;60(6):660–7.

32. Seeley WW. Selective functional, regional, and neuronal vulnerability in frontotemporal dementia. Curr Opin Neurol 2008;21(6):701–7.

33. Schroeter ML, Raczka K, Neumann J, et al. Neural networks in frontotemporal dementia–a meta-analysis. Neurobiol Aging 2008;29(3):418–26.

34. Seeley WW, Menon V, Schatzberg AF, et al. Dissociable intrinsic connectivity networks for salience processing and executive control. J Neurosci 2007; 27(9):2349–56.

35. Seeley WW, Zhou J, Kim EJ. Frontotemporal dementia: what can the behavioral variant teach us about human brain organization? Neuroscientist 2012;18(4): 373–85.

36. Kfoury N, Holmes BB, Jiang H, et al. Trans-cellular propagation of Tau aggregation by fibrillar species. J Biol Chem 2012;287(23):19440–51.

37. Walker LC, Jucker M. Neurodegenerative diseases: expanding the prion concept. Annu Rev Neurosci 2015;38:87–103.

38. Kramer JH, Jurik J, Sha SJ, et al. Distinctive neuropsychological patterns in frontotemporal dementia, semantic dementia, and Alzheimer disease. Cogn Behav Neurol 2003;16(4):211–8.

39. Tekin S, Cummings JL. Frontal-subcortical neuronal circuits and clinical neuropsychiatry: an update. J Psychosom Res 2002;53(2):647–54.

40. Tranel D, Bechara A, Denburg NL. Asymmetric functional roles of right and left ventromedial prefrontal cortices in social conduct, decision-making, and emotional processing. Cortex 2002;38(4):589–612.

41. Diehl-Schmid J, Perneczky R, Koch J, et al. Guilty by suspicion? Criminal behavior in frontotemporal lobar degeneration. Cogn Behav Neurol 2013; 26(2):73–7.

42. Liljegren M, Naasan G, Temlett J, et al. Criminal behavior in frontotemporal dementia and Alzheimer disease. JAMA Neurol 2015;72(3):295–300.

43. Rankin KP, Baldwin E, Pace-Savitsky C, et al. Self awareness and personality change in dementia. J Neurol Neurosurg Psychiatr 2005;76(5):632–9.

44. Chow TW, Binns MA, Cummings JL, et al. Apathy symptom profile and behavioral associations in frontotemporal dementia vs dementia of Alzheimer type. Arch Neurol 2009;66(7):888–93.

45. Merrilees J, Hubbard E, Mastick J, et al. Rest-activity and behavioral disruption in a patient with frontotemporal dementia. Neurocase 2009;15(6):515–26.

46. Holroyd CB, Yeung N. Motivation of extended behaviors by anterior cingulate cortex. Trends Cogn Sci 2012;16(2):122–8.

47. Rosen HJ, Gorno-Tempini ML, Goldman WP, et al. Patterns of brain atrophy in frontotemporal dementia and semantic dementia. Neurology 2002;58(2):198–208.

48. Mendez MF, Shapira JS. Loss of emotional insight in behavioral variant fronto-temporal dementia or "frontal anosodiaphoria". Conscious Cogn 2011;20(4):1690–6.

49. Rankin KP, Gorno-Tempini ML, Allison SC, et al. Structural anatomy of empathy in neurodegenerative disease. Brain 2006;129(Pt 11):2945–56.

50. Ames D, Cummings JL, Wirshing WC, et al. Repetitive and compulsive behavior in frontal lobe degenerations. J Neuropsychiatry Clin Neurosci 1994;6(2):100–13.

51. Josephs KA, Whitwell JL, Jack CR Jr. Anatomic correlates of stereotypies in frontotemporal lobar degeneration. Neurobiol Aging 2008;29(12):1859–63.

52. Perry DC, Whitwell JL, Boeve BF, et al. Voxel-based morphometry in patients with obsessive-compulsive behaviors in behavioral variant frontotemporal de-mentia. Eur J Neurol 2012;19(6):911–7.

53. Rosso SM, Roks G, Stevens M, et al. Complex compulsive behaviour in the tem-poral variant of frontotemporal dementia. J Neurol 2001;248(11):965–70.

54. Miller BL, Darby AL, Swartz JR, et al. Dietary changes, compulsions and sexual behavior in frontotemporal degeneration. Dementia 1995;6(4):195–9.

55. Woolley JD, Gorno-Tempini ML, Seeley WW, et al. Binge eating is associated with right orbitofrontal-insular-striatal atrophy in frontotemporal dementia. Neurology 2007;69(14):1424–33.

56. Whitwell JL, Sampson EL, Loy CT, et al. VBM signatures of abnormal eating be-haviours in frontotemporal lobar degeneration. Neuroimage 2007;35(1):207–13.

57. Piguet O. Eating disturbance in behavioural-variant frontotemporal dementia. J Mol Neurosci 2011;45(3):589–93.

58. Gregory CA, Serra-Mestres J, Hodges JR. Early diagnosis of the frontal variant of frontotemporal dementia: how sensitive are standard neuroimaging and neu-ropsychologic tests? Neuropsychiatry Neuropsychol Behav Neurol 1999;12(2):128–35.

59. Kipps CM, Hodges JR, Hornberger M. Nonprogressive behavioural frontotem-poral dementia: recent developments and clinical implications of the 'bvFTD phenocopy syndrome'. Curr Opin Neurol 2010;23(6):628–32.

60. Khan BK, Yokoyama JS, Takada LT, et al. Atypical, slowly progressive behaviou-ral variant frontotemporal dementia associated with C9ORF72 hexanucleotide expansion. J Neurol Neurosurg Psychiatr 2012;83(4):358–64.

61. Ranasinghe KG, Rankin KP, Lobach IV, et al. Cognition and neuropsychiatry in behavioral variant frontotemporal dementia by disease stage. Neurology 2016;86(7):600–10.

62. Suarez J, Tartaglia MC, Vitali P, et al. Characterizing radiology reports in patients with frontotemporal dementia. Neurology 2009;73(13):1073–4.

63. Mesulam MM. Primary progressive aphasia: differentiation from Alzheimer's dis-ease. Ann Neurol 1987;37:1448–553.

64. Gorno-Tempini ML, Dronkers NF, Rankin KP, et al. Cognition and anatomy in three variants of primary progressive aphasia. Ann Neurol 2004;55(3):335–46.

65. Mesulam M, Wicklund A, Johnson N, et al. Alzheimer and frontotemporal pathol-ogy in subsets of primary progressive aphasia. Ann Neurol 2008;63(6):709–19.

66. Rabinovici GD, Jagust WJ, Furst AJ, et al. Abeta amyloid and glucose metabolism in three variants of primary progressive aphasia. Ann Neurol 2008; 64(4):388–401.
67. Seeley WW, Bauer AM, Miller BL, et al. The natural history of temporal variant frontotemporal dementia. Neurology 2005;64(8):1384–90.
68. Hodges JR, Mitchell J, Dawson K, et al. Semantic dementia: demography, familial factors and survival in a consecutive series of 100 cases. Brain 2010;133(Pt 1):300–6.
69. Flanagan EP, Baker MC, Perkerson RB, et al. Dominant frontotemporal dementia mutations in 140 cases of primary progressive aphasia and speech apraxia. Dement Geriatr Cogn Disord 2015;39(5–6):281–6.
70. Goldman JS, Farmer JM, Wood EM, et al. Comparison of family histories in FTLD subtypes and related tauopathies. Neurology 2005;65(11):1817–9.
71. Hodges JR, Patterson K, Ward R, et al. The differentiation of semantic dementia and frontal lobe dementia (temporal and frontal variants of frontotemporal dementia) from early Alzheimer's disease: a comparative neuropsychological study. Neuropsychology 1999;13(1):31–40.
72. Miller BL, Chang L, Mena I, et al. Progressive right frontotemporal degeneration: clinical, neuropsychological and SPECT characteristics. Dementia 1993;4(3–4): 204–13.
73. Rosen HJ, Perry RJ, Murphy J, et al. Emotion comprehension in the temporal variant of frontotemporal dementia. Brain 2002;125(Pt 10):2286–95.
74. Miller BL, Boone K, Cummings JL, et al. Functional correlates of musical and visual ability in frontotemporal dementia. Br J Psychiatry 2000;176:458–63.
75. Miller BL, Cummings J, Mishkin F, et al. Emergence of artistic talent in frontotemporal dementia. Neurology 1998;51(4):978–82.
76. Miller BL, Ponton M, Benson DF, et al. Enhanced artistic creativity with temporal lobe degeneration [letter]. Lancet 1996;348(9043):1744–5.
77. Liu A, Werner K, Roy S, et al. A case study of an emerging visual artist with frontotemporal lobar degeneration and amyotrophic lateral sclerosis. Neurocase 2009;15(3):235–47.
78. Rohrer JD, Rosen HJ. Neuroimaging in frontotemporal dementia. Int Rev Psychiatry 2013;25(2):221–9.
79. Ogar J, Willock S, Baldo J, et al. Clinical and anatomical correlates of apraxia of speech. Brain Lang 2006;97(3):343–50.
80. Gorno-Tempini ML, Ogar JM, Brambati SM, et al. Anatomical correlates of early mutism in progressive nonfluent aphasia. Neurology 2006;67(10):1849–51.
81. Lomen-Hoerth C, Anderson T, Miller B. The overlap of amyotrophic lateral sclerosis and frontotemporal dementia. Neurology 2002;59(7):1077–9.
82. McGeer PL, Schwab C, McGeer EG, et al. Familial nature and continuing morbidity of the amyotrophic lateral sclerosis-parkinsonism dementia complex of Guam. Neurology 1997;49(2):400–9.
83. Lomen-Hoerth C. Clinical phenomenology and neuroimaging correlates in ALS-FTD. J Mol Neurosci 2011;45(3):656–62.
84. Geevasinga N, Loy CT, Menon P, et al. Awaji criteria improves the diagnostic sensitivity in amyotrophic lateral sclerosis: a systematic review using individual patient data. Clin Neurophysiol 2016;127(7):2684–91.
85. Brooks BR. El Escorial World Federation of Neurology criteria for the diagnosis of amyotrophic lateral sclerosis. Subcommittee on Motor Neuron Diseases/ Amyotrophic Lateral Sclerosis of the World Federation of Neurology Research Group on Neuromuscular Diseases and the El Escorial "Clinical limits of

amyotrophic lateral sclerosis" workshop contributors. J Neurol Sci 1994; 124(Suppl):96–107.

86. Carvalho MD, Swash M. Awaji diagnostic algorithm increases sensitivity of El Escorial criteria for ALS diagnosis. Amyotroph Lateral Scler 2009;10(1):53–7.

87. Olney RK, Murphy J, Forshew D, et al. The effects of executive and behavioral dysfunction on the course of ALS. Neurology 2005;65(11):1774–7.

88. Mackenzie IR, Feldman HH. Ubiquitin immunohistochemistry suggests classic motor neuron disease, motor neuron disease with dementia, and frontotemporal dementia of the motor neuron disease type represent a clinicopathologic spectrum. J Neuropathol Exp Neurol 2005;64(8):730–9.

89. Arai T, Hasegawa M, Akiyama H, et al. TDP-43 is a component of ubiquitin-positive tau-negative inclusions in frontotemporal lobar degeneration and amyotrophic lateral sclerosis. Biochem Biophys Res Commun 2006;351(3):602–11.

90. Mackenzie IR, Neumann M, Baborie A, et al. A harmonized classification system for FTLD-TDP pathology. Acta Neuropathol 2011;122(1):111–3.

91. Neumann M, Sampathu DM, Kwong LK, et al. Ubiquitinated TDP-43 in frontotemporal lobar degeneration and amyotrophic lateral sclerosis. Science 2006; 314(5796):130–3.

92. Kwiatkowski TJ Jr, Bosco DA, Leclerc AL, et al. Mutations in the FUS/TLS gene on chromosome 16 cause familial amyotrophic lateral sclerosis. Science 2009; 323(5918):1205–8.

93. Neumann M, Bentmann E, Dormann D, et al. FET proteins TAF15 and EWS are selective markers that distinguish FTLD with FUS pathology from amyotrophic lateral sclerosis with FUS mutations. Brain 2011;134(Pt 9):2595–609.

94. Vance C, Rogelj B, Hortobagyi T, et al. Mutations in FUS, an RNA processing protein, cause familial amyotrophic lateral sclerosis type 6. Science 2009; 323(5918):1208–11.

95. Mackenzie IR, Rademakers R, Neumann M. TDP-43 and FUS in amyotrophic lateral sclerosis and frontotemporal dementia. Lancet Neurol 2010;9(10): 995–1007.

96. Neumann M, Rademakers R, Roeber S, et al. A new subtype of frontotemporal lobar degeneration with FUS pathology. Brain 2009;132(Pt 11):2922–31.

97. Snowden JS, Hu Q, Rollinson S, et al. The most common type of FTLD-FUS (aFTLD-U) is associated with a distinct clinical form of frontotemporal dementia but is not related to mutations in the FUS gene. Acta Neuropathol 2011;122(1): 99–110.

98. Urwin H, Josephs KA, Rohrer JD, et al. FUS pathology defines the majority of tau- and TDP-43-negative frontotemporal lobar degeneration. Acta Neuropathol 2010;120(1):33–41.

99. Hosler BA, Siddique T, Sapp PC, et al. Linkage of familial amyotrophic lateral sclerosis with frontotemporal dementia to chromosome 9q21-q22. JAMA 2000;284(13):1664–9.

100. DeJesus-Hernandez M, Mackenzie IR, Boeve BF, et al. Expanded GGGGCC hexanucleotide repeat in noncoding region of C9ORF72 causes chromosome 9p-linked FTD and ALS. Neuron 2011;72(2):245–56.

101. Renton AE, Majounie E, Waite A, et al. A hexanucleotide repeat expansion in C9ORF72 is the cause of chromosome 9p21-linked ALS-FTD. Neuron 2011; 72(2):257–68.

102. Rebeiz JJ, Kolodny EH, Richardson EP Jr. Corticodentatonigral degeneration with neuronal achromasia. Arch Neurol 1968;18(1):20–33.

103. Armstrong MJ, Litvan I, Lang AE, et al. Criteria for the diagnosis of corticobasal degeneration. Neurology 2013;80(5):496–503.
104. Boeve BF, Maraganore DM, Parisi JE, et al. Pathologic heterogeneity in clinically diagnosed corticobasal degeneration. Neurology 1999;53(4):795–800.
105. Josephs KA, Petersen RC, Knopman DS, et al. Clinicopathologic analysis of frontotemporal and corticobasal degenerations and PSP. Neurology 2006; 66(1):41–8.
106. Lee SE, Rabinovici GD, Mayo MC, et al. Clinicopathological correlations in corticobasal degeneration. Ann Neurol 2011;70(2):327–40.
107. Ling H, O'Sullivan SS, Holton JL, et al. Does corticobasal degeneration exist? A clinicopathological re-evaluation. Brain 2010;133(Pt 7):2045–57.
108. Hassan A, Whitwell JL, Boeve BF, et al. Symmetric corticobasal degeneration (S-CBD). Parkinsonism Relat Disord 2010;16(3):208–14.
109. Kertesz A, Davidson W, McCabe P, et al. Primary progressive aphasia: diagnosis, varieties, evolution. J Int Neuropsychol Soc 2003;9(5):710–9.
110. Kertesz A, McMonagle P, Blair M, et al. The evolution and pathology of frontotemporal dementia. Brain 2005;128(Pt 9):1996–2005.
111. Wadia PM, Lang AE. The many faces of corticobasal degeneration. Parkinsonism Relat Disord 2007;13(Suppl 3):S336–40.
112. Myers AJ, Pittman AM, Zhao AS, et al. The MAPT H1c risk haplotype is associated with increased expression of tau and especially of 4 repeat containing transcripts. Neurobiol Dis 2007;25(3):561–70.
113. Rabinovici GD, Rosen HJ, Alkalay A, et al. Amyloid vs FDG-PET in the differential diagnosis of AD and FTLD. Neurology 2011;77(23):2034–42.
114. Whitwell JL, Jack CR Jr, Boeve BF, et al. Imaging correlates of pathology in corticobasal syndrome. Neurology 2010;75(21):1879–87.
115. Boxer AL, Geschwind MD, Belfor N, et al. Patterns of brain atrophy that differentiate corticobasal degeneration syndrome from progressive supranuclear palsy. Arch Neurol 2006;63(1):81–6.
116. Rankin KP, Mayo MC, Seeley WW, et al. Behavioral variant frontotemporal dementia with corticobasal degeneration pathology: phenotypic comparison to bvFTD with Pick's disease. J Mol Neurosci 2011;45(3):594–608.
117. Steele JC, Richardson JC, Olszewski J. Progressive supranuclear palsy. Arch Neurol 1964;10(April):333–60.
118. Chambers CB, Lee JM, Troncoso JC, et al. Overexpression of four-repeat tau mRNA isoforms in progressive supranuclear palsy but not in Alzheimer's disease. Ann Neurol 1999;46(3):325–32.
119. Osaki Y, Ben-Shlomo Y, Lees AJ, et al. Accuracy of clinical diagnosis of progressive supranuclear palsy. Mov Disord 2004;19(2):181–9.
120. Hughes AJ, Daniel SE, Ben-Shlomo Y, et al. The accuracy of diagnosis of parkinsonian syndromes in a specialist movement disorder service. Brain 2002; 125(Pt 4):861–70.
121. Litvan I, Agid Y, Calne D, et al. Clinical research criteria for the diagnosis of progressive supranuclear palsy (Steele-Richardson-Olszewski syndrome): report of the NINDS-SPSP international workshop. Neurology 1996;47(1):1–9.
122. Donker Kaat L, Boon AJ, Kamphorst W, et al. Frontal presentation in progressive supranuclear palsy. Neurology 2007;69(8):723–9.
123. Williams DR, Lees AJ. Progressive supranuclear palsy: clinicopathological concepts and diagnostic challenges. Lancet Neurol 2009;8(3):270–9.
124. Kertesz A, McMonagle P. Behavior and cognition in corticobasal degeneration and progressive supranuclear palsy. J Neurol Sci 2010;289(1–2):138–43.

125. Lu CH, Macdonald-Wallis C, Gray E, et al. Neurofilament light chain: a prognostic biomarker in amyotrophic lateral sclerosis. Neurology 2015;84(22): 2247–57.

126. Meeter LH, Dopper EG, Jiskoot LC, et al. Neurofilament light chain: a biomarker for genetic frontotemporal dementia. Ann Clin Transl Neurol 2016;3(8):623–36.

127. Rohrer JD, Woollacott IO, Dick KM, et al. Serum neurofilament light chain protein is a measure of disease intensity in frontotemporal dementia. Neurology 2016; 87(13):1329–36.

128. Rojas JC, Karydas A, Bang J, et al. Plasma neurofilament light chain predicts progression in progressive supranuclear palsy. Ann Clin Transl Neurol 2016; 3(3):216–25.

129. Kim YE, Kang SY, Ma HI, et al. A visual rating scale for the hummingbird sign with adjustable diagnostic validity. J Parkinsons Dis 2015;5(3):605–12.

130. Mackenzie IR, Neumann M, Bigio EH, et al. Nomenclature for neuropathologic subtypes of frontotemporal lobar degeneration: consensus recommendations. Acta Neuropathol 2009;117(1):15–8.

131. Mackenzie IR, Neumann M, Bigio EH, et al. Nomenclature and nosology for neuropathologic subtypes of frontotemporal lobar degeneration: an update. Acta Neuropathol 2010;119(1):1–4.

132. Weingarten MD, Lockwood AH, Hwo SY, et al. A protein factor essential for microtubule assembly. Proc Natl Acad Sci U S A 1975;72(5):1858–62.

133. Mandelkow EM, Mandelkow E. Biochemistry and cell biology of tau protein in neurofibrillary degeneration. Cold Spring Harb Perspect Med 2012;2(7): a006247.

134. Jenkins SM, Johnson GV. Tau complexes with phospholipase C-gamma in situ. Neuroreport 1998;9(1):67–71.

135. Leugers CJ, Lee G. Tau potentiates nerve growth factor-induced mitogen-activated protein kinase signaling and neurite initiation without a requirement for microtubule binding. J Biol Chem 2010;285(25):19125–34.

136. Morris M, Maeda S, Vossel K, et al. The many faces of tau. Neuron 2011;70(3): 410–26.

137. Clark LN, Poorkaj P, Wszolek Z, et al. Pathogenic implications of mutations in the tau gene in pallido-ponto-nigral degeneration and related neurodegenerative disorders linked to chromosome 17. Proc Natl Acad Sci U S A 1998;95(22):13103–7.

138. Hutton M, Lendon CL, Rizzu P, et al. Association of missense and 5'-splice-site mutations in tau with the inherited dementia FTDP-17. Nature 1998;393(6686):702–5.

139. Poorkaj P, Bird TD, Wijsman E, et al. Tau is a candidate gene for chromosome 17 frontotemporal dementia. Ann Neurol 1998;43(6):815–25.

140. Spillantini MG, Murrell JR, Goedert M, et al. Mutation in the tau gene in familial multiple system tauopathy with presenile dementia. Proc Natl Acad Sci U S A 1998;95(13):7737–41.

141. Wilhelmsen KC, Lynch T, Pavlou E, et al. Localization of disinhibition-dementia-parkinsonism-amyotrophy complex to 17q21-22. Am J Hum Genet 1994;55(6): 1159–65.

142. Ghetti B, Oblak AL, Boeve BF, et al. Invited review: frontotemporal dementia caused by microtubule-associated protein tau gene (MAPT) mutations: a chameleon for neuropathology and neuroimaging. Neuropathol Appl Neurobiol 2015;41(1):24–46.

143. Zhukareva V, Mann D, Pickering-Brown S, et al. Sporadic Pick's disease: a tauopathy characterized by a spectrum of pathological tau isoforms in gray and white matter. Ann Neurol 2002;51(6):730–9.

144. Tacik P, DeTure M, Hinkle KM, et al. A novel tau mutation in exon 12, p.Q336H, causes hereditary pick disease. J Neuropathol Exp Neurol 2015;74(11): 1042–52.

145. Graff-Radford NR, Damasio AR, Hyman BT, et al. Progressive aphasia in a patient with Pick's disease: a neuropsychological, radiologic, and anatomic study. Neurology 1990;40:620–6.

146. Irwin DJ. Tauopathies as clinicopathological entities. Parkinsonism Relat Disord 2016;22(Suppl 1):S29–33.

147. Irwin DJ, Brettschneider J, McMillan CT, et al. Deep clinical and neuropathological phenotyping of Pick disease. Ann Neurol 2016;79(2):272–87.

148. Dickson DW, Bergeron C, Chin SS, et al. Office of rare diseases neuropathologic criteria for corticobasal degeneration. J Neuropathol Exp Neurol 2002;61(11): 935–46.

149. Josephs KA, Hodges JR, Snowden JS, et al. Neuropathological background of phenotypical variability in frontotemporal dementia. Acta Neuropathol 2011; 122(2):137–53.

150. Litvan I, Hauw JJ, Bartko JJ, et al. Validity and reliability of the preliminary NINDS neuropathologic criteria for progressive supranuclear palsy and related disorders. J Neuropathol Exp Neurol 1996;55(1):97–105.

151. Dickson D. Neurodegeneration: the molecular pathology of dementia and movement disorders. 2nd edition. Chichester, West Sussex: Wiley-Blackwell; 2011. p. 1. online resource (xvii, 477 pages).

152. Lee VM, Goedert M, Trojanowski JQ. Neurodegenerative tauopathies. Annu Rev Neurosci 2001;24:1121–59.

153. Bigio EH, Brown DF, White CL. Progressive supranuclear palsy with dementia: cortical pathology. J Neuropathol Exp Neurol 1999;58(4):359–64.

154. Feany MB, Dickson DW. Neurodegenerative disorders with extensive tau pathology: a comparative study and review. Ann Neurol 1996;40(2):139–48.

155. Ahmed Z, Bigio EH, Budka H, et al. Globular glial tauopathies (GGT): consensus recommendations. Acta Neuropathol 2013;126(4):537–44.

156. Fujino Y, Wang DS, Thomas N, et al. Increased frequency of argyrophilic grain disease in Alzheimer disease with 4R tau-specific immunohistochemistry. J Neuropathol Exp Neurol 2005;64(3):209–14.

157. Thal DR, Schultz C, Botez G, et al. The impact of argyrophilic grain disease on the development of dementia and its relationship to concurrent Alzheimer's disease-related pathology. Neuropathol Appl Neurobiol 2005;31(3):270–9.

158. Grinberg LT, Wang X, Wang C, et al. Argyrophilic grain disease differs from other tauopathies by lacking tau acetylation. Acta Neuropathol 2013;125(4):581–93.

159. Ishihara K, Araki S, Ihori N, et al. Argyrophilic grain disease presenting with frontotemporal dementia: a neuropsychological and pathological study of an autopsied case with presenile onset. Neuropathology 2005;25(2):165–70.

160. Tsuchiya K, Mitani K, Arai T, et al. Argyrophilic grain disease mimicking temporal Pick's disease: a clinical, radiological, and pathological study of an autopsy case with a clinical course of 15 years. Acta Neuropathol 2001;102(2):195–9.

161. Baralle M, Buratti E, Baralle FE. The role of TDP-43 in the pathogenesis of ALS and FTLD. Biochem Soc Trans 2013;41(6):1536–40.

162. Polymenidou M, Lagier-Tourenne C, Hutt KR, et al. Long pre-mRNA depletion and RNA missplicing contribute to neuronal vulnerability from loss of TDP-43. Nat Neurosci 2011;14(4):459–68.

163. Buratti E, Baralle FE. The molecular links between TDP-43 dysfunction and neurodegeneration. Adv Genet 2009;66:1–34.

164. Cairns NJ, Neumann M, Bigio EH, et al. TDP-43 in familial and sporadic fronto-temporal lobar degeneration with ubiquitin inclusions. Am J Pathol 2007;171(1): 227–40.

165. Mackenzie IR. The neuropathology of FTD associated With ALS. Alzheimer Dis Assoc Disord 2007;21(4):S44–9.

166. Snowden JS, Adams J, Harris J, et al. Distinct clinical and pathological pheno-types in frontotemporal dementia associated with MAPT, PGRN and C9orf72 mutations. Amyotroph Lateral Scler Frontotemporal Degener 2015;16(7–8): 497–505.

167. Cairns NJ, Bigio EH, Mackenzie IR, et al. Neuropathologic diagnostic and noso-logic criteria for frontotemporal lobar degeneration: consensus of the Con-sortium for Frontotemporal Lobar Degeneration. Acta Neuropathol (Berl) 2007; 114(1):5–22.

168. Baloh RH. How do the RNA-binding proteins TDP-43 and FUS relate to amyotro-phic lateral sclerosis and frontotemporal degeneration, and to each other? Curr Opin Neurol 2012;25(6):701–7.

169. Mackenzie IR, Neumann M. FET proteins in frontotemporal dementia and amyo-trophic lateral sclerosis. Brain Res 2012;1462:40–3.

170. Munoz DG, Neumann M, Kusaka H, et al. FUS pathology in basophilic inclusion body disease. Acta Neuropathol 2009;118(5):617–27.

171. Mackenzie IR, Munoz DG, Kusaka H, et al. Distinct pathological subtypes of FTLD-FUS. Acta Neuropathol 2011;121(2):207–18.

172. Neumann M, Roeber S, Kretzschmar HA, et al. Abundant FUS-immunoreactive pathology in neuronal intermediate filament inclusion disease. Acta Neuropathol 2009;118(5):605–16.

173. Lee EB, Russ J, Jung H, et al. Topography of FUS pathology distinguishes late-onset BIBD from aFTLD-U. Acta Neuropathol Commun 2013;1(9):1–11.

174. Holm IE, Isaacs AM, Mackenzie IR. Absence of FUS-immunoreactive pathology in frontotemporal dementia linked to chromosome 3 (FTD-3) caused by mutation in the CHMP2B gene. Acta Neuropathol 2009;118(5):719–20.

175. Skibinski G, Parkinson NJ, Brown JM, et al. Mutations in the endosomal ESCRTIII-complex subunit CHMP2B in frontotemporal dementia. Nat Genet 2005;37(8):806–8.

176. Chow TW, Miller BL, Hayashi VN, et al. Inheritance of frontotemporal dementia. Arch Neurol 1999;56(7):817–22.

177. Malamud N, Waggoner RW. Geneaologic and clinicopathologic study of Pick's disease. Arch Neur Psych 1943;50(3):288–303.

178. Sjogren H. Alzheimer's disease-Pick's disease; a clinical analysis of 72 cases. Acta psychiatrica et neurologica Scandinavica. Supplementum 1951;(74): 189–92.

179. Wilhelmsen KC, Lynch T, Pavlou E, et al. Localization of disinhibition-dementia-parkinsonism-amyotrophy complex to 17q21-22. Am J Hum Genet 1994;55: 1159–65.

180. Grover A, Houlden H, Baker M, et al. 5' splice site mutations in tau associated with the inherited dementia FTDP-17 affect a stem-loop structure that regulates alternative splicing of exon 10. J Biol Chem 1999;274(21):15134–43.

181. Rohrer JD, Warren JD. Phenotypic signatures of genetic frontotemporal demen-tia. Curr Opin Neurol 2011;24(6):542–9.

182. Yasuda M, Nakamura Y, Kawamata T, et al. Phenotypic heterogeneity within a new family with the MAPT p301s mutation. Ann Neurol 2005;58(6):920–8.

183. Whitwell JL, Jack CR Jr, Boeve BF, et al. Voxel-based morphometry patterns of atrophy in FTLD with mutations in MAPT or PGRN. Neurology 2009;72(9): 813–20.
184. Conrad C, Andreadis A, Trojanowski JQ, et al. Genetic evidence for the involvement of tau in progressive supranuclear palsy [see comments]. Ann Neurol 1997;41(2):277–81.
185. Coppola G, Chinnathambi S, Lee JJ, et al. Evidence for a role of the rare p.A152T variant in MAPT in increasing the risk for FTD-spectrum and Alzheimer's diseases. Hum Mol Genet 2012;21(15):3500–12.
186. Baker M, Mackenzie IR, Pickering-Brown SM, et al. Mutations in progranulin cause tau-negative frontotemporal dementia linked to chromosome 17. Nature 2006;442(7105):916–9.
187. Cruts M, Gijselinck I, van der Zee J, et al. Null mutations in progranulin cause ubiquitin-positive frontotemporal dementia linked to chromosome 17q21. Nature 2006;442(7105):920–4.
188. Petkau TL, Leavitt BR. Progranulin in neurodegenerative disease. Trends Neurosci 2014;37(7):388–98.
189. Ward ME, Miller BL. Potential mechanisms of progranulin-deficient FTLD. J Mol Neurosci 2011;45(3):574–82.
190. Coppola G, Karydas A, Rademakers R, et al. Gene expression study on peripheral blood identifies progranulin mutations. Ann Neurol 2008;64(1):92–6.
191. Van Damme P, Van Hoecke A, Lambrechts D, et al. Progranulin functions as a neurotrophic factor to regulate neurite outgrowth and enhance neuronal survival. J Cell Biol 2008;181(1):37–41.
192. Mackenzie IR. The neuropathology and clinical phenotype of FTD with progranulin mutations. Acta Neuropathol 2007;114(1):49–54.
193. Le Ber I, Camuzat A, Hannequin D, et al. Phenotype variability in progranulin mutation carriers: a clinical, neuropsychological, imaging and genetic study. Brain 2008;131(Pt 3):732–46.
194. van Swieten JC, Heutink P. Mutations in progranulin (GRN) within the spectrum of clinical and pathological phenotypes of frontotemporal dementia. Lancet Neurol 2008;7(10):965–74.
195. Smith KR, Damiano J, Franceschetti S, et al. Strikingly different clinicopathological phenotypes determined by progranulin-mutation dosage. Am J Hum Genet 2012;90(6):1102–7.
196. Mann DM. Dipeptide repeat protein toxicity in frontotemporal lobar degeneration and in motor neurone disease associated with expansions in C9ORF72—a cautionary note. Neurobiol Aging 2015;36(2):1224–6.
197. Mackenzie IR, Arzberger T, Kremmer E, et al. Dipeptide repeat protein pathology in C9ORF72 mutation cases: clinico-pathological correlations. Acta Neuropathol 2013;126(6):859–79.
198. Mackenzie IR, Neumann M. Molecular neuropathology of frontotemporal dementia: insights into disease mechanisms from postmortem studies. J Neurochem 2016;138(Suppl 1):54–70.
199. Vatsavayai SC, Yoon SJ, Gardner RC, et al. Timing and significance of pathological features in C9orf72 expansion-associated frontotemporal dementia. Brain 2016;139(Pt 12):3202–16.
200. Baborie A, Griffiths TD, Jaros E, et al. Accumulation of dipeptide repeat proteins predates that of TDP-43 in frontotemporal lobar degeneration associated with hexanucleotide repeat expansions in C9ORF72 gene. Neuropathol Appl Neurobiol 2015;41(5):601–12.

201. Proudfoot M, Gutowski NJ, Edbauer D, et al. Early dipeptide repeat pathology in a frontotemporal dementia kindred with C9ORF72 mutation and intellectual disability. Acta Neuropathol 2014;127(3):451–8.
202. Boeve BF, Boylan KB, Graff-Radford NR, et al. Characterization of frontotemporal dementia and/or amyotrophic lateral sclerosis associated with the GGGGCC repeat expansion in C9ORF72. Brain 2012;135(Pt 3):765–83.
203. Sha SJ, Takada LT, Rankin KP, et al. Frontotemporal dementia due to C9ORF72 mutations: clinical and imaging features. Neurology 2012;79(10):1002–11.
204. Whitwell JL, Weigand SD, Boeve BF, et al. Neuroimaging signatures of frontotemporal dementia genetics: C9ORF72, tau, progranulin and sporadics. Brain 2012;135(Pt 3):794–806.
205. Lee SE, Khazenzon AM, Trujillo AJ, et al. Altered network connectivity in frontotemporal dementia with C9orf72 hexanucleotide repeat expansion. Brain 2014; 137(Pt 11):3047–60.
206. Neumann M, Mackenzie IR, Cairns NJ, et al. TDP-43 in the ubiquitin pathology of frontotemporal dementia with VCP gene mutations. J Neuropathol Exp Neurol 2007;66(2):152–7.
207. Watts GD, Thomasova D, Ramdeen SK, et al. Novel VCP mutations in inclusion body myopathy associated with Paget disease of bone and frontotemporal dementia. Clin Genet 2007;72(5):420–6.
208. Johnson JO, Mandrioli J, Benatar M, et al. Exome sequencing reveals VCP mutations as a cause of familial ALS. Neuron 2010;68(5):857–64.
209. Borghero G, Floris G, Cannas A, et al. A patient carrying a homozygous p.A382T TARDBP missense mutation shows a syndrome including ALS, extrapyramidal symptoms, and FTD. Neurobiol Aging 2011;32(12):2327.e1–e5.
210. Kovacs GG, Murrell JR, Horvath S, et al. TARDBP variation associated with frontotemporal dementia, supranuclear gaze palsy, and chorea. Mov Disord 2009; 24(12):1843–7.
211. Mosca L, Lunetta C, Tarlarini C, et al. Wide phenotypic spectrum of the TARDBP gene: homozygosity of A382T mutation in a patient presenting with amyotrophic lateral sclerosis, Parkinson's disease, and frontotemporal lobar degeneration, and in neurologically healthy subject. Neurobiol Aging 2012;33(8):1846.e1–e4.
212. Freischmidt A, Wieland T, Richter B, et al. Haploinsufficiency of TBK1 causes familial ALS and fronto-temporal dementia. Nat Neurosci 2015;18(5):631–6.
213. Pottier C, Bieniek KF, Finch N, et al. Whole-genome sequencing reveals important role for TBK1 and OPTN mutations in frontotemporal lobar degeneration without motor neuron disease. Acta Neuropathol 2015;130(1):77–92.
214. Pottier C, Ravenscroft TA, Sanchez-Contreras M, et al. Genetics of FTLD: overview and what else we can expect from genetic studies. J Neurochem 2016; 138(Suppl 1):32–53.
215. Fecto F, Yan J, Vemula SP, et al. SQSTM1 mutations in familial and sporadic amyotrophic lateral sclerosis. Arch Neurol 2011;68(11):1440–6.
216. Deng HX, Chen W, Hong ST, et al. Mutations in UBQLN2 cause dominant X-linked juvenile and adult-onset ALS and ALS/dementia. Nature 2011; 477(7363):211–5.
217. Narvid J, Gorno-Tempini ML, Slavotinek A, et al. Of brain and bone: the unusual case of Dr. A. Neurocase 2009;15(3):190–205.
218. Kimura T, Takamatsu J. Pilot study of pharmacological treatment for frontotemporal dementia: risk of donepezil treatment for behavioral and psychological symptoms. Geriatr Gerontol Int 2013;13(2):506–7.

219. Mendez MF, Shapira JS, McMurtray A, et al. Preliminary findings: behavioral worsening on donepezil in patients with frontotemporal dementia. Am J Geriatr Psychiatry 2007;15(1):84–7.

220. Boxer AL, Knopman DS, Kaufer DI, et al. Memantine in patients with frontotemporal lobar degeneration: a multicentre, randomised, double-blind, placebo-controlled trial. Lancet Neurol 2013;12(2):149–56.

221. Vercelletto M, Boutoleau-Bretonniere C, Volteau C, et al, French research network on frontotemporal, dementia. Memantine in behavioral variant frontotemporal dementia: negative results. J Alzheimers Dis 2011;23(4):749–59.

222. Herrmann N, Black SE, Chow T, et al. Serotonergic function and treatment of behavioral and psychological symptoms of frontotemporal dementia. Am J Geriatr Psychiatry 2012;20(9):789–97.

223. Ikeda M, Shigenobu K, Fukuhara R, et al. Efficacy of fluvoxamine as a treatment for behavioral symptoms in frontotemporal lobar degeneration patients. Dement Geriatr Cogn Disord 2004;17(3):117–21.

224. Mendez MF, Shapira JS, Miller BL. Stereotypical movements and frontotemporal dementia. Mov Disord 2005;20(6):742–5.

225. Swartz JR, Miller BL, Lesser IM, et al. Frontotemporal dementia: treatment response to serotonin selective reuptake inhibitors. J Clin Psychiatry 1997; 58(5):212–6.

226. Lebert F, Stekke W, Hasenbroekx C, et al. Frontotemporal dementia: a randomised, controlled trial with trazodone. Dement Geriatr Cogn Disord 2004; 17(4):355–9.

227. Pijnenburg YA, Sampson EL, Harvey RJ, et al. Vulnerability to neuroleptic side effects in frontotemporal lobar degeneration. Int J Geriatr Psychiatry 2003; 18(1):67–72.

228. Chow TW, Mendez MF. Goals in symptomatic pharmacologic management of frontotemporal lobar degeneration. Am J Alzheimers Dis Other Demen 2002; 17(5):267–72.

229. Cruz M, Marinho V, Fontenelle LF, et al. Topiramate may modulate alcohol abuse but not other compulsive behaviors in frontotemporal dementia: case report. Cogn Behav Neurol 2008;21(2):104–6.

230. Finger EC. New potential therapeutic approaches in frontotemporal dementia: oxytocin, vasopressin, and social cognition. J Mol Neurosci 2011;45(3):696–701.

231. Jesso S, Morlog D, Ross S, et al. The effects of oxytocin on social cognition and behaviour in frontotemporal dementia. Brain 2011;134(Pt 9):2493–501.

232. Merrilees J. A model for management of behavioral symptoms in frontotemporal lobar degeneration. Alzheimer Dis Assoc Disord 2007;21(4):S64–691.

233. Cheng ST, Chow PK, Song YQ, et al. Mental and physical activities delay cognitive decline in older persons with dementia. Am J Geriatr Psychiatry 2014;22(1): 63–74.

234. Kortte KB, Rogalski EJ. Behavioural interventions for enhancing life participation in behavioural variant frontotemporal dementia and primary progressive aphasia. Int Rev Psychiatry 2013;25(2):237–45.

235. Karakaya T, Fusser F, Prvulovic D, et al. Treatment options for tauopathies. Curr Treat Options Neurol 2012;14(2):126–36.

236. Schneider A, Mandelkow E. Tau-based treatment strategies in neurodegenerative diseases. Neurotherapeutics 2008;5(3):443–57.

237. Tsai RM, Boxer AL. Therapy and clinical trials in frontotemporal dementia: past, present, and future. J Neurochem 2016;138(Suppl 1):211–21.

238. Boxer AL, Gold M, Huey E, et al. Frontotemporal degeneration, the next thera-peutic frontier: molecules and animal models for frontotemporal degeneration drug development. Alzheimers Dement 2013;9(2):176–88.

239. Boxer AL, Gold M, Huey E, et al. The advantages of frontotemporal degenera-tion drug development (part 2 of frontotemporal degeneration: the next thera-peutic frontier). Alzheimers Dement 2013;9(2):189–98.

240. Lagier-Tourenne C, Baughn M, Rigo F, et al. Targeted degradation of sense and antisense C9orf72 RNA foci as therapy for ALS and frontotemporal degenera-tion. Proc Natl Acad Sci U S A 2013;110(47):E4530–9.

Index

Note: Page numbers of article titles are in **boldface** type.

A

Acculturation
     in cognitive impairment evaluation in Hispanics, 212
AD. *See* Alzheimer's disease (AD)
AGD. *See* Argyrophilic grain disease (AGD)
Aging
     changes in cognition associated with, 196–197
Alzheimer's disease
     late-onset, **283–293** *See also* Late-onset Alzheimer's disease (LOAD)
Alzheimer's disease (AD)
     amyloid cascade hypothesis in, 175–176
          synaptic loss and elaborations on, 176–177
     APOE in, 179–182
     APs in, 171–172
     astrocytes in, 184–185
     characteristics of, 232, 234
     cholesterol in, 179–180
     early-onset, **263–281** *See also* Early-onset Alzheimer's disease (EOAD)
     inflammation in, 181–185
     innate immune system in, 181–185
     introduction, 263–264
     microglia in, 182–184
     neuropathology of, 171–172
     NFTs in, 171–172
     prevalence of, 171
     rapidly evolving basic science in, **175–190**
     spread of tau pathology in, 177–179
     update on, **171–174**
Amyloid cascade hypothesis, 175–176
     synaptic loss and elaborations on, 176–177
Amyloid imaging
     by PET
          in cognitively impaired elderly assessment, 249–252
Amyloid PET biomarkers
     in EOAD, 270–271
Amyloid plaques (APs)
     in AD, 171–172
APOE. *See* Apolipoprotein E *(APOE)*
Apolipoprotein E *(APOE)*
     in AD, 179–180
          inflammation and, 181–182
APs. *See* Amyloid plaques (APs)

Neurol Clin 35 (2017) 375–386
http://dx.doi.org/10.1016/S0733-8619(17)30019-1
0733-8619/17

Moving?

Make sure your subscription moves with you!

To notify us of your new address, find your **Clinics Account Number** (located on your mailing label above your name), and contact customer service at:

Email: journalscustomerservice-usa@elsevier.com

800-654-2452 (subscribers in the U.S. & Canada)
314-447-8871 (subscribers outside of the U.S. & Canada)

Fax number: 314-447-8029

Elsevier Health Sciences Division
Subscription Customer Service
3251 Riverport Lane
Maryland Heights, MO 63043

*To ensure uninterrupted delivery of your subscription, please notify us at least 4 weeks in advance of move.

Printed and bound by CPI Group (UK) Ltd, Croydon, CR0 4YY

14/10/2024

01773622-0001